the pregnancy quiz Try the quiz at the
start of your pregnancy and then again at the end, and see how
far you've come.

1 Colostrum is:
a) a very attractive ruin in Rome
b) stuff that comes out of
   your bosoms before you
   breastfeed
c) that strange blue goo that
   newborn babies are covered in
d) a thrash-trance band

**2 Can you retain fluid and
be dehydrated at the same
time?**
a) don't be ridiculous
b) oh, lordy, yes
c) it depends on what star sign
   you are

**3 Should you try to get time
off before the baby arrives,
rather than work until the
due date?**
a) yes
b) uh-huh
c) ooh, yeah
d) ab-so-lutely

**4 Which is the most relaxing
birth support team:**
a) a midwife and your partner,
   sister or friend
b) a film crew, a live Internet
   webcam support team,
   a stills photographer,
   your children, parents and
   second cousins, all the girls
   from work and somebody
   called Arthur who took a
   wrong turn on the way to
   the canteen
c) nobody at all

5 Inducement is:
a) a very large diamond ring and
   a holiday in the Bahamas
b) an artificial medical process to
   stimulate labour
c) holding a hobnob at the end
   of the vagina to coax the baby
   out
d) a technical term for the
   placement of the placenta

6 Braxton Hicks is:

a) that lantern-jawed bloke who slept with his aunty on 'The Bold and the Beautiful'

b) a term coined by NASA astronauts for a false alarm, named after an over-excited engineer on the Apollo 12 mission

c) practice labour contractions

d) a combination of the two most popular baby names in Kentucky in 1897

7 Palpation is:

a) what happens to your cervix when you have an orgasm

b) a pretentious word for 'having a feel of your baby'

c) the medical term for the faster heart rate you attain towards the end of a pregnancy

d) the opposite of temptation or craving: something that makes you nauseated

8 Placenta is:

a) the most popular girl's name after Emma, Rebecca and Sophie

b) the geographical location where you have your baby

c) a big gloopy item that looks like a liver and keeps the baby alive with nutrients and oxygen

d) a terrific marketing opportunity if you put it through a blender, whack it in a moisturiser and give it a French name

9 The easiest way of giving birth is by:

a) taking all the drugs you can get your hands on and shouting a lot at random

b) imagining you're in a perfectly charming wheat field having sex with Brad Pitt

c) having a general anaesthetic and paying someone to look after the baby for the first ten years

d) whatever means are necessary at the time

e) just like they do it in the movies

10 **Women who say childbirth doesn't really hurt are:**

a) lucky

b) deluded

c) insane

d) men

11 **A primigravida is:**

a) one of those ballerinas who doesn't eat enough

b) a woman giving birth for the first time

c) the first time you feel the baby move inside you

12 **Living with a newborn baby is:**

a) just like a lovely holiday

b) exhausting

c) what was the question again?

13 **If you don't have a husband, you can:**

a) get help from relatives and friends

b) just go straight to hell, you flaunty Miss Jezebel person

c) claim benefits and be involved in special re-employ-ment and study programmes provided by the government

14 **Postpartum means after the birth. Antenatal means:**

a) prenatal, or before the birth

b) you're against the whole idea of pregnancy, or being in any way slightly natal

c) another word for childbirth

15 **Sex is:**

a) really a tremendously heightened sensual experience all through pregnancy

b) just asking for trouble

c) apparently something that single, childless people do in their spare time

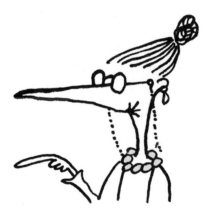

MRS FANNY BRAXTON HICKS

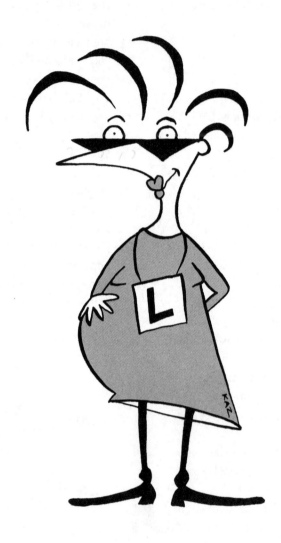

THE **ROUGH GUIDE** TO

Pregnancy
and birth

by
Kaz Cooke

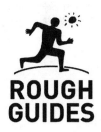

**ROUGH
GUIDES**

for Geoffrey and Oofty Goofty

While every care has been taken in researching and compiling the medical information in this book, it is in no way intended to replace or supersede professional medical advice. Neither the author nor the publisher may be held responsible for any action or claim howsoever resulting from the use of this book or any information contained in it. Readers must obtain their own professional medical advice before relying on or otherwise making use of the medical information contained in this book.

This revised second edition published by Rough Guides, London, May 2006

An earlier and very Australian edition of this book was published under
the very Australian title "Up The Duff" by Penguin Books Australia

10 9 8 7 6 5 4 3 2

Designed by Sandy Cull and Leonie Stott
Typeset in Shannon and Minion 11.5pt
Printed by Biddles Ltd, Guildford & Kings

Cataloguing-in-Publication data:

Cooke, Kaz, 1962– .
The Rough Guide to Pregnancy and birth.

432 pages, includes index.
ISBN 10: 1-84353-684-6.
ISBN 13: 978-1-84353-684-0.

1. Pregnancy – Popular works. I. Title

contents

Intro

The world is not short of pregnancy gurus – and (I promise) I'm not trying to join their ranks. When I got pregnant, one of the first friends who I told had just one piece of advice: 'Whatever you do, don't read any of the books.'

Of course, I disregarded this at once (disregarding advice comes even more naturally when you're pregnant) and went out and bought a squillion pregnancy books and sat down to discover about the miracle of new life. Which was when I started to see what she had meant. Many of the books were quite mad, making such suggestions as 'get a sink installed in your child's bedroom' (I ask you), or pushing the theory of giving birth in a wading pool full of lavender water. Even the sane ones were a bit weird, with their ways of describing the size of the developing foetus in terms of food. One week it's a brazil nut, then a plum, then an aubergine. Scary, huh? And another thing. Most of the books finished at week 40, when the baby is due. In real life, while you're pregnant, you can't think any further than the birth. But the very minute you have a baby you can hardly remember a thing about the pregnancy. It's suddenly entirely irrelevant and you have to deal IMMEDIATELY with a tiny person who depends on you completely (and also do stuff with your bosoms they don't even ask from exotic dancers).

For some reason I had always imagined that being pregnant would just be like being me with a big bump out the front. It hadn't occurred to me that the reality of being pregnant eventually would be felt constantly in every physical part of my body, and in every recess of what I fondly used to call my mind. Even though I had heard about nausea and fluid retention and vagueness and a ferzillion other things, for some dumb reason I thought they were part of an old-fashioned pregnancy, relegated to history along with the concept of 'confinement' and Mrs Spinoza's mechanical home-perm-and-gherkin-bottling machine.

I'm a career woman, I thought. I'm over 30. I've always pretended to be in control of my life, and that doesn't have to stop just because I'm pregnant. I'll just live my life the way it has always been (without getting pissed and having a few fags at the weekend). Work will go on as normal, life at home will be just the same, only I'll need bigger shirts at some point. My life will only completely change once the baby comes out.

WELL.

Apparently not.

I had not bargained on the body taking control of itself. The power of the mind? Pah. As far as my body was concerned, its major priority was growing a healthy baby. Several times I felt my legs going off along the corridor for a lie down when I thought my torso should have been elsewhere. I woke up in the middle of the night compelled to eat banana sandwiches and drink glasses of soy milk. I had become a host organ.

My first thoughts every morning and my last thoughts at night were about being pregnant, and there was a fair whack of it in between. Would I be a good mother? What if something went wrong? Was it too late to have second thoughts? Should I feel guilty about having second thoughts? Where do we stand on third and subsequent thoughts? Where the hell are my keys? Why is the marmite in the freezer? Did I do that? What the hell has happened to my HAIR? What's that weird bump forming on my gums? Do stretch marks stay that fetching shade of royal purple forever? Will I ever want to have sex again? What do people mean when they say 'pregnancy hormones'? Is it true some aromatherapy can make you have a miscarriage? Isn't this uncomfortable? Isn't this terrifying, and wonderful, and fascinating, and boring as batshit, all at the same time? Am I supposed to feel serene, or just seasick? If you don't do your pelvic-floor exercises will your fanny fall out? Why can't I feel the baby move yet? Could the baby stop moving for a while and give me a rest? What about those cigarettes I had before I realised I was pregnant?

And so it went on: Will I ever be able to be alone again? How can I tell people I don't want my career back? How can I get my career back? When does a foetus become a baby? Does that mean if it's born then it will survive? Could I get any fatter? What's pre-eclampsia and how do you get it? What can you see on an ultrasound screen? What if labour goes on forever and nothing comes out? Could somebody get me a cup of tea?

And then when I had a baby the questions really started.

So to find out what's what, I wrote this Rough Guide. The researchers and I went to work, and then experts checked everything written about their special area and suggested new bits, and then the editor asked a gadzillion questions and in the normal course of events I would have had a huge tantrum but I was too tired because by that time I'd had a baby, so instead we checked it all over again and took bits out and put bits in and waved it all about, and now here it is.

If you read everything in the book you might think pregnancy is a terrible minefield of bizarre health complaints. Don't freak out: lots of the pregnancy problems are rare – they're included 'just in case'. If you do have a special interest or problem, though, this book will give you the basics. And if there's something you need to know more about, you can find an organisation or book that will point you in the right direction recommended in the 'Help' section (that's the bit at the back).

_ Kaz

PS: Oh, yeah. The Diary scattered through this book includes many aspects of my own experience but it is not quite my story and incorporates lots of stuff from other people's pregnancies. Actually, if truth will out, I'm not really an orphan, nor a fashion designer (I'm not too sure about the exact nature of a kitten heel). But a girl has to try to cling to some sense of mystery, especially when she's got baby vomit up her nose. (Don't ask.)

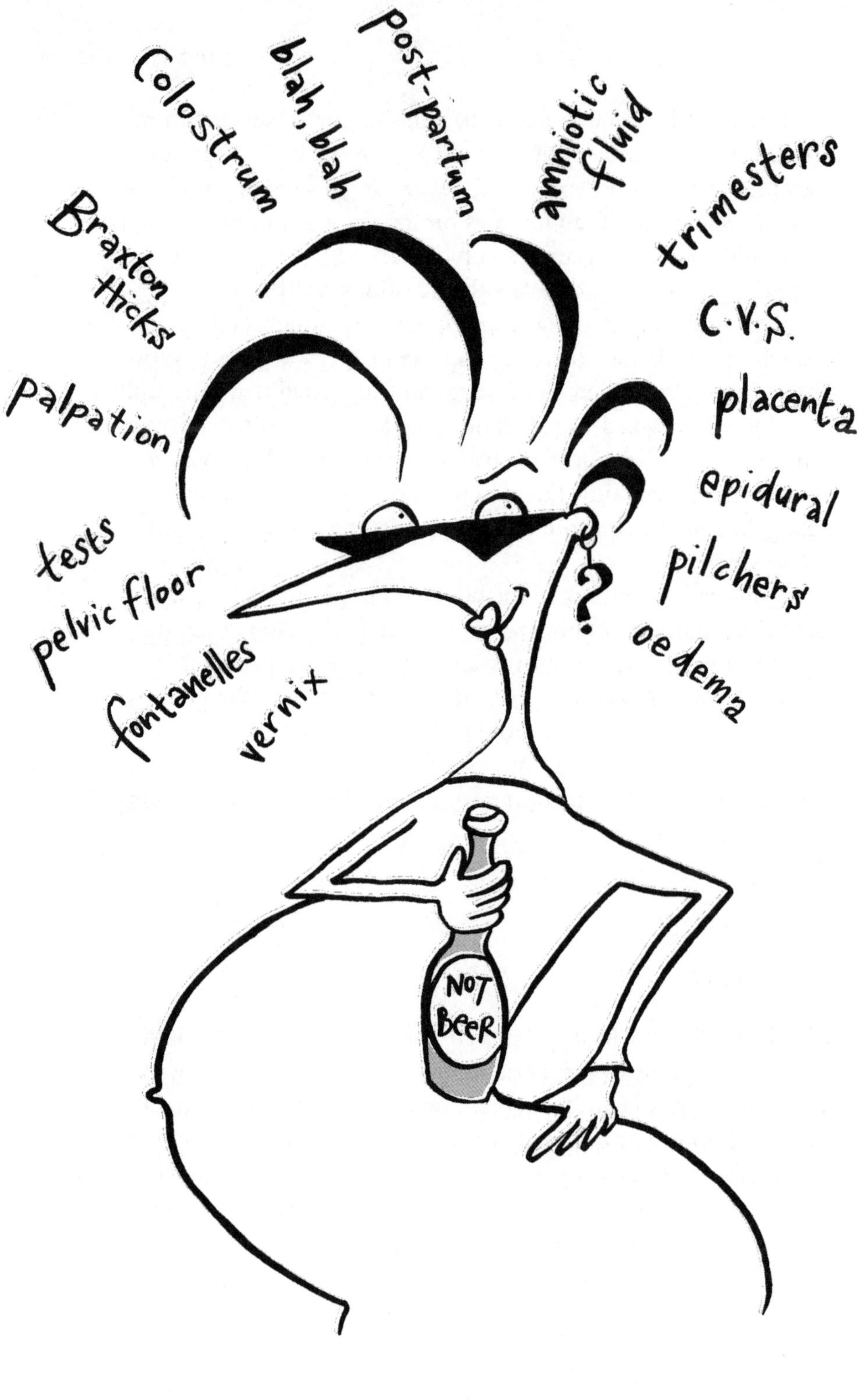
Colostrum
blah, blah
post-partum
amniotic fluid
trimesters
Braxton Hicks
C.V.S.
placenta
palpation
epidural
tests
pilchers
pelvic floor
?
oedema
fontanelles
vernix
NOT BEER

TeRmS of ENdeARMeNt

From conception we call the developing baby an EMBRYO, even in its earliest, cell-dividing days. At ten weeks, the embryo becomes a FOETUS (or FETUS), although you'll find that the term is often used for the unborn baby at all stages from conception to birth. All its organ systems are formed by then, and it's ready to expend most of its energy on maturing and growing.

At twenty-eight weeks the foetus becomes a BABY, even though a lot of medical staff still call it a foetus right up until it's born. We've called it a baby from week 28 because most premature babies born at this stage are likely to survive with modern, teaching-hospital care. (Many babies survive an earlier birth, although very premature babies often have continuing health problems.)

Pregnancy speak

The trimesters
'Trimester' means three months, so:

◎ The first trimester is up to the end of week 13.

◎ The second trimester is week 14 to the end of week 26.

◎ The third trimester is week 27 until birth.

Dates
This book, like most doctors, counts a pregnancy from the first day of your last period. So even if technically you conceived two weeks ago, you're 'four weeks pregnant'.

what's going on Not much. By the end of the week, you've just finished the last period you'll have for a while. You're into the 'follicular' phase of the menstrual cycle, which means the egg-making and dispatch phase ('follicle' is the name for the tiny sac in which the egg matures). One of your two ovaries is deciding which of the eggs developing in this menstrual cycle will be the one to go forth. (An egg is also known as an ovum, if you want to get medical and Latin about it.) Your ovaries release 400–500 mature eggs during your 'fertile' years. It only takes one to get pregnant.

Your body is going about its usual hormonal carry-on. Lots of oestrogen (actually several oestrogens but called 'oestrogen' as an umbrella term) is being produced by your ovaries. This stimulates the uterus to grow more lining, called the endometrium, to replace the lining that has just left as your last period. This new endometrium is the welcoming surface for the egg if it's fertilised. The egg is extremely weeny: about a tenth of a millimetre in diameter).

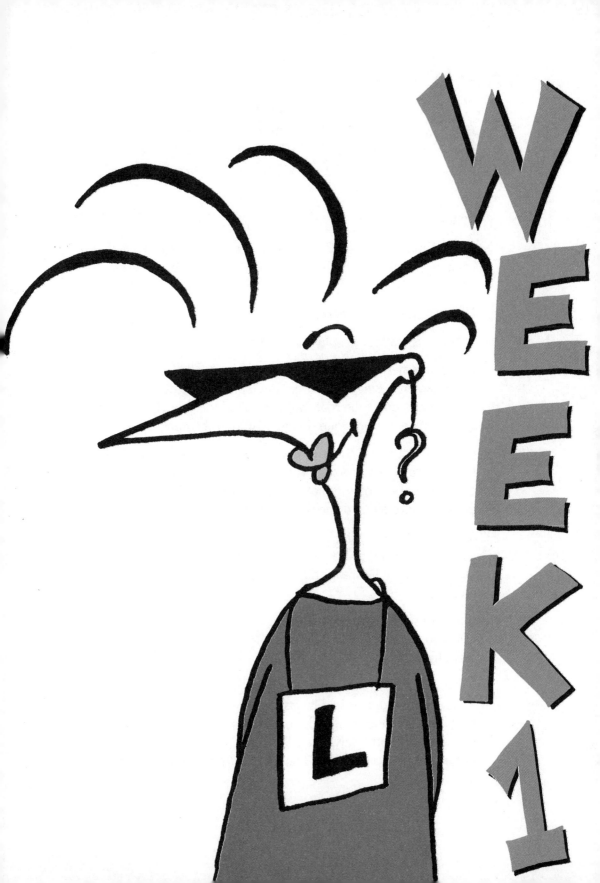

DiARY

I took an inventory of my life recently, and wrote it down with an eyebrow pencil on the back of a brown paper bag that used to have a muffin in it. It pretty much came out this way:

✳ Kaz Cooke.

✳ Age: 32.

✳ Unglamorous designer for small south London fashion company, Real Gorgeous Ltd (we make the Real Women Wear label, sizes 8–18).

✳ Sagittarius (tactless and jovial).

✳ Hobbies: eating, sleeping, buying shoes.

✳ Accoutrements: perfectly decent boyfriend called Geoff, who has a garden business. Small flat in Clapham (and about to move into a house down the road, with crippling mortgage). Nice couch. Some ageing white goods. £1600 in the bank.

✳ Shape: not unlike the fruit known colloquially as a pear. With legs. Unusually fat knees. Never mind. Rest of self reasonably overweight, but nothing that a lot of exercise and a little less reliance on chocolate and cheese wouldn't cure.

✳ Medical history: long tussle with endometriosis, a menstrual condition that can cause infertility, which I have controlled by taking the Pill full-time without a break. Haven't had a period for four years.

✳ Doctor's advice last time I went: if you want to get pregnant, come off the Pill and start shagging for your country (or words to that effect).

So Geoff and I had a talk. Six months before, I'd said I wanted to have kids and he'd said it was too soon (he's only 31; my toy-boy). This time though, he'd thought about it and was as ready as he'd ever be, particularly since I told him that, given my medical history, nothing at all might happen, or it might take two years to get everything working again. I told Geoff there were a few things to sort out: like what would we do if a test during pregnancy showed that the baby had Down's syndrome? And how would he feel if the kid grew up to be a gay man?

Geoff put his head on the side and thought for a moment. 'As long as he plays midfield for Palace I can't see the problem.'

We each made a list of stuff we'd have to do before I got pregnant. Mine said:

✳ Go off Pill, and see Beck (that's my herbalist and medical adviser and fellow champagne admirer) about what else I should be on instead.

✳ Lose weight.

✳ Get fit.

✳ Lottery ticket.

✳ Stop smoking.

✳ Stop drinking.

✳ Get driver's licence.

✳ Don't roll about in pesticide-soaked paddocks, stop eating junk food, cook magnificently cunning little low-fat dishes from primary food sources, stop saying 'fuck' so much, get legs waxed, organise the sanding of the floor of our new house without breathing in any of that polyurethane topcoat. (The sanders, who breathe it in all day long, seem to have the IQ of amoebas.)

✳ I sellotaped the list of things to do onto the fridge. Then I took it off and replaced it with a note on a small piece of the muffin bag saying, 'Change entire life immediately', and threw my packet of Pills in the bin in a rather melodramatic fashion.

There was absolutely nothing on Geoff's list except:

✳ Buy milk and bread.

✳ Have sex.

info

getting ready for pregnancy

This is the time – before you get pregnant – to tackle any relationship problems or sort out any mixed feelings you have about life, and pregnancy. Why do you want to have a baby? Do you want a toddler and a teenager (that's what babies become)? Have you talked it all out with your partner, if you have one? Will the father be involved after the baby is born? How can you protect yourself from sexually transmitted diseases while trying to get pregnant? Is pregnancy going to spoil your chances of getting that part in Babewatch UK?

Some people think that having a baby will bring them closer together. These people should take a powder and lie down. Having a baby is probably the most stressful thing you'll ever do. Everyone quotes Nora Ephron: 'A baby is a hand grenade thrown into a marriage'. And there's all the practical stuff to think about before you get up the duff:

⑥ Are you really ready to make the transition from ready-for-anything-at-a-moment's-notice to 'slave-to-baby'-Mummy-who-hasn't-had-time-to-shower-in-two-days-and-whose-every-outing-must-be-planned-with-a-military-precision-that-needs-to-be-totally-flexible-if-the-baby-wakes-up/won't-wake-up/cries/vomits/needs-feeding/poos-on-the-mobile-phone? But if you do

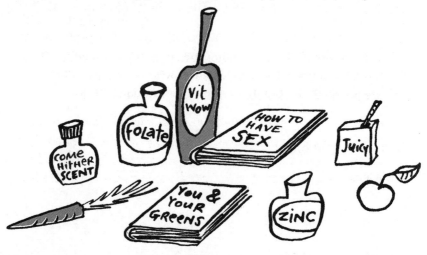

postpone the decision, does that mean you might later be trying to get pregnant when your fertility is declining rapidly?

◎ If you have a partner, this is a very fine time to share your ideas about parenting, to avoid heartache further down the track. Do you need to move in together? Are you both going to stop smoking during the pregnancy? What are your views on antenatal (also referred to as 'prenatal') screening tests? What would you do if you found out your child had a severe abnormality or a disabling condition? How would you cope with the idea of terminating the pregnancy, or living with a baby who will grow up always having special needs? Will the baby be part of a religious group? If it's a boy, will you have him circumcised? (Many of these issues are explored in this book and you can look up topics such as screening tests and circumcision in the Index.)

◎ What child-care arrangements do you see as ideal? What's going to be possible, or affordable? How about education? Who does most of the housework and other unpaid jobs around the house, and would that need to change? Do you share the same feelings about the possibility of your child growing up to be gay, or a stockbroker? What are your views on discipline and the issue of smacking children? Do you have a good support network of family and friends? Have any of them had recent experience with babies? Do you have Plan B for any of this stuff?

◎ Do you have private health insurance? If so, find out exactly what your policy covers in respect of pregnancy. Many policies cover very little in the way of 'routine' care, while others might pay for the cost of a caesarean birth (if recommended by your GP and obstetrician) and/or after care in a private hospital. If you are thinking about using a private midwife (£1000 to £4000), or a private hospital birth, start looking at the costs right now.

◎ See your GP and announce that you've decided you're going to try to get pregnant. Hopefully, they can give you a clean bill of health and peace of mind. They may recommend you start taking a special pre-pregnancy multi-vitamin supplement that includes zinc, folic acid (folate), calcium and magnesium, and excludes Vitamin A. The doses will have to be modified once you are pregnant because your baby will have different needs. Pregnant women are often deficient in zinc, which is important for the baby's development. All GPs advise taking folic acid, which can reduce your risk of having a baby with spina bifida or a related problem; to be effective, you need to start taking a folic supplement at least a month before conception. With any supplement, check with your doctor that it is compatible with any other drugs you are taking. (See 'Week 2' for more on supplements.)

⑥ Tell your doctor and pharmacist you are trying to be, or may be pregnant, before you buy any prescription or over-the-counter drug, vitamin, herbal treatment or tea. Don't take any painkillers based on ibuprofen or aspirin (under various brand names). If in doubt, don't take anything on anybody's advice until you can ask a medical professional with up-to-date knowledge.

⑥ If you don't have immunity to it (you can have a test done for this), get vaccinated against rubella (German measles), which can harm an unborn baby. Be careful not to conceive until three months after the shot – and if you think you could already be pregnant, check with your doctor before having any kind of vaccination as some can cause damage to an unborn baby.

⑥ If you suffer from a chronic health problem (for example, asthma, heart disease, liver problems, thyroid disease, diabetes, epilepsy, multiple sclerosis or mental illness), you should discuss with your GP medications and the management of your condition during pregnancy before you conceive.

⑥ If you or your partner has a family history of hereditary disorders, speak to your GP about seeing a genetic counsellor before conceiving (see Genetic Counselling in 'Week 10').

⑥ Family Planning Association clinics, like your doctor, can advise you on all sorts of things, from termination to where to get support through your pregnancy, at the birth and afterwards.

⑥ The fitter and healthier you are going into conception and pregnancy, the better. Growing another human being is a huge workload and it's a job that goes on twenty-four hours a day for about nine months. If you're trying to get pregnant, the following are things you really should do: eat healthy food and take the right supplements, after consulting your GP (see Eating and Supplements in 'Week 2'); take reasonable exercise; stop smoking, drinking and taking recreational drugs (see Looking After Your Embryo in 'Week 4').

⑥ Also, aim to increase or decrease your weight so that it's within the recommended range for your height and build. This is not the weight your mum or Cosmopolitan magazine thinks you should be. It's called the Body Mass Index calculation and it's only relevant if you're over 18 and have completely finished growing. Ask your doctor about it. All local hospitals have a dietician service and if you want to discuss your weight and diet before or during pregnancy, it may be possible to be referred by your GP to one of these advice centres.

⑥ If you have a partner, encourage him to adopt a healthy diet and lifestyle so he will be producing healthy sperm when you conceive (in other words, try not to have unprotected sex with a drug fiend who chainsmokes and won't eat his greens).

⑥ Go to the dentist. You may as well get any dental work that includes X-rays, anaesthetics or medication out of the way before conception (though bear in mind that dentistry is free for women during pregnancy and for the first year after the baby's life). If you do have dental work during pregnancy or while breastfeeding, ask about alternatives to mercury fillings, which may be harmful.

⑥ If you're in employment, check your entitlement to maternity leave. In a large company you may be able to do this anonymously by phone. You have a standard legal entitlement of 26 weeks' paid maternity leave, and are also entitled to time off for antenatal appointments. Dads in employment can take up to two weeks paid leave following the birth of the baby. These are the minimum entitlements. Some employers offer more benefits including extra leave, flexible working hours when you return to work, and work-based childcare. Your employer is legally required to offer you the same job or an equivalent level job on your return from leave.

⑥ If you have recently left work, changed jobs or are self employed you are still entitled to a Maternity Allowance based on your National Insurance contribution. If you are unemployed, you are entitled to a range of benefits during pregnancy and after the birth. Get advice as soon as you know you're pregnant. Your local social security office is the best first stop and there is excellent advice on the ACAS 'Tiger' website (*www.tiger.gov.uk*).

⑥ If one parent is taking time off paid work to look after the baby, how are your family finances going to be reorganised? (How do you spell 'budget'?) How would you feel about a joint account? Or about an automatic transferral of money from the income of the paid partner to the account of the one at home with the bub? Would it be a good idea to rob a bank at this point?

⑥ If you plan to renovate your home, make sure jobs that could be harmful to the pregnancy – such as stripping old, lead-based paint or sealing floorboards with polyurethane – are carried out before you conceive, or stay somewhere else while they are being done. Consider paints and DIY products that are baby-safe.

⑥ Make sure items around the house are environmentally friendly and avoid fumes or other foetus-threatening situations: have gas fires, microwaves and appliances serviced to make sure they're not leaking carbon monoxide, radiation, or anything else spooky.

LAST CHANCE SALOON ...

Before you decide to have a baby:

● Spend time with friends who already have a baby, or older children, and have a good, hard look at their life.

● Spend at least a full day from dawn until late with a mother and a small baby; it's impossible to imagine just how much work is involved until you are in the thick of it.

⊚ If you're buying a car, make sure it has rear fitted seat belts (rear seats are useful too), or can have them fitted safely and cheaply. Don't buy a four-wheel-drive CO_2 monster – especially one with a bullbar. A kid hit by a four-wheel-drive – and/or by a bullbar – is statistically very much more likely to die. So if you do have a bullbar, remove it, for everyone's sake. Be aware, too, that research shows four wheel-drives are also over-represented in accidents where children are hit in their own driveway, and that all vehicles have blind spots, especially close to the ground. Proximity alarms, lenses and video systems are no guarantee of safety and can promote false confidence.

⊚ Buy a lottery ticket. If you win, buy a great washing machine, a dryer, and a fridge with the freezer at the bottom. If you can afford a good central heating system, install one. You might also consider engaging a private midwife (see p.97) to look after your concerns right through the pregnancy and in the first couple of weeks at home. If there's any money left over, get yourself a holiday and an emerald tiara.

trying to get pregnant

If you're trying to get pregnant, make absolutely sure you know which times of the month are most fertile for you: cycles vary greatly but it is commonly about day 14 if you have a twenty-eight day cycle, counting the first day of your last period as day 1. Your doctor can help you with discussions about ovulation, fertile mucus and the other nitty-gritties.

According to many fertility specialists, you shouldn't 'keep trying' forever. If you're not pregnant after a year of having unprotected sex, get a referral from your GP to a medical fertility specialist. If you're approaching 40, don't leave it as long as a year. Generally speaking, your fertility declines steadily after 35 and plunges after 40.

If you have particular concerns about your fertility, it may be a good idea to see someone even before you start trying. Your GP or a gynaecologist can talk to you about ways to maximise your chances of conception based on your individual situation. (Conception rates for your age group, for example, could be irrelevant to you if you have a medical condition that's preventing conception.)

Do-it-yourself home fertility tests are now available for both men and women at chemists. The male one can be a useful first stop – and saves the poor lads the embarassment of producing a sperm sample at the clinic. But even with a positive result on either test, if you don't have any luck getting pregnant within a few months, take yourselves off to the doctors for a more comprehensive look at your chances. The ability to become pregnant can be based on many factors, not just those considered in a home test.

 If you're having trouble, see Fertility in 'Help' (p.405), and talk to your GP.

BOOKS FOR PRE-PREGNANCY

 **Healthy Parents, Better Babies: A Couple's Guide to Natural Preconception Health Care** by Francesca Naish and Janette Roberts, Crossing Press, UK, 1999.
Natural ways and various theories to improve your health and fitness – and perhaps, for some people, fertility – before getting pregnant.

Drugs in Conception, Pregnancy and Childbirth by Judy Priest with Kathy Attawell, Rivers Oram Press/Pandora List, UK, 1996.

A clear, practical guide to the benefits and risks (for the mother and baby) of everything from caffeine, alcohol and aspirin to prescribed drugs.

REALITY CHICKS

Life after Birth: What Even Your Friends Won't Tell You About Motherhood by Kate Figes, Penguin, 2000.

Despite the sunny cover image of mum and baby on the beach, this is essentially a book about the unglamorous side of having a child – the exhaustion, worries and passions. Readers seem to divide strongly: some find it the best book about babies, full stop, with unpatronising advice; others find it overly negative and a real downer, especially if read early in pregnancy. The list of contents tells the story: 'Childbirth: Just the Beginning', 'Emotions', 'Exhaustion', 'Relations with the Father', 'Friends and the Outside World'. The author is a British novelist and editor, and resources listed are all geared to the UK.

The Mask of Motherhood by Susan Maushart, Penguin Books, UK, 2000.

Maushart is an Australian mother and social scientist and in this book – subtitled 'How Motherhood Changes Everything and Why We Pretend It Doesn't – she, too, addresses the negative side of mothering: the loss of self, the chaos and confusion, the pain, the difficulty of juggling relationships, the lot. Again, you may find this either inspiring or offputting.

In addition, you could browse through any of the books about how to care for a baby (see 'Week 43'); these will also give you an inkling of what you're in for.

Your record

You may find it useful to record (and will almost certainly find it amazing to look back on) your thoughts during your pregnancy. Here are some things you might want to address on page one of your journal.

✳ The changes you made to get ready for pregnancy.
✳ Why do you want to have a baby?
✳ What do you imagine looking after a baby will be like?
✳ How do you think your life will change after the baby?
✳ What do you think you will do about work?

WEEK 2

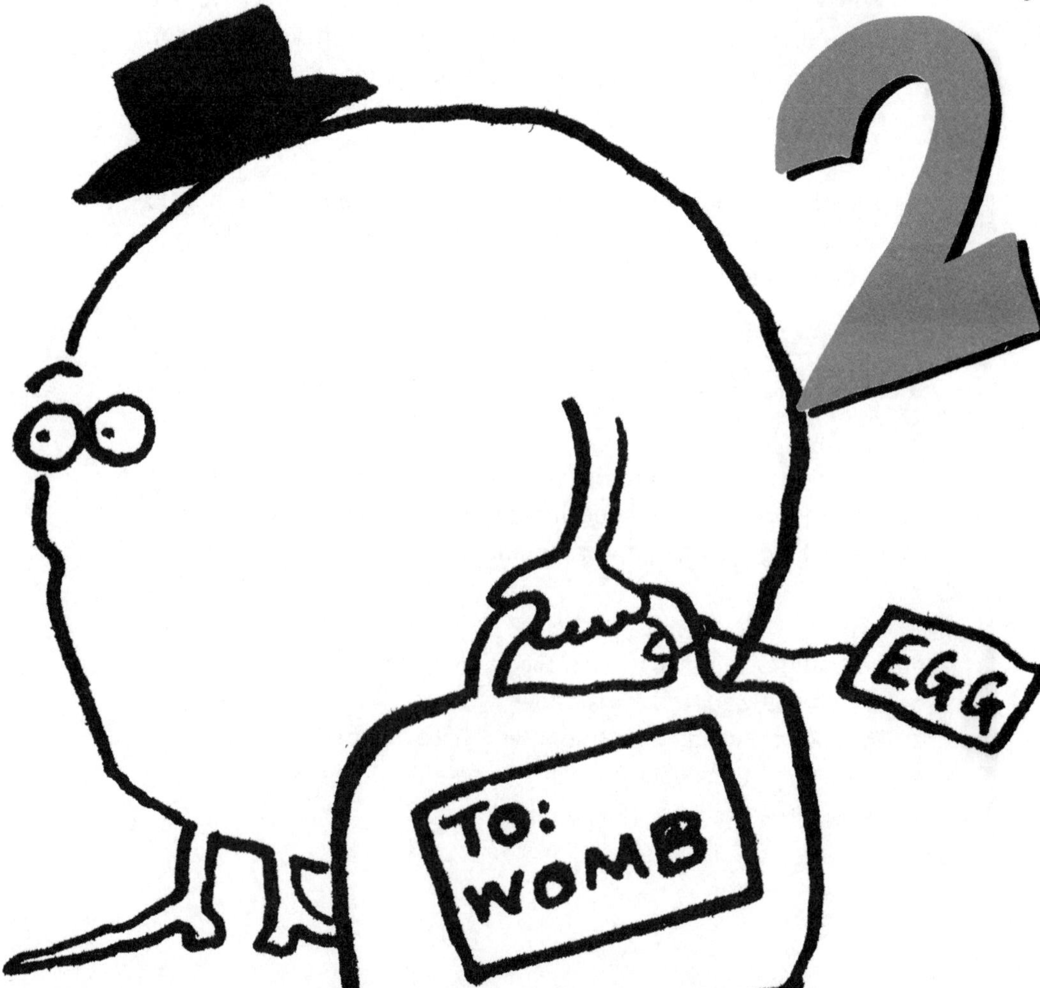

what's going on

By about day 14 (day 1 is the first day of your last period), you've reached the dispatch stage and your body is ready to ovulate. This means this month's 'dominant' egg is released from one of your ovaries, and 'waved' into the nearby opening of a fallopian tube by tentacly-looking bits on the end of the tube. You have two fallopian tubes, one on each side of the uterus, providing the link between each ovary and the uterus. At the time of ovulation, your vaginal mucus (look, you're going to hear a lot worse words and concepts than vaginal mucus in the next nine months so pull yourself together) will usually look like raw egg-whites, and is known as 'fertile mucus'. And at some point you'll have to get some sperm up there. Most women do this by having sex with a bloke: this is usually the easiest way.

After this week, you'll be into the 'proliferative' part of your menstrual cycle. This means the endometrium (the lining of the uterus) is 'proliferating' – growing like mad.

DiARY

I decide to blow our savings and take Geoff away to a Greek island for a week to ravish him constantly. Before we go I see my herbalist friend, Beck, who's also had years of experience as a hospital midwife. She gives me a tonic and some vitamins that include something called folic acid and heaven knows what other baby-friendly stuff, in preparation for the great shag-fest. Geoff and I both need a holiday to fortify us anyway, having been working like demons to raise the deposit for the new house.

I believe there are many ways you can pinpoint the moment of ovulation, involving thermometers, ropes and pulleys, and other implements. I should have got out the calculator and a protractor and a slide rule and a sextant and a sexton and half a sundial to work out when I might ovulate. (Don't know what a sexton is, but it sounds rather raunchy.) I haven't enough endometrium to have a period yet, but that's how it is when you come off the Pill after four years on it non-stop. A menstrual chart's about as much use to me as a metal detector.

Instead I just guess.

So ten days after I've come off the Pill, I am poised for Operation Up The Duff. Geoff keeps looking up from his beach towel and science fiction novel and saying, 'Hello, is it that time again?', when he sees the look in my eye.

But in between ravishings and drinking champagne, I start to have second thoughts about being pregnant. This could be a big year for me at work; even the chance of designing my own small range of clothes. I'm in line for promotion to head designer of Real Women Wear (stuff sold to people you or I might know, in things called 'shops', as opposed to what's known rather unkindly in the industry as 'Sluts on Stilts Wear' – the flashier end of the collections called 'couture' that end up only on catwalk models).

I go over and over the decision, obsessing about all the things I couldn't have if I had a baby: independence, a disposable income, velvet shoes, the chance of being able to walk out the door and catch a plane or go to the shops by myself, vomit-free shoulders, bosoms I can call my own. And I know women whose partners say they'll 'help' instead of 'I'll do half', and house husbands (primary caregivers, thank you very much) who play with the kids but don't cook the dinner or do any washing.

I keep double-checking with Geoff that he really wants to stay home the first year of the baby's life while I go out to work, and that he'll also do the washing. Then I start panicking – as I'm sure most blokes do – that I've got to bring home the bacon and stay employed for the next twenty years. We have long conversations about changing my mind, what it will do to the career, how being childless would be so much easier.

After a particularly well-executed ravishing on the Tuesday morning I lie there looking at the languid ceiling fan with the definite feeling that *that* was exactly the sort of behaviour that would get one pregnant, if one were able to get pregnant. Which of course triggers the decision to go back on the Pill as soon as I get home and postpone the whole thing.

'It's all right, Kaz,' Geoff the Ravishee reassures. 'Plenty of time. It's up to you.'

Then he says something terribly sensible, which is that there is never an ideal time to have a baby unless you're the sort of person who has nothing to do all day, vats of money and a spare teddy bear. Neither of us falls into this category, but really it could be worse. We're both in work, we've got somewhere to live and a car and neither of us has a conviction for aggravated assault. And even if things were not so good, we'd work it out somehow.

Still, it might be better to just wait and see if I get the promotion before I spend any more energy swinging from the chandelier in the nude making diverting remarks about likely ovulation days. Metaphorically speaking.

info

eating and supplements

You usually need more than the standard
requirements of energy, protein and certain
vitamins and minerals when you're pregnant.
Basically, you've got to pay attention to your overall
intake of everything to sustain the healthy growth and
development of your baby. Not to mention getting
through pregnancy without fainting around the
joint and being all gaunt and frazzled.

How many calories you need will depend on
your age, height, build, weight at the time of conception, current diet, and whether you're a couch
potato. Remember that for almost everyone it's
important to put on weight during pregnancy. This is
no time to go on a weight-loss diet or a fast. Either could
be very dangerous for your baby and you.

Although some women won't need to increase their energy
intake at all, the average recommended increase is 50 calories a
day. You need to add more than this if you were underweight to
start with; you're a teenager; or you're carrying more than one
baby. Your individual diet should be discussed with your midwife,
doctor, obstetrician or the dietician at your local hospital.

To keep your weight within recommended limits while giving
your baby all the goodies it needs, and so you don't get madly hungry,
you need to eat quality calories. Fresh, seasonal food provides far more
nutrients than processed 'convenience' and junk foods. Choosing a
variety of foods and eating regularly each day gives a healthy balance.
Aim for three meals plus two snacks during the day to avoid long gaps
without food. And think about buying organic, if you don't already.

Most people can get all the nutrients, vitamins and minerals
necessary for a healthy pregnancy from a well-planned, balanced
and varied diet. And the vitamins and nutrients you eat are always
better value than ones in tablets or capsules.

But who always eats a perfectly balanced diet? Probably no one unless they've got a private chef or a seriously leisured, foodie partner. You could be frantically busy and not quite eating what you should. Or throwing up could be leaving you depleted of vital nutrients. Or you might be trying to get through pregnancy on a vegan diet (no animal products), which is just not adequate for foetal development. (You may want to reconsider your vegan status during pregnancy.)

Taking some supplements during pregnancy can be a good way of improving your intake of nutrients if your diet isn't perfect. Your individual needs for certain supplements and doses will be different from those of anyone else, so talk about them with your doctor, midwife, dietician, obstetrician or natural therapist. Special multi-vitamin and mineral supplements designed for pregnant women are available in most pharmacies, but read all labels carefully and consult (or avoid them) if at all doubtful. Some multi-vitamin supplements (see below) are not suitable during pregnancy.

WARNING 1: VITAMIN A
Excessive levels of vitamin A are associated with birth defects, including cleft palate and heart malformation. Don't take any vitamin A supplement while pregnant, and make sure any multi-vitamin you are taking doesn't contain it: vitamin A can turn up in unexpected places like a B-group vitamin supplement. Avoid eating pâté or liver (which is full of vitamin A and may be full of chemicals, such as cadmium.)

WARNING 2: PEANUTS
More and more children are diagnosed with peanut allergies. At time of writing, there is no proven link that eating peanuts during pregnancy increases the risk of an allergy, however many women choose not to do so, especially if they (or a family member) suffer from a peanut allergy, or from hayfever, asthma or eczema. (It is commonly recommended that children are not given a taste of peanuts until four years old, in case of violent reaction).

protein

You'll usually need an extra 6 grams of protein a day on top of your non-pregnant requirement. That means a total of 5–6 portions of protein a day: one portion could be a glass of low-fat milk (unless you need the fat); 30g (1oz) of hard cheese; 150g (5.25oz) of yoghurt; 100g (3.5oz) of lean meat; 200g (7oz) of fish; or 200g (7oz) of cooked beans or lentils.

Vegetarians need to be really strict about combining grains with legumes – to maximise the quality of their protein intake. Protein-rich foods include miso, tofu, eggs and dairy foods, seaweeds, nuts and seeds. Vegans will need to pay special attention to their protein requirements. If you've been vegetarian or vegan and crave meat while you're pregnant, listen to your body and answer the call for extra protein with other foods (or, if your diet is a health choice rather than belief, by adding some meat or fish).

STAYING VEGGIE

Many medical professionals assert that a vegetarian diet is inadequate for pregnant women, women who are breastfeeding, and for babies and children. If you're determined to stick to your guns you'll need to know your stuff, so that you and your child get the right amounts of protein (see above) and other nutrients. Feeling full and healthy may still mean you are deficient in some areas, as pregnant women have a need for more vitamins and minerals than usual. (And many, if not most, women are deficient in some vitamins and nutrients before they're pregnant).

While not advocating a vegetarian or vegan diet for babies and children, it's important for those who choose that way to be as well-informed as possible. Some vitamins are only found in meat, or only found in useful quantities in meat, so must be supplemented in a veggie diet. Children can appear healthy but not be growing as much as they would with some meat in their diet, and may not be getting all the nutrients needed for brain development (and of course all of this also applies to non-vegetarians who may be giving their child a meat-including diet devoid of enough vitamins and minerals available in a varied selection of fruit and veg.)

calcium

Your tiny offspring is growing bones and teeth, and will pinch the very calcium out of your bones if you don't step up your intake. This might mean you're more likely to get osteoporosis later in life. Many natural therapists say that calcium and magnesium deficiency is one known cause of cramp, while many doctors say this is a fallacy and there's no scientific proof. If supplements help your cramps, take them.

You'll probably need to have at least 1,200 milligrams of calcium a day during pregnancy (3 or 4 glasses of low-fat milk or the equivalent yoghurt or cheese). This is about a third more again than your non-pregnant requirement. Teenage mothers who are still growing will need a higher calcium allowance: check with your dietician or doctor.

Some examples of calcium-rich foods are dairy foods (milk, yoghurt and parmesan cheese in particular), broccoli or other leafy green vegetables, spinach, tofu and tinned fish. Some people want to get all their calcium needs from dairy products, not least because 600 grams (1lb 5oz) of cooked spinach or 1 kilo (2lb 3oz) of cooked broccoli yield the same amount as a glass of milk. (This doesn't mean you can just drink litres of milk and never eat your greens!) But if you want or need to avoid dairy products, your other calcium-packed options include baked beans and red kidney beans, sardines, tinned salmon with the little bones in it, tahini made from unhulled sesame seeds, apricots and oranges.

It's a good idea to maintain a calcium supplement (which ideally contains magnesium and zinc as well) after giving birth if you are breastfeeding, as this also makes substantial demands on your body's calcium supplies.

Vitamin D

Vitamin D is needed to absorb calcium in you and the baby, and to help prevent health problems in the baby. The best way of getting Vitamin D is to get out in the sunlight each day, or at least every second day, when you can (you don't have to take all your kit off, but some exposed skin is needed to absorb the vitamin). Women with dark skin who live far from the equator tend to have a much higher risk of Vitamin D deficiency. A person with dark skin will need to spend about an hour to an hour and a quarter in sunlight to absorb the required amount of vitamin D – a pale person needs only 10 to 15 minutes. Being under full cloud cover, or in the shade, means you need to double those times. Remember to pop on the sunscreen after that, or come inside, as sunburn won't help anything. Anybody who wears a full veil or otherwise keeps most of their body covered should think about finding some private time to expose their skin to sunlight.

If you know you can't get enough sun, talk to your doctor about a supplement, but don't "prescribe" one for yourself or get it off the shelf. Too much of this vitamin can be bad for you and the baby. (Beware of cod liver oil, which has very high concentrations of Vitamin D.)

magnesium

You need magnesium or you don't get the full effect of the calcium and protein you take in. Some good sources of magnesium are whole-wheat flour, muesli, wheat germ, beetroot leaves, spinach and raw parsley.

⊘ It's important to have magnesium included in a calcium supplement because of its crucial role in helping retain calcium in bones and because normal diets are often deficient in magnesium.

zinc

Zinc needs to be increased during pregnancy and lactation (breast-feeding). Zinc is needed for enzyme production, brain and nerve formation and to help build an immune system in the foetus. Proper zinc levels have been linked to safer birth weights and less-premature babies. This mineral is often really low in pregnant women's diets. It's found in wheat bran, wheat germ, dried ginger root, brazil nuts, hazel nuts, dried peas and other legumes, red meat, chicken, fish, wholegrains and cheeses – especially parmesan.

🔅 A zinc supplement is even more important if you're taking an iron supplement because iron may interfere with the body's absorption of zinc. Vegetarians and vegans especially may need a zinc supplement. A zinc supplement during breastfeeding is also often recommended.

folic acid (folate)

This B-group vitamin is universally acknowledged as a supplement every woman should take for one month before pregnancy and for three months after conception. It has been proved dramatically effective in reducing neural tube defects (the main one is spina bifida) that affect one in 600 pregnancies. Although folic acid is naturally available in green leafy and yellow vegetables and whole-grain cereal, up to half of it can be lost in cooking or storage.

⊘ Just to cover yourself, it's best to take a supplement rather than try to make up the folic acid requirement in food every day. A daily dose of at least 400 micrograms (µg) – not 400 milligrams (mg), the more common measurement of many supplements – is the recommended daily dose. Higher doses may be recommended if you've already had a pregnancy with a neural tube problem, are taking medication for epilepsy, are diabetic or have coeliac disease. If you're already taking a vitamin or mineral supplement that includes folic acid, check that it has at least 400 micrograms – it probably doesn't, so you'll be better off with a specific pre-pregnancy vitamin supplement (but check these contain enough folic acid, too).

other B-group vitamins

Vegetarians and vegans will need to take vitamin B_{12} supplements or drink plenty of soya milk fortified with B_{12}. B_{12} only occurs naturally in animal products and is crucial in developing the baby's nervous system, brain and red blood cells.

🔅 A supplement containing B-group vitamins can be good for keeping up energy levels during pregnancy.

iron

Your iron requirement increases during the pregnancy: up to 20 per cent of women become iron deficient during pregnancy. Extra blood volume – yours and the baby's – means more iron is needed to make more haemoglobin. The placenta gives first priority to the baby's iron requirements, taking it from your blood, and you risk anaemia if you don't make up for it. You're considered to be at higher risk from iron deficiency if you're having a multiple pregnancy, you've had children quickly one after another, you've been vomiting a lot during pregnancy or you're a vegetarian or vegan.

You need 20–30 milligrams per day during the last six months of pregnancy compared to a non-pregnant requirement of 12–16 milligrams. Iron absorption is helped by vitamin C and hindered by tea, coffee and antacid medicines. Some examples of iron content in 100-gram (3.5 oz) servings of food are lean beef (3.4 mg); sardines (2.4 mg); eggs (2 mg); wheat bran (12.9 mg); raw parsley (8 mg); spinach (3.4 mg); lentils (2.4 mg); dried peaches (6.8 mg); dried figs (4.2 mg); and dried apricots (4.1 mg). (If you want a quick boost of iron, have a drink of Ovaltine.)

⊘ Iron supplements are sometimes recommended from about the thirteenth week of pregnancy to keep up that daily requirement of 20–30 milligrams after the first trimester. Vegetarians who are not careful about their diet, and vegans, will need an iron supplement. Vegetarians will also find it very helpful when they don't feel like eating a mountain of spinach.

Supplements may cause constipation, or sometimes diarrhoea, and this should be discussed with your midwife, GP or dietician, who can suggest an alternative form. Floradix is a popular organic supplement that can be bought from most healthshops.

fats

You gotta have 'em for proper foetal development, but steer clear of saturated fats. Use mono-unsaturated vegetable oils, such as extra virgin olive oil, for cooking and salad dressings. You also need fatty acids, found in linseeds or linseed oil, pumpkin seeds, walnuts and pecan nuts, and oily fish; and linoleic acid, found in seeds, seed and vegetable oils, nuts and dark green vegetables. Avoid high-fat cooking methods such as frying and roasting in fat: better to grill, steam and stir-fry.

sugar and salt

Going for nine months without any sugar is, of course, deeply weird, but do steer clear of refined sugars where possible, for all the usual reasons. (You probably already know that eating a block of chocolate the size of your head is not considered healthy.)

A completely salt-free diet isn't recommended, but there's enough natural salt in food without shaking on extra.

fluids

Get onto them! You'll have more blood pumping around and the amniotic fluid surrounding the developing baby is constantly being replaced. (Not to mention all that sweating and crying that can go on.) Drinking at least two litres (3.5 pints) of water a day will help you avoid constipation and urinary tract infection. Steer clear of diuretics such as caffeine and alcohol. Diuretic drugs are unsafe during pregnancy, even if you have fluid retention: plain dandelion-leaf tea is okay (this is not the same as dandelion-root coffee substitute: dandelion-leaf tea looks more like a bag of bad marijuana or lawn clippings).

more info on eating and supplements

The dieticians at your hospital or GP clinic will be able to help you with diet information, and you may want to consult the Health Service web-site (http://www.eatwell.gov.uk), the Vegetarian and Vegan Foundation (www.vegetarian.org.uk), or one of the following books:

BOOKS ON FOOD AND PREGNANCY

NCT Book of Safe Foods by Hannah Hume and Rosemary Dodds, Thorsons, UK, 2003.

A no-nonsense guide from the National Childbirth Trust to what you should and shouldn't be eating during pregnancy.

Vegetarian Pregnancy: The Definitive Nutritional Guide to Having a Healthy Baby by Sharon Yntema, Windrush, UK, 1994.

Sensible and well-researched, this tells you exactly what you need to know to maintain a vegetarian diet during pregnancy – and even has a section for self-defence against tutting grandparents.

PREGNANCY BOOKS

 A lot of books are handed to you when you're pregnant. Don't take them. When a friend recommends a book, buy the latest edition of it yourself. Some pregnancy books with out-of-date and even dangerous medical and safety info are passed around. And do your friends a favour: don't lend yours when you've finished with them. Here's a brief critical look at the main ones in circulation.

See also the **Pregnancy websites**, detailed on p.412–414.

Pregnancy and Birth: Your Questions Answered by Christoph C. Lees, Karina Reynolds, Grainne McCartan, Dorling Kindersley, UK, updated 2002.

This is a good supplement to the book you are holding, with info in easy-to-look-up, bite-size bits. Two obstetricians and a midwife come up with the the answers on just about everything likely (or unlikely) to happen during pregnancy.

The National Childbirth Trust Complete Book of Pregnancy by Daphne Metland, Thorsons, UK, 2000.

Drawing on the NCT's bank of experience, this novel book informs by following the course of three pregnancies: a young mother (20–25), an older mother (35–40), and a second-time mother. The experiences are accompanied by comments, tips and advice. A good complement to the manuals above, though don't assume your age will dictate your pregnancy.

Conception, Pregnancy and Birth by Dr Miriam Stoppard, Dorling Kindersley, UK, updated 2005.

Miriam Stoppard has become the bestselling pregnancy and childcare author in the UK, aided and abetted by the clear Dorling

Kindersley illustration-heavy approach. This is a well-researched, informative book, taking you from thoughts of conceiving through to the realities of early parenthood (there's a chapter for fathers, too), although I personally could have got through pregnancy quite happily without the emphasis on body and beauty concerns.

What to Expect When You're Expecting by Arlene Eisenberg, Heidi E. Murkoff and Sandee E. Hathaway, Workman, updated 2002.

This is the topselling US pregnancy guide. The UK edition tends to lag behind and, though it is partially adapted from its home country, its tone and sometimes content (buttermilk pancakes, anyone?) remain distinctly American. That said, this is a valuable and encyclopedic look-it-up-when-you-need-to guide.

The New Pregnancy and Childbirth by Sheila Kitzinger, Penguin, UK, updated 2003.

Sheila the guru, Sheila the natural birth pioneer, Sheila the psycho-sexual water birth advocate: this is the (British) voice of the 1970s birth revolution – one of the pregnancy 'bibles' that gets handed on most. It is a major tome, covering pretty much every subject in depth, including the emotional side of pregnancy and birth, the dad's experience, and the newborn's first days. It includes photos of births, and lots of pictures of baby in the uterus, yoga, and sex during pregnancy (Good LORD!).

New Natural Pregnancy: Practical Wellbeing from Conception to Birth by Janet Balaskas, Gaia Books, UK, updated 2004.

A holistic look at pregnancy with informative, well-illustrated sections on nutrition, yoga and exercise, massage, natural therapies and holistic healing. There are suggestions for natural remedies for most common pregnancy complaints.

Home Birth by Nicky Wesson, Vermilion, UK, updated 2006.

Packed with good advice and inspirational case studies, this title has become an essential guide for the growing number of women choosing a home birth. As well as outlining practical issues and safety, Wesson provides good advice on how to hose down concerned friends and family.

what's going on
Fertilisation! Inside you your single-cell egg is tootling slowly down the fallopian tube when it is rather suddenly accosted by an insistent sperm, which wriggles inside it. The cell splits in two, then those two new cells split in two, and so on, within a surrounding jellylike coat. This fertilised egg or embryo takes about four days to languidly drift down the tube and into the uterus. A couple of days after arriving it finally sheds its jellylike coating and decides where to park itself, usually in the top, front part of the uterus. By now it's made up of about 200 cells. There's an inner bit that is the embryo; and an outer bit that will become the placenta (which will sustain the developing baby) and the amniotic sac (which contains the nice, warm amniotic fluid 'bath' the growing baby will float around in).

The embryo sends out roots to anchor it in the endometrium surface and draw in goodies from your blood-stream. It's this system that develops into the placenta.

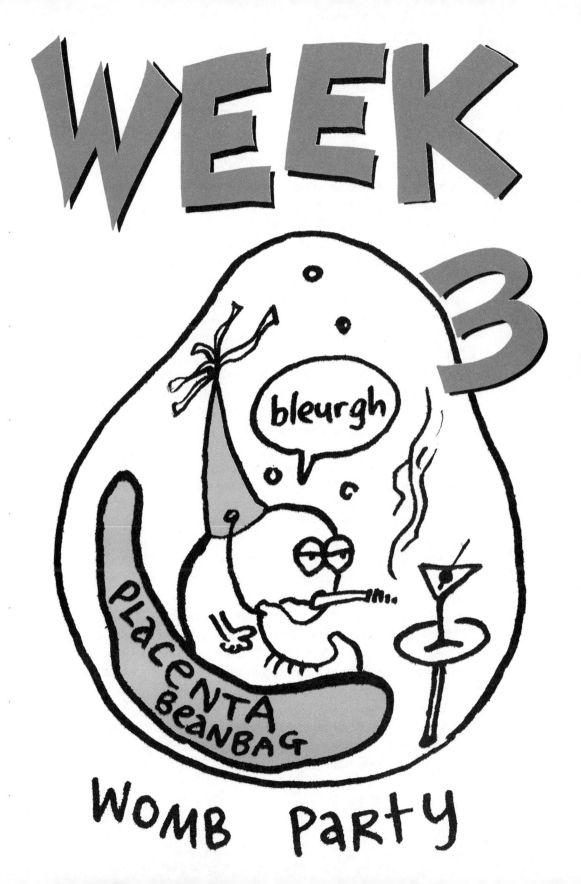

DiARY

We're getting ready to move house. I want everything in its place. Tidy, tidy, tidy. I've been collecting boxes and putting things in them and pretending this means I'm an organised person with a streamlined life. Actually it just means that I'm a disorganised person in possession of a number of boxes.

Geoff bought a Bedford Rascal to transport his azaleas, bay trees and, on really tasteful gardening jobs, small statues of weeing cherubs. This new van, along with moving to a larger house, has led to much unseemly speculation. Combine house purchase, larger car and a hint of an enigmatic smile, which one cultivates to cover a whirling sense of nothing-to-speak-of going on in the brain region, and there is an immediate 'she's pregnant' calculation on the part of bystanders.

Some people, almost always the ones who have their own kids and often plenty of them, bang on about it constantly. 'Are you pregnant yet?', 'When are you going to start a family?', as if a baby's just something you send off for with a stamped-addressed envelope.

Luckily we don't have the sort of parents who pressure us, given that Mum died before I could remember her, nobody knows who my Dad was, and Geoff's parents are usually off studying lichen on Welsh mountain ranges, rather than demanding that we have some grandchildren to keep them amused. I am constantly amazed by the parents of friends who think it's their perfect right to insist that their offspring hurry up and 'give them grandchildren'.

I'm sure Aunt Julie, who raised me with the help of Uncle Mike before he moved out to live with his secretary, would be chuffed to bits, but at least she isn't leaning on me. Uncle Mike, who has since become a born-again eco-nut, would no doubt go all new-age on me. And he ought to know by now I'm not the earth-mother type.

Just for fun, Geoff and I have been playing mummies and daddies with a Tamagotchi baby we found in a car-boot sale – it's one of those tiny Japanese digital games that look like key rings.

We turned the game on, called our electronic-screen baby Fred and pressed Start. There was a button to be pressed when Fred produced what the instructions called 'dung'. And buttons to press to see Fred's weight and age; to play paper, scissors, rock with him; to give him rice or a bottle; and to 'discipline' him. (Unfortunately there seemed to be no ChildLine button.)

Every night Geoff bounds in from a day of demanding clients saying things like, 'What about a water feature by the shed?' and 'I've never liked agapanthus' and 'Can't we just patio that bit?' and 'No, I've changed my mind', and he asks breathlessly and tenderly, 'How's Fred?'.

And each time, flushed with the bloom of mothering a newborn, baby-purple extruded-plastic capsule with digital liquid-crystal output screen thingie, I report, 'Haven't seen him all day. Busy', 'Try the cutlery drawer' or 'I left him in a café.' Or more often, the simply poignant diagnosis, 'Well . . . Fred's dead.' Bloody depressing game, if you ask me.

No, it has to be said: motherhood is the hardest and most honourable job in the world. Oh well. With my medical history it might take years to get pregnant. If at all. Probably just as well. Let's face it, I'm not likely to get a reference from Fred.

I suppose if I'm going to stay off the Pill, I had better find a friend with a baby and spend a day or so with them. I was off wearing miniskirts in foreign parts when my old mate Amanda's babies were small, and not that interested really. Now that I am, I realise most of my friends are lesbians or career women who are only just starting to wonder how they might manage it. The only one who's already launched her kayak into the creek is Susanne, and she's only four months pregnant. I guess I can practise on her baby when it arrives. I had better find an instructional DVD called something like 'A New Baby: Which End Up?'.

We just don't live any more in a tribal society surrounded by a million kids of varying ages and great scads of extended families. My second cousin Chris has six of the blighters, but they live in Spain, there's not much practising to be had there. There should be some kind of library service.

info

sense of smell

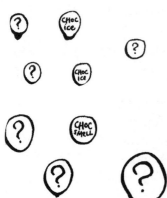

Your sense of smell may be far more acute than usual during pregnancy, especially in the first three months. You may even notice it before you know you're pregnant. Perfumes or food smells that previously seemed downright scrumptious may now send you heaving to the bathroom. What's really annoying is that none of the experts seem to be able to say why. Maybe the nausea is a defence mechanism so you're more likely to identify 'off' foods that could harm you or your baby. Maybe it's to compensate for the last two-thirds of a pregnancy often being accompanied by a blocked nose (due to a general increase in bodily secretions you don't want to have to think about yet). Or maybe it's just a meaningless side effect of one of the 'pregnancy hormones'.

aromatherapy

Aromatherapy, the therapeutic use of essential oils, can make you feel nurtured and relaxed during pregnancy, but some essential oils can harm your unborn baby or bring on labour or miscarriage. Any oils you consider using should be checked carefully – and diluted in a carrier oil if used during a bath or massage.

Qualified aromatherapists advise against any aromatherapy applied directly to the skin during pregnancy, especially during the first trimester, without advice from an aromatherapist specialising in pregnancy. Some oils are not even recommended for burning to scent a room when you're pregnant.

Unfortunately some masseurs who use essential oils with-out being qualified aromatherapists are simply unaware of any risks and will tell you anything they use is quite safe at whatever concentration they feel like squirting on you. And even the oils considered 'safe' for massage or in the bath should be used at half-strength during pregnancy.

It can be confusing for a layperson to decide what is safe. For example, despite spearmint used directly on the skin being in the 'banned during pregnancy' list given below, some pregnancy magazines recommend it to relieve nausea when used as an infusion to breathe in or to scent a room.

Oils generally considered safe for use during pregnancy include lavender, grapefruit, orange, lemon, tangerine, mandarin, neroli, sandalwood, rose, ylang-ylang, geranium (after the fifth month), bergamot, ginger and tea-tree.

Oils that can induce miscarriage (abortifacients) or bring on a period (emmenagogues) must be avoided during pregnancy. Many of them are obscure and it is always advisable to consult a qualified aromatherapist. These oils include, but not exclusively confined to, basil, cinnamon, clove, origanum, hyssop, pennyroyal, spearmint, parsley, sage, rosemary, Roman chamomile, German chamomile, myrrh, juniper, clary sage, sage, bay, pine, thyme, and jasmine.

Remember that you may be supersensitive to smell, but your nose can also be blocked up during pregnancy and therefore less sensitive to smell. So always follow the recipes given by a qualified aromatherapist rather than your schnozz. And obviously, for your own comfort, don't use anything that makes you feel queasy.

Here are some safe aromatherapy ideas.

⑥ Aches and pains – throw a couple of drops of (dilute in oil) lavender in the bath, and maybe a drop of geranium or rose.

⑥ Fatigue – in a burner to send the smell wafting through the room, 2 drops of lavender oil, 1 drop of mandarin oil and 1 drop of ylang-ylang oil; or 1 drop of lavender oil, 1 drop of rose oil and 2 drops of bergamot oil.

⑥ Nausea – in a burner, 1–2 drops of lemon oil or lemongrass oil; or make some ginger tea (see Nausea in 'Week 4') – drink the tea and breathe in the aroma as you go. You could also try a drop of peppermint oil in some water. This can be repeated every hour until you feel a little better.

⑥ Insomnia – put 3 dilute drops of lavender, mandarin or ylang-ylang oil, or a mixture of the three, in the bath; scent your bedroom with 2–3 drops of lavender or ylang-ylang oil, or a mixture of the two.

⑥ Stuffy nose – make an inhalation by adding 2 drops of eucalyptus or tea-tree oil to a bowl of hot water, then stick a towel over your head and breathe in the vapour for a couple of minutes. (You can't use many 'cold remedy' drugs during pregnancy so this is a good one to remember. Steam on its own works, too.)

⑥ Bad circulation – in a burner, 2 drops of grapefruit oil, eucalyptus oil or frankincense.

Many women burn lavender oil when giving birth – but wherever there are oxygen tanks a naked flame is banned. An electric burner can be used for essential oils during labour in the hospital environment. Alternatively, hot compress or essential oils in a base massage oil can be a treat in labour. Aromatherapy won't actually help physically with pain relief but many women find it a useful aid for their overall state of mind.

herbal teas

Herbal teas should not be confused with essential oils: an oil extracted from a plant contains very large quantities of components that could be dangerous, whereas a tea made from the plant might not. However, many herbs can bring on a period, or cause miscarriage or birth defects and even with teas you should always check with a trained herbalist. (No more than three cups of any kind of herbal tea should be consumed every day as a habit.)

Herbal teas generally considered safe during pregnancy include: peppermint, fresh ginger, lemon balm, chamomile, and dandelion leaf (which is a safe diuretic) but not dandelion root.

medicine and natural therapies

Remember, don't take medicines, herbs or vitamins without consulting a properly trained doctor or herbalist. Just because your friend swears by something she took during her pregnancy doesn't mean it's safe for you or your baby. Some preparations can be taken at different times during the pregnancy; others are dangerous at different times, or at any stage. Some preparations are safe except during pregnancy. Don't assume because something is 'natural' it is 'safe'. And always tell your doctor and natural therapist what the other one has prescribed.

Beware of dippy 'natural therapy' or 'diet' advice. Most diets that involve restriction of certain food types are not suitable for pregnancy, and fasting is compleeeeetely out of the question as it could damage the developing baby or even cause miscarriage. (See Eating and Supplements in 'Week 2' for the lowdown on eating properly during pregnancy.)

BOOKS ON NATURAL PREGNANCY AND AROMA-THERAPY

Natural Pregnancy by Zita West, Dorling Kindersley, UK, 2002. Written by a practising midwife who is also a nutritionist and acupuncturist (presumably she never sleeps), this well-presented book covers a whole range of complementary therapies useful during pregnancy and the post-natal period. Organised into trimesters, with five-point action plans, it includes everything from acupuncture and aromatherapy to shiatsu massage and yoga.

Aromatherapy For Women by Maggie Tisserand, Thorsons, UK, 1999. This enthusiastic guide to aromatherapy includes a good section on pregnancy, with warnings on oils to avoid, as well as directions for those you can use safely for relief.

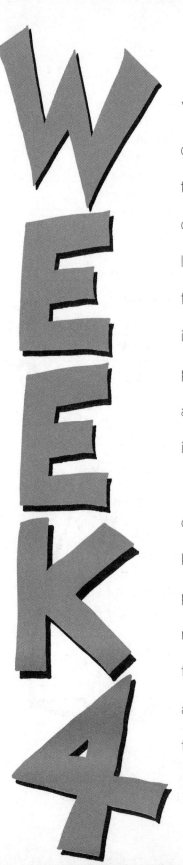

WEEK 4

what's going on

Your period is due. Maybe you've started going wee, wee, wee all the way home. Perhaps you've gone off the smell of alcohol and cigarettes, and foods that you usually like. Now or in the next few weeks, you might start feeling slightly queasy, which in bad cases results in vomiting. (According to one pregnancy book photo, this is when you will wear a hideous smock and an Alice band, and stare out the window holding a cup and saucer like a demented fool.)

The tiny embryo burrows into the wall of the uterus until it's completely embedded, and keeps getting bigger every day. The ovaries are pumping out the hormone progesterone to make the endometrium tough. The sex of your baby, the colour of its hair and eyes, how tall it can grow and whether it has natural footy talent – all these factors have been genetically programmed from the start, and can't be altered. By the end of this week the

embryo's about a fifth of a millimetre – still too little to see with-

out using magnifying instruments.

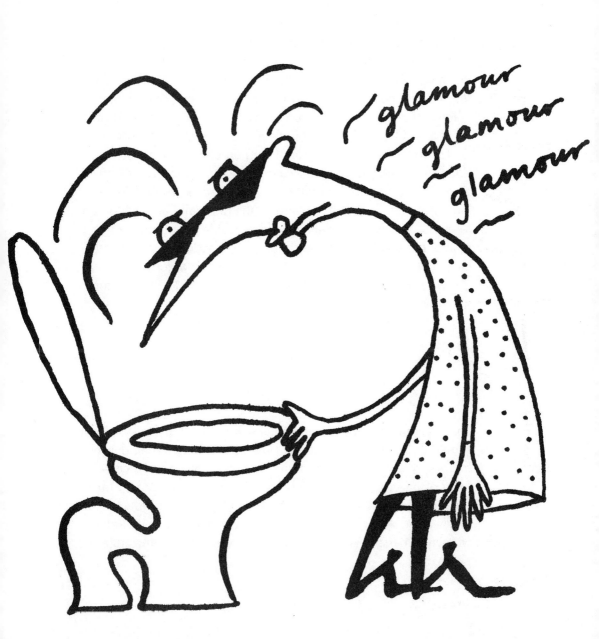

DiARY

Went for a drink with Jon from work, whose wife has been at home with the kids for four years and is now dashing her head against a plywood wall trying to get into the workforce again – the restaurant industry wants her to work split shifts for approximately £6.50 a day. He says apart from this whole work problem, and vomit and poo, motherhood is INCREDIBLY GLAMOROUS.

I also meet with the boss about becoming head designer of Real Women Wear and agree to a schedule of sacred weekly meetings with the new buyers. I sign on the dotted line for my first range. Off to Michelle's party with the girls and smoke about seven cigarettes – and have two glasses of some hideous home-made cocktail. For some reason I don't want to get drunk. Have a bit of a half-hearted dance. I'm feeling tired and out of sorts.

For some reason I've started being absolutely vile to Geoff. I don't know why. I'm quite aware I'm doing it but I can't stop myself. He comes in the front door and I narrow my eyes look-ing for a fault. I swear if he came in the door with a bunch of red roses and tickets to the Bahamas I'd probably say, 'Wipe those muddy boots!', for all the world as if I had suddenly developed a passion for clean floors. I think I'm turning into a gorgon.

Oh, how could I be so STUPID? It must be PMT. I've just for-gotten what it's like after four years on the Pill.

info

nausea

Some people still call it morning sickness, but it isn't, so they shouldn't. It can get you at any time of the day, even all day. Not everybody gets it, but most pregnant women experience some form of nausea, usually in the first trimester, and half will throw up at least once. It can range from a slightly queasy feeling to full-on, head-in-a-bucket, serious vomiting. For some very unlucky women, it persists after the fourteenth week, even all through the pregnancy.

The cause has not been absolutely identified, and may even vary from person to person. The culprits are thought to include any or all of the following: high levels of the hormone HCG; a fall in blood pressure resulting from progesterone-induced relaxation of muscles, which causes dilation of the blood vessels; less efficient digestion due to less stomach acid in the gut; an increase in oestrogen challenging the liver to break it down, so the liver works overtime; and altered senses, which means that some smells and tastes make you feel sick. (For more information see Pregnancy Hormones in 'Week 12'.)

Here are some things that may help.

⑥ Eat small, frequent snacks to avoid an empty tummy or a low blood-sugar level – keep a handbag or briefcase 'pantry' of dried fruit, dry biscuits and raw nuts, fruit or vegetables.

⑥ Have four or five smaller meals a day instead of three biggies (this can also be useful in the third trimester when your tummy is squished up).

⑥ Eat something bland before you get out of bed in the morning, such as dry toast or a dry biscuit, or have a small amount of fruit juice.

⑥ Have a snack just before bedtime.

⑥ Avoid the fish market or perfume counter or anything else that makes you feel queasy; this can include fatty or fried foods, cigarette smoke, coffee and alcohol.

⑥ Maintain your intake of protein (chicken soup is good) and complex carbohydrates (potato, rice and pasta).

⑥ Avoid getting tired or stressed.

⑥ Try ginger tea – infuse 1–2 teaspoons of grated fresh ginger (or a piece of ginger, about the size of your little finger and chopped into four or five bits) in a small teapot of boiling water for 5 minutes; strain; add honey or a squeeze of lemon to taste, breathing in the steam as you go.

⑥ Sniff a fresh lemon.

⊚ If you've been vomiting, drink lots of water so you don't become dehydrated.

⊚ Try 50 to 100mg of vitamin B_6 per day, which may be recommended by natural therapists and doctors for severe sickness. Foresight, the organisation for pre-conceptual care, recommend zinc (20mg) and vitamin B_6 as a supplement to prevent sickness.

It's not common for vomiting to be so bad that it needs medical intervention, but if you are vomiting more than once a day for days in a row, or any aspect of your vomiting is distressing, tell your doctor straight away. The main risks are that you'll become dehydrated, especially if you can't keep down fluids, or that the baby will miss out on nutrients.

Nausea is often said to be a good sign – evidence that the hormones are pumping, indicating a strong, stable pregnancy. Some people claim first-trimester nausea lowers the risk of miscarriage. (Others point out that nausea affects only half of all pregnant women, so it's hardly a prerequisite for a healthy pregnancy.) More severe nausea is associated with a twin or multiple pregnancy because the hormone levels in the bloodstream are higher.

Morning Sickness by Nicky Wesson, Vermilion, UK, 1997.
If you think you're going to strangle the next person who offers you a dry cracker, this is the book for you. Full of reassuring advice, case studies and remedies.

looking after your embryo – teratogens

Teratogens are infections, substances or environmental factors that can damage an embryo or foetus at certain stages of development – the biggest danger being in the first three months of pregnancy. (In usual tactless-doctor language, 'teratogen' is derived from the ancient Greek teras meaning 'monster'.) The effect of teratogens can range from impaired growth or increased risk of a miscarriage through to serious birth defects.

The impact on the developing baby depends on the teratogen – some are much more dangerous than others – and your level of exposure, as well as what stage of pregnancy you're at when exposed, and individual susceptibility, and luck. (Even if you know somebody who drank vodka like a mad thing through their pregnancy and had a 'normal' baby, it doesn't mean the same will apply for you.)

It's believed that not much damage is likely to be done between conception and when the egg implants itself in the wall of the uterus six to eight days later. The most dangerous time is from implantation to the tenth week after conception, when major organs and limbs are being formed. But some teratogens can affect major parts of the developing baby throughout the whole pregnancy, including the brain, eyes and sex organs.

scary illnesses

Hyperthermia (overheating) Any illness that causes a high temperature (39°C/102°F or more) for an extended time, especially in the first three months of pregnancy, can cause damage to an embryo or foetus. If you are running a temperature, take a cool bath or a shower to try to lower your body temperature, go to bed and drink lots of fluid. Saunas and hot tubs can also raise your body temperature and are best avoided while you're pregnant.

Toxoplasmosis This infection causes an illness that can be symptomless or feel like mild flu. It's caused by a parasite commonly found in raw or undercooked meat (meat should be cooked to an internal temperature of at least 60°C/140°F), including game birds; unpasteurised goat's milk products; and the poo from cats and, more rarely, dogs. The infection can cause brain and eye damage in the foetus, and miscarriage.

Many people come into contact with the toxoplasmosis parasite at some point and therefore have developed an immunity to it. However, avoid close contact with cats (get someone else to empty

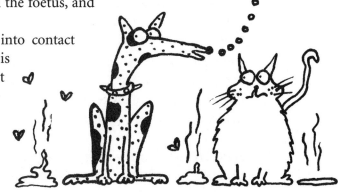

litter trays) and wear gloves when-gardening. Wash all raw, garden-grown produce thoroughly before eating.

Listeriosis This relatively rare bacterial infection is transmitted through foods. Its symptoms include fever, headache, tiredness, aches and pains. It may cause miscarriage or stillbirth. High-risk foods are raw, insufficiently cooked and prepared, 'ready-to-eat' seafood, such as smoked fish and mussels (but tinned fish should be safe); premixed salad vegetables; precooked meats and pâtés; thickshakes and soft-serve ice-cream; and unpasteurised milk or milk products, especially soft cheeses such as brie, blue vein and camembert. Sheep also carry this bacterium so avoid all contact with (live!) sheep or lambs during your pregnancy.

Rubella (German measles) Rubella can cause such a high incidence of abnormalities in babies (congenital rubella syndrome includes blindness and deafness), particularly when mothers are exposed to it in the first trimester, that routine immunisation is offered to all girls in the UK. Often you need a booster shot, so before trying to get pregnant it's a good idea to have your doctor organise a blood test to check your immunity. If you need to be vaccinated, wait three months afterwards before trying to conceive. Your midwife or GP will organise a blood test to check your immunisation status in the first trimester when pregnant.

Syphilis and Gonorrhea This is now a very rare sexually transmitted disease (STD) that can cross the placenta and cause premature birth and stillbirth, or long-term effects in children such as dental abnormalities. It can be detected in routine pregnancy tests and safely treated in early pregnancy with a course of antibiotics. Gonorrhoea is usually tested for at the same time as syphilis and it, too, can be safely treated in pregnancy.

HIV HIV is a virus which attacks the body's immune or defence system so that it cannot fight infections. Pregnant women with

HIV will not automatically pass it on to their babies. However the Department of Health recommends HIV testing in all pregnant women so that measures can be taken in the case of a positive result. These can reduce the transmission rate to babies from an average of 15 per cent to around 1 per cent. For example, highly effective drug treatments can be prescribed in pregnancy and the baby could be delivered by an elective caesarean section. Avoiding breast feeding also reduces the risk of passing on the virus.

Genital herpes An active case of herpes at the time of birth creates a small risk of infection for the baby. Obviously it depends on where the lesion is and a caesarean delivery may be necessary to protect the baby. If you have an infection of genital herpes during your pregnancy or a recurrance of symptoms, tell your GP or midwife so they can decide on treatment and recommend ways to reduce the risk of transmission to the baby.

Cytomegalovirus An infectious cause of mental retardation and congenital deafness, cytomegalovirus is another virus in the herpes group, but fortunately rarely affects babies, as most women have developed immunity (ie had the infection) by the time they become pregnant. A blood test can check whether you have immunity.

Hepatitis Hepatitis B is an infection spread by contact with infected blood and body fluids, usually from sexual contact or from sharing needles. If you get it when you are pregnant it can be passed on to the baby. Many hospitals screen for hepatitis B infection with a blood test. Babies who are at risk can be immunised at birth.

Other diseases and conditions There are various other diseases and conditions that can affect your embryo or foetus. Some of these have 'silent' symptoms so you may not be aware of any risk or problem. Tell your doctor about any high fever, rash, sweats or fluid retention or any other symptom that worries you.

what goes in (1): pills, herbs, vitamins and caffeine

No prescription or over-the-counter drug, herbal or natural remedy or vitamin or mineral supplement should be taken during pregnancy without consulting a doctor or midwife who knows you're pregnant. If you're buying an over-the-counter drug, always go to a chemist and ask for a recommendation, telling them that you are pregnant; and if you're unsure, check with your GP. Don't use drugs, vitamins, or other supplements without up-to-date professional advice.

Painkillers Anti-inflammatory painkillers containing ibuprofen or aspirin (they come under different brand names) should not be taken by pregnant women without medical supervision, as they could lower hormone levels vital for a continued pregnancy.

Herbs Many herbs, herbal supplements and herbal teas and juice bar additives are unsafe for pregnant women and their developing babies. Never assume that "natural" or "herbal" means it's okay to take during pregnancy and seek up-to-date professional advice, no matter what you're told by friends.

Vitamin A Although this vitamin is needed in small quantities by the body, too much can be harmful during pregnancy. Any supplement or acne or skin treatment containing vitamin A should be stopped while you're pregnant, and avoid liver or liver products such as pâté.

Caffeine Recent study results vary on the effects of caffeine in pregnancy. Small amounts are not thought to be harmful but there is some evidence that an intake of five cups of tea or coffee or cola a day can increase the risk of miscarriage. If you are reading this after a diet of a couple of cups a day through your pregnancy, there seems no need to worry.

what goes in (2): alcohol, cigarettes and drugs

No recreational or street drugs are safe to use during pregnancy, and it's a good idea to get 'clean' before you conceive – and get help to stay that way. Many people think that knowing they're having a baby will get them to quit cigarettes or drugs or alcohol, but that's rarely enough. Everyone needs help to quit an addiction, and it's available. If you don't entirely succeed, be sure to tell your GP or midwife about any drugs you've used during pregnancy: they're not allowed to tell the police, and their priority is you and your baby.

Alcohol There is no evidence that light or occasional drinking in pregnancy will harm your baby. But research shows that heavy or frequent drinking can seriously harm your baby's development. Excessive drinking can cause foetal alcohol syndrome: mental retardation, slow growth, and a variety of physical abnormalities and behavioural problems. To be on the safe side, stop drinking altogether or limit your intake to no more than one or two units of alcohol once or twice a week.

Cigarettes Cigarette smoking stunts the growth of the foetus and inhibits the growth of the placenta. So the baby is more likely to be born early, have complications during labour and additional breathing problems at birth. Smoking is also believed to be linked to miscarriage, sudden infant death syndrome (SIDS), childhood asthma and other respiratory traumas for babies and children. All local NHS hospitals offer 'Stop Smoking' services to help pregnant women and their partners quit smoking, and your GP or midwife will be able to give you further information and support.

Dope Cannabis, marijuana and hash are linked to premature birth and low birth weight. There is no known 'safe' amount.

LSD and other hallucinogens LSD carries the risk of miscarriage and chromosomal damage. There is little research on other hallucinogens but it's safest to assume any amount is dangerous.

Ecstasy There isn't much detailed research yet on Es but the drug has been associated with placental bleeding, and the effects on the baby's brain are not known. It is definitely not a good idea.

Amphetamines (speed) Speed is associated with premature babies, and possibly baby heart problems.

Heroin and methadone These drugs can cause prematurity, low birth weight, mental problems and stillbirth. Babies share their mother's addiction and so suffer withdrawal symptoms when they are born, although this can be managed by medical staff. Prescribed methadone is preferable to heroin in pregnancy because it provides a regulated dose to the foetus. The baby must be weaned from its methadone addiction after birth. Coming off heroin suddenly while pregnant is a cause of miscarriage: don't stop abruptly without talking to your doctor.

Cocaine Even a single, one-off hit can damage a foetus. A baby born to a habitual user will need to be weaned off its own addiction and may suffer dangerous health problems.

what goes in (3): environmental hazards
If your job or workplace is unsafe during pregnancy, you have the legal right to be given duties that don't expose you to the hazards. Avoid any of the following.

Radiation X-rays can cause malformations in a foetus. Tell any doctor or dentist who wants to X-ray you that you're pregnant. If you had an x-ray before you knew you were pregnant, ask your obstetrician about the risk to the foetus. It's usually not bad news. Low-level radiation emitted by computer visual display units has not been proven to have an effect on a developing baby.

Overheating As with overheating caused by illness, your body temperature should not be above 39°C/102°F for an extended time.

Poisons and pesticides There are heaps of potentially harmful substances at home and in the workplace, and even in the food you eat (another good reason to buy organic). Read labels and avoid using toxins. Definitely avoid 'fumy' cleaning products, like oven

TELL YOUR DOCTOR
STRAIGHT AWAY ABOUT ANY:

- bleeding from the vagina
- vomiting, if you can't keep down fluids
- abdominal pain
- fainting spells
- high temperature
- major fluid retention
- nagging worries
- instruction or information they gave you that you don't fully understand.

cleaners and drycleaning solvents, most paints, lacquers, thinners, paint strippers, pesticides, herbicides, petrol, glue, many manufacturing chemicals and waste products. Beware of lead in the air in heavy traffic areas and nearby soil, in old house paint and in some water, particularly in houses with old lead pipes or lead-soldered pipes. Lead can also leach into food or drink from very old or handmade china or earthenware pottery.

People in high-risk jobs include health-care workers, farmers, gardeners, factory workers, printing or photographic processing workers, artists, chemists, hairdressers, nail artists, beauty therapists, drycleaners, cleaners, and people who work with petrol. Exposure to air pollution – such as carbon monoxide from car exhausts and smoke from cigarettes – may be a problem, too.

If you are concerned that substances or practices specific to your circumstances are harmful during pregnancy, check with your doctor, midwife, health-and-safety officer or your union. And don't just rely on your employer as the only source of information about what's in your workplace and what the risks are to you.

And don't worry too much: most babies turn out fine.

1
2
3
4
5
6
7
8
9
10
11
12
13
14
15
16
17
18
19
20
21
22

what's going on
Your period hasn't turned up. You might feel premenstrual, with slightly swollen breasts, as well as weeing more often and feeling queasy.

The embryo is still very tiny but starting to form into a tube shape and growing very quickly. The head and tail ends become obvious. The heart and blood vessels are only just starting to form so the embryo doesn't have its independent circulation yet. At this stage the placenta consists of lots of 'tentacles' called chorionic villi. Eventually they will grow into the big, temporary organ that runs the exchange between you and your developing baby, which sends in nutrients and oxygen and takes out waste products and carbon dioxide, using the vein and two arteries in the umbilical cord that connects it to the baby. You'll find that pregnancy books disagree on the size of the developing baby, partly because some measure from head to bum, and some from head to feet.

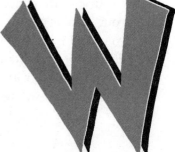

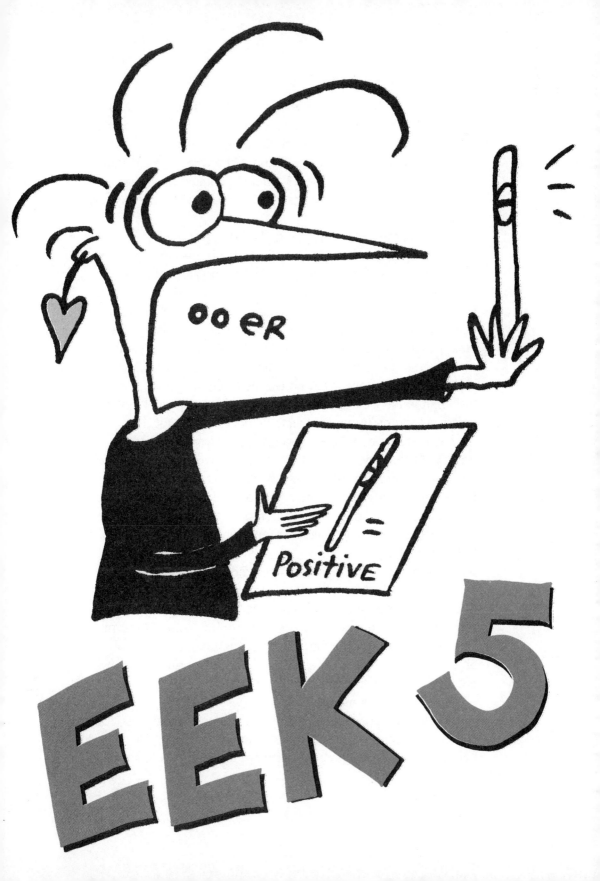

DiARy

We move house and my thirty-third birthday party on Sunday is conducted amid towers of cardboard boxes and tea-chests full of stuff we didn't even open at the last house. My advice to anyone under 27 is don't blink or you'll be 33 before you know what happened. Kind of like Rumpelstiltskin. (Only your beard isn't usually *quite* that bad.)

People at the party keep asking, 'Kaz, do you want another drink?', and I keep saying no. Just like that. No, meaning no, I don't want a drink, which means people keep looking at me strangely. Or I say yes and then leave the drink somewhere under a tree. And it is really flash champagne too, being my birthday and everybody being nice about it. And normally, although I don't smoke – except other people's (oh all right, and those times when I buy a packet for a party, or a sales conference) – I will have the odd puff at a social extravaganza, even one involving tea-chests. But this time I just don't feel like it in the slightest. I begin to feel quite snappy and restless, in fact. All sort of 'It's my party and I'll pout if I want to'.

Then I get scared. I start to think: 33. Thirty-three and I don't want to party any more. It's over. It's been over since Geoff bought that new van. What was I thinking – that I could live in a house with a perfectly nice man who owns a Bedford Rascal and has a steady job and earns his own money and doesn't expect me to pay for everything and isn't some kind of frustrated troll of a tortured artiste?

What happened to my life? When did I get sensible? How can I escape? Maybe I should run through the streets in the nicky-noo-nar shooting out streetlights. Or I could just go to bed. I'm a wee bit on the nod and I've been squirgly again. Must be coming down with something. Need a good night's rest, probably. Nightie-night everyone. Please. Don't stop drinking on my account. I'll just zzzzzzzz.

4am Hang on a minute.

9.10am Pop down to the chemist. Need some dental floss, some cotton balls, some orange nail polish, naturally, and oh, what the hell, I'll take that £7.99 home pregnancy test kit on a whim.

Pregnancy tests from the chemist have obviously changed since last I was a careless idiot. You used to have to wee into some sort of container (yoghurt pot, jam jar, plastic tub with 'Sainsbury's Cottage Cheese' written on the side of it, that kind of thing), and then dip a white plastic magic wand, which was a bit like a flat biro, into it. The most useful instruction was always 'Use the midstream urine for the test'. What that meant was that you did some wee, then you stopped, if you had pelvic-floor muscles like a steel trap, and neatly did a mighty bull's-eye midstream wee into the jar, then stopped (steel trap again), removed the jar and finished the wee.

What always happened was more like sticking a thimble under a waterfall and then snatching it out again and finding that, although you had wee on your hand, the outside of the jar, your hair, the cuffs of your trousers and some articles in another room entirely, you'd managed to miss the jar.

Now you're supposed to hold the magic wand in one hand and – I'm sorry, but basically you just piss on it for a minute or so. This seems such an incredibly male thing to do. I almost feel like trying to write my name in the snow with my own wee. But there is no snow. Only a thin, blue line showing in the 'window', which the instructions say means you're pregnant. And I'm not talking a baby blue, a wimpy sort of a 'We think it's within the realms of possibility that you might conceivably have conceived'. No, it is almost a luminous, pulsating navy blue indicating 'YOU, madam, are *utterly* UP THE DUFF good and proper!'.

I always thought I might cry a tiny tear of feminine, yet sensible joy. Instead, I stare at the wall thinking 'Oh . . . Woo.'

Ring Geoff and tell him to come straight home after his five-a-side football, don't even have one drink, there is something I have to tell him. 'Ooohhhh,' he says, 'Woo,' sounding like he knows what it might be.

I tell him at the front door. He looks pretty shocked. We just start laughing, with tears in our eyes, and then we can't stop laughing. It just seems so ridiculously UNLIKELY. Geoff says he is happy, and then talks about the finer points of five-a-side footie really fast for about 25 minutes. I think he's in shock.

'You told me it would probably take two years to get pregnant,' he says later, quietly.

'Ooops. Woo,' I concur.

Geoff commences to grin for two days straight, the grin punctuated by an expression of profound bewilderment. I begin to refer to him as the bewilderbeest. Luckily he's an optimist whose most remarkable traits include a 'she'll be right' attitude to almost anything. If you told Geoff there was a hurricane coming, he'd be dead interested from a meteorological point of view.

info

pregnancy tests

Pregnancy tests can be done for you by a GP or Family Planning Clinic; many chemists also offer the test, usually for a small fee. Or for about a tenner you can buy a home pregnancy test kit at any chemist and do the test yourself. Whichever path you take, you will get an instant result. All the tests are basically the same. You take a sample of your urine and the test looks for the presence of HCG (human chorionic gonadotrophin hormone). It used to be that you needed to test the first wee of the day (which will have the greatest concentration of HCG) but modern tests can give reliable results for any sample.

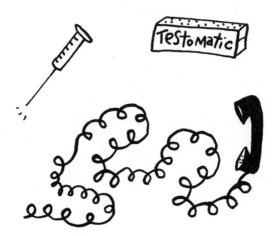

You can do the test as early as fourteen days after conception, about when your period would be due. Results of these tests are almost always accurate, especially if they're positive. A false negative result can happen if the levels of HCG being produced by a pregnant body are low. So if your period doesn't start, and you still suspect you are pregnant, you can wait a few days and do the test again, or go to the doctor for a blood test, which can measure HCG levels as early as one week after conception.

The problem with getting a positive test in the two weeks after you may have conceived, is that the fertilised egg may not implant in your womb, and instead will come out naturally as part of your next period. (This is not generally considered to be a miscarriage, or needing treatment, but part of the body's natural processes.) If you are keen to be pregnant, and an early test gives a positive result, you can be sadly disappointed when it turns out not to be a continuing pregnancy. To avoid this, doctors suggest that you only use a pregnancy test when you have definitely missed a period.

After a positive home test, or other signs of early pregnancy such as a missed period, tender breasts, nausea, frenzied weeing, a funny metallic taste in your mouth, tiredness or moodiness, you should go to your GP. The doctor will discuss a pregnancy plan with you, and may possibly give you a physical examination. If that takes place, the doctor may check for further signs to confirm the pregnancy, such as an enlarged uterus and the changed texture and colour of the cervix (the small opening, and surrounding tissue, between the uterus and the vagina).

It is important to see your GP as soon as possible when you know you are pregnant, to discuss your medical history, and it is crucial if you are currently being treated for a chronic disease such as diabetes or epilepsy. If your medical history gives reason, your doctor might refer you to an obstetrician (a specialist pregnancy doctor). If you have had a previous baby with spina bifida, Down's syndrome, or you have a family history of a genetic disorder, additional tests will be available. These are generally carried out early in pregnancy, from nine to twelve weeks, so the sooner your doctor can refer you to the specialist centre the better (see p.114).

Your GP will be able to give you information about maternity services in your area so that you can decide where to have your baby and choose what sort of antenatal (pregnancy) care would be appropriate for you (see 'Week 9' on Choosing Your Birth Place). Your doctor will also be able to put you in contact with a midwife if you'd like, and will write a referral letter to your chosen hospital, birth centre or maternity unit. You will be invited for your first visit there at around 10–12 weeks and will usually be offered a routine ultrasound scan on this visit.

ectopic pregnancy scan

When the pregnancy is confirmed, an early ultrasound scan might be recommended, especially if you have ever had a miscarriage, you have a medical history that might indicate a blockage in a fallopian tube, or the doctor suspects you have an ectopic pregnancy, which happens when the egg implants itself outside the uterus, usually in a tube. Sadly, an ectopic pregnancy can't be saved and turned into a viable pregnancy. Unless the body naturally aborts the embryo very early, it is a very serious medical problem and must be resolved by surgery as soon as it is diagnosed. Be aware that it's possible to have an ectopic pregnancy even if you think you can't conceive because you're on the Pill or Minipill.

Risk factors include a previous ectopic pregnancy; pelvic inflammatory disease; damage to or scarring of the fallopian tubes caused by infection or surgery; endometriosis; an intra-uterine device (IUD) in place when you conceived; or malformed reproductive organs (there is a history of malformations among women whose mothers took a miscarriage drug called DES – diethylstilboestrol – to combat recurrent miscarriage).

Symptoms of ectopic pregnancy, which usually occur at about six weeks, may include abdominal pain, either on one side of the abdomen or more generalised, that can come and go; spotting or bleeding; dizziness, faintness, paleness and sweating; nausea and vomiting; sometimes shoulder pain; and sometimes a feeling of pressure in the bum. Tell your doctor or obstetrician immediately about these symptoms. Early treatment improves your chances of saving the tube and maintaining fertility. (One in ten ectopic pregnancies ends in infertility.)

If a fallopian tube bursts, the pain is terrible: go straight to hospital because you'll need emergency surgery.

your first antenatal visit

Antenatal care varies around the UK. In some areas, the first appointment is at your local hospital, then all or most subsequent appointments are with your GP or midwife, unless the pregnancy is complicated, when all appointments are at the hospital. In other areas, all care is given by the GP and/or midwife unless there is a reason for referral to the hospital antenatal clinic. If you are referred for specialist monitoring or advice, you will be seen by a hospital-based obstetrician.

Your first antenatal visit is usually your longest, as a detailed medical history will be taken by a midwife. There will be a set of notes recording all this, which you should be given a copy of: these become a record of your pregnancy and you should keep them with you at home or on any trip away; should you need medical assistance you will have all the information that's needed. Antenatal notes will include details of: previous illnesses and surgery; allergies; prescription medications or alternative treatments you're taking; gynaecological and obstetric history, including the pattern of your menstrual cycle; past pregnancies, miscarriages or pregnancy terminations (abortions); any family history of twins or genetic disorders; any STDs; your lifestyle, particularly diet, smoking, drinking, drugs, work and fitness habits; your family's medical history, and possibly your mum's obstetric history (though most doctors nowadays know this is neither here nor there).

At this first visit, the midwife will also ask about your plans for antenatal classes. This is a good time to get information about what is available in your area and to get further referral names and addresses, leaflets and recommended groups. If you are interested in joining the NCT (National Childbirth Trust) classes, for instance, you should sign up fairly soon as in many areas they are oversubscribed (see the following page).

routine tests

The routine antenatal tests carried out by your midwife or doctor at your first visit will probably include:

⊚ A basic all-round 'physical' with the emphasis on questions about your general health and a check of blood pressure.

⊚ You may be weighed, and perhaps your pelvis will be measured with a tape measure.

⊚ Urine test (this is mainly to look for any urinary tract infection, which if left untreated might increase the risk of having a premature baby).

⊚ Routine blood tests to establish various standard things, such as your blood group, and checks on whether you have any immunities or problems – including anaemia, rubella, hepatitis, syphilis, HIV, or any genetic disorders which could be passed on to the baby. (See Help – Screening and Blood Tests on p.410).

The midwife will also have a discussion with you about whether you would like to breast feed, how you can get help with this, and what will happen if you can't, or don't want to. They may also discuss screening tests that will be offered (see Week 11 – p.114).

further antenatal visits

Usually you will continue to have antenatal checks every three to four weeks throughout your pregnancy. These give you the opportunity to discuss issues and ask questions. You'll need to bring a urine sample to each visit to be tested for protein (a possible sign of urine infection or high blood pressure) and glucose (which can indicate high blood sugar). Small plastic specimen jars are usually provided and can be reused throughout your pregnancy. You need to bring your notes to each visit.

At each visit your blood pressure will be checked and your tummy examined to measure the growth of the uterus, and you may be weighed. Your baby's heartbeat will also be monitored, using a handheld doppler (ultrasound tool) or a pinard (stethoscope). After about sixteen weeks you'll be able to hear the baby's heartbeat when the midwife puts a doppler on your tummy.

TWINS AND MULTIPLE BIRTHS

Twins happen about once in every 80 pregnancies – although the incidence is higher if you have had IVF or other fertility treatment. Triplets (or more) are very rare unless you have had multiple embryos implanted as part of a fertility treatment. In an ordinarily conceived pregnancy, you will normally find out you have twins at your first ultrasound scan – probably at twelve weeks. Of course, if for any reason you have an earlier scan, you will find out then. Whenever you make that discovery, nothing can quite prepare you for the shock.

Your pregnancy, antenatal care and birth options will be different in many ways with a multiple birth. Nothing is quite straightforward in a twin pregnancy and you will receive more frequent antenatal check-ups, generally with an obstetrician as well as a midwife. The babies are scanned regularly to measure their growth and monitor their development. Your health will also be monitored because certain complications of pregnancy are more common with twins – pre-eclampsia, preterm labour, anaemia and, not least, sheer exhaustion.

Some mothers find the old saying of double the trouble is a very accurate way to describe a twin pregnancy. Extra tiredness, extra weight gain and more movements from the growing babies are all guaranteed. The most important advice in carrying twins is rest. The second is to re-think your timeframe (including maternity leave). Twins are generally born early – at 37 rather than 40 weeks on average. You will probably be advised to slow down towards 18–20 weeks and, if you're working, you should think about negotiating part-time hours at that stage. The work of carrying two babies is very tiring and the reality of caring for them in the first few months is so exhausting it is worth spoiling yourself whilst pregnant and taking some time off.

Your labour may also be different with a multiple birth. If the babies are lying in good positions, then there is no reason not to have labour and a normal hospital birth. But they often lie awkwardly in the last few weeks of pregnancy in which case the safest way for them to be delivered will be by a caesarean birth.

It's easy to forget something you've been meaning to ask the doctor or midwife – list your questions somewhere in your diary or with your notes as they occur to you, and jot down the answers while you're there, too, because sometimes your head's in a whirl with all the new info and emotions and you can't remember afterwards exactly what was said.

back to the classroom: the nct

Now is a good time to be thinking about the classes you and your partner might want to inflict upon yourselves in the run-up to the birth. The NHS hold some parenting skills classes, and all over the country independent teachers offer everything from 'active birth' (which promotes the use of yoga during pregnancy, 'active' labour and delivery in the upright position) to 'aqua natal' (basically swimming during pregnancy), but the most popular classes are those offered by the NCT (National Childbirth Trust).

Set up forty years ago, the NCT is a charitable organisation that offers educational advice and support for parents during pregnancy and birth, and on through the toddler years. The NCT has campaigned successfully to ensure that fathers have the right to attend their baby's birth and that babies are not separated from their mothers immediately after birth. They continue to push for more women-centred postnatal care and a positive breastfeeding culture.

For its users, the NCT offers a wealth of well-researched information, maternity sales (equipment, books, bras, etc), and most crucially, a network of antenatal courses – which offer you not only knowledge about pregnancy and babycare but a local support group with other women and couples in the same boat. This may not sound like what you want right now but when a baby turns your life over, you may well find it invaluable.

The structure of NCT classes depends on your local branch (there are 380 across the UK – see p.409 for contact addresses), and the content is often determined by particular concerns of group members. Most classes start toward the end of the second trimester (Week 26 or 27) and continue with weekly sessions for the next eight weeks. By then, you've probably made a network of new friends, with whom you'll be in surprisingly close contact before and after the birth.

twins and multiple births

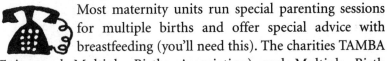 Most maternity units run special parenting sessions for multiple births and offer special advice with breastfeeding (you'll need this). The charities TAMBA (Twins and Multiple Births Association) and Multiple Birth Foundation are an excellent source of information and run support groups (see Twins and Multiple Births in 'Help', p.411).

Twins and Multiple Births: The Essential Parenting Guide by Dr Carol Cooper, Vermilion, UK, 2004.

This really is an essential guide (and by far the best book of its kind) if you are expecting more than one baby – a compendium of good, sensible advice for you and your partner covering every aspect of antenatal care and preparation. Should you get any free time after the birth there is a really good section on practicalities of feeding and sleeping arrangements for the siblings and how to survive and enjoy their first year. Written by a GP and mother of twins, the book is based on experience as well as sound evidence. There is even a section exploring what it is like to be a twin and the relationship that developes between twins and how you can influence this.

your record

☀ Do you know exactly where and when you got pregnant?

☀ After a party, on holiday, while recreational boating perhaps? Have a guess!

☀ What date did you find out you were pregnant?

☀ What mix of emotions did you experience?

☀ If you have a partner, how did you break the news?

WEEK

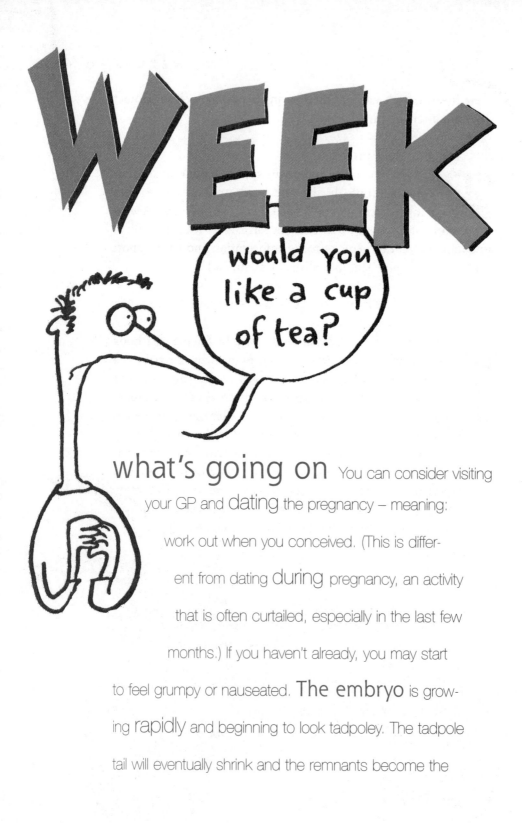

would you like a cup of tea?

what's going on You can consider visiting your GP and dating the pregnancy – meaning: work out when you conceived. (This is different from dating during pregnancy, an activity that is often curtailed, especially in the last few months.) If you haven't already, you may start to feel grumpy or nauseated. The embryo is growing rapidly and beginning to look tadpoley. The tadpole tail will eventually shrink and the remnants become the

6 baby's coccyx. In the centre of the embryo

is the start of the digestive system, lungs and

bladder. This is surrounded by a layer that will

develop into muscles, skeleton, heart, kidneys and

genitals, and this is wrapped up in what will become the skin,

nervous system, ears and eyes. Tiny bumps are appearing

that will grow into arms. The immature heart starts to beat

and pump blood around the embryo and into the chorionic

villi (the pre-placenta) and can be clearly seen as a pulsation

on an ultrasound

screen. Really, the whole

thing looks like some tiny

thing that might come out if you

sneezed.

yeah?
You and
whose
army?

DiARy Work is hotting up. We sign up to produce new fashion ranges for a couple of big department stores. The spicy earth colours of winter! The divine madness of spring! You know the sort of thing. Will we get it all done before the baby arrives? I can't even tell anyone I'm pregnant yet. The convention is to wait until after thirteen weeks, when they reckon the biggest risk of miscarriage is over.

We tell some close friends of Geoff's, quietly, at a wedding. They scream. I have to pretend there is a spider down my knickers to explain the kerfuffle.

Beck, of course, has known about the pregnancy even before the sperm got going, and is taking the adviser role seriously. She says I need to get my GP to refer me to a pregnancy clinic right away because of my endometriosis, which can cause an ectopic pregnancy. She says that an early ultrasound would check that the pregnant bit of me is where it should be – in the uterus – instead of ectopic (stuck in a fallopian tube), which can be very danger-ous. My GP, Dr Fisher is quite reassuring and refers me directly to the early pregnancy clinic at the local hospital, where he says I'll meet the midwife team who will provide most of my pregnancy care. Before I leave, he asks me to fill in a few details on the hos-pital referral form to take with me.

Who is your family doctor? (Dr Fisher)

Last period? (Well, in my case about four years, but surely that's going to take too long to explain.)

Number of previous pregnancies? (One. This pregnancy business sure flicks open the clasps on your emotional baggage. When I get to the hospital clinic, I look at the posters on the wall of a foetus developing week by week. It was so long ago. I can't remember now whether I terminated at six weeks or eight weeks. So many of us women having babies in our thirties had abortions when we were younger, vowing that we would only become mothers when we could be good at it. I'm glad I waited. I didn't even know who I really was then. But I really don't want to look at that poster.)

Previous surgery: how many operations? (Can't remember so compromise by writing 'Loads'. That should give an idea.)

Husband's name? (Well, I have got a boyfriend, but what is a single girl supposed to write? 'Missing In Action'? Not Available'?

The day of my ultrasound appointment, I am shown into a small room and lie on a flat, hard, raised couch. The ultrasound operator, Dr Donaldson, sits next to me at about hip level with a screen in front of him.

If I crane my neck, I can just about make out a tiny dot on the screen pulsating incredibly quickly and rhythmically. That's the embryo's heartbeat. And it's all in the right spot: the uterus. I feel incredibly relieved.

Then Dr Donaldson launches into a speech that is like a parody of the detached medical consultant, saying I should realise that there might be 'wastage'. It takes me a beat or two until I realise he's warning me that it's very early days and I could have a miscarriage – in typically sensitive medical parlance.

I go to see Dr Fisher again a couple of days later – I made a bit of an excuse for the visit but he didn't seem to mind, in any case. 'Everything's absolutely fine,' he grins.

Now that's what I call a doctor.

info

miscarriage

About one in eight confirmed pregnancies ends in miscarriage. It's believed the actual figure might be one in six of all pregnancies, but many miscarriages occur very early and are mistaken for a period. As you get older your risk increases; you're also more likely to miscarry if you have already had a miscarriage.

About three-quarters of all known miscarriages happen in the first trimester (the first 13 weeks). Loss of a baby after twenty-four weeks is called a preterm stillbirth. You may hear a doctor refer to a miscarriage by the medical term 'spontaneous abortion' and when a pregnancy ends in miscarriage because the embryo does not develop the embryo is often called a 'blighted ovum'. These medical terms do not help your feelings.

After a miscarriage you may need to have a small operation to prevent infection, which makes sure the uterus is free of all the tissue that should come out. The endometrium will grow back as good as new. The operation is known as a curette, or a D and C (dilatation and curettage), and is performed under general anaesthetic in hospital. If you miscarry before six weeks you probably won't need a D and C.

bleeding

By far the most common symptom of miscarriage is bleeding from the vagina. If this happens, it is important to contact your GP immediately. You will need to be ready to describe the colour, quantity and time frame of the bleeding. Light spotting might not be a cause for alarm and the doctor might tell you to rest for a couple of days. A heavy flow could mean the doctor will tell you that you need to go straight to hospital. Don't use a tampon for any bleeding during pregnancy, and keep the pad you do use until you have spoken to your GP. And don't have penetrative sex until the bleeding has been checked by the doctor.

Vaginal bleeding occurs in about a quarter of pregnant women, but most of them go on to have healthy babies. This can be a very worrying time and many maternity units run early pregnancy clinics where ultrasound scans are offered. The baby's heart beat can be checked and this can be very reassuring.

I know this sounds a bit gross and depressing but, if you can, keep any clots and tissue from a miscarriage in a clean plastic bag or container, so they can be examined. This can help your obstetrician decide whether the miscarriage is complete.

causes of miscarriage

Possible causes of miscarriage include 'nature rejecting a problem with a pregnancy', such as foetal abnormality; exposure to certain chemicals, illnesses or medications; problems with the uterus, placenta, cervix, sperm, or egg implantation; and hormonal imbalances. Occasionally, recurrent miscarriage is a sign of an auto-immune condition. The mother produces antibodies that cause blood clots in the placenta. Low doses of aspirin throughout pregnancy may help these women.

An 'incompetent cervix' (another charming medical term) is sometimes diagnosed when miscarriage occurs. It means that the cervix gets over-eager and opens too soon. This may be the cause of up to a quarter of miscarriages in the second trimester (week 14 until the end of week 26). Previous gynaecological surgery or laser treatments, abortions or miscarriages could increase your risk of this condition – another reason to give your doctor and midwife your full medical history. A misbehaving cervix can be stitched closed during your next pregnancy until the baby is due.

After you've had a miscarriage, get all the information you can from your obstetrician – make sure all your questions are answered – and review the possible risk factors that could be avoided or treated in future pregnancies. If you have more than two miscarriages, you'll usually be tested for uterine problems and hormonal imbalances and have your immune system evaluated.

Miscarriage is no less distressing because it's common. Friends and family can make things worse by well-meaning but insensitive remarks, such as 'Hurry up and have another one', or 'You'll soon get over it'. It's important to allow yourself time to talk over and mourn the loss with your partner, who may grieve differently from you, causing friction. It can be really helpful to find a support group so you can talk to other people who have been through it. But take some comfort: you now know you can get pregnant.

 You can ask to be put in touch with a support group (see Grief and Loss in 'Help' – p.406).

1
2
3
4
5
6
7
8
9
10
11
12
13
14
15
16
17
18
21
22

what's going on
Your breasts may be bigger and more sensitive, and the nipples and surrounding areolae may have started to look bigger and bumpier. (The little bumps on each areola are officially called Montgomery's tubercles but who cares about Montgomery, whoever he was: 'little bumps' sounds a lot cuter.) You could have continuing nausea and need to wee a lot. Foods may taste different, and you may go off the smell of things you previously liked.

Teeny buds that will grow into legs are appearing on the embryo. Everything continues growing at a cracking pace. The heart is going strongly inside a developing chest but the lungs have only just started to form. Embryonic kidneys begin to develop and function (the finished kidneys come later). The head bulge is getting more like the right shape. The chorionic villi are making more and longer tentacles into

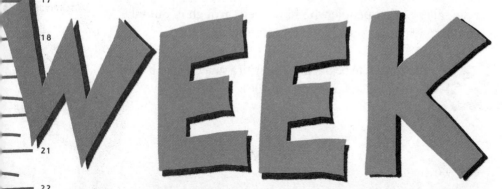

WEEK

the uterus. Some books say the embryo is about the size of

a brazil nut or an olive ('Shall I compare thee to a cocktail party

nibble?'), but we are officially going with coffee bean.

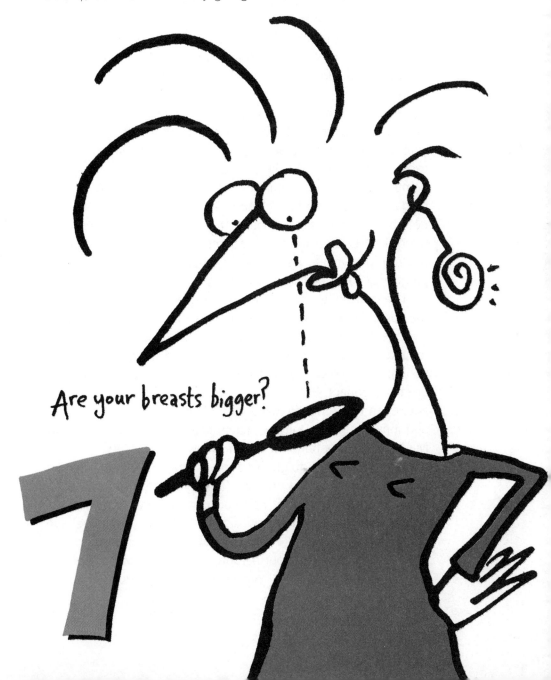

DiARy

I couldn't be less interested in sex if my private parts had been packed away in a shoe box in the back of the wardrobe. This will not do. Where is the surge of lascivious sex-kittenry the books promise and the magazines go on about?

Take the pregnancy special issue of this month's *She* magazine, and I quote: 'In the middle of your pregnancy, your libido soars. You're not too enormous but you're round enough not to be concerned about maintaining the missionary position in the quest for a flat stomach and no chins. You bounce about with abandon.' Oh bollocks.

Apart from the fact that the last thing you want to be thinking about when you're having fun is whether he's thinking about your double chin – and anyway what bloke is thinking anything except 'Bingo!' with a girlie on top of him? – apart from a few pointers on that kind of palaver, I'd just like to know where these magazine writers get off, telling us how we're going to feel. As if everybody is the same as them – that is, wanders around saying things like 'Beige is the new black, essentials this summer include platform pantyliners with a daisy motif, and in the middle of your pregnancy you'll be rutting like a farmyard animal.'

I've been reflecting on Dr Donaldson at the ultrasound using the appalling word 'wastage' to warn me about a possible miscarriage. It must be his regular spiel to everybody. Anyway it has reminded us again not to tell anyone in case something goes wrong. So we've only told Deborah, Tania, Susanne cos she's already pregnant, Beck because, let's face it, she is my medical adviser and I'll probably need a bit of advice, Liz and John, Jo and Jonathan, Pete, Duncan, Helen, Kate, Richard, Teresa, Nat and Mark. Less than a hundred people, anyway.

Apart from that I might have to tell some people at work so they don't think I've lost my mind. (I go around with this permanent off-the-air expression, which actually indicates I'm talkin' sales figures and thinkin', 'Creature inside me! Creature inside me! Size of a Tic Tac. I feel seasick right now and I have to pretend I don't! Bleeeeuuurghhh! I beg your pardon, I appear to have thrown up on your shoes', or simply 'I know something YOU don't know.')

We don't want to tell everyone we're 'expecting' and then have to say, 'Oh we lost it', as if we'd been a bit careless in the Safeway car park and left the little bundle in the returned trolleys section by mistake. I heard that one in eight pregnancies ends in miscarriage.

'Oh no, that's not right,' says Beck.

'Thank God I've got you to calm my fears with proper medical facts, Beck,' I say.

'I think it's one in six, or maybe even five,' she explains helpfully.

So much of pregnancy seems to be about odds. It automatically turns you into a gambler. The statistics mean everything and nothing at the same time. One in four is high, even if some of those are miscarriages you wouldn't know about because they would be just like having a period. And if you do have a miscarriage, your own personal chance was 100 per cent. And if you don't have a miscarriage, your individual risk was zero per cent. But you can't help brooding on 'one in four' and every other percentage risk they tell you about.

We go to a birthday do at Geoff's mum's – we don't tell. The next night, Geoff has a work dinner do that is full of pregnant gardening associates. Geoff wants to tell everyone and has to be sternly restrained.

Poor Geoff. He's got a seasick, exhausted girlfriend who'd rather stick peas up her nose than have sex, and he's going to be a daddy. I think we're both feeling kind of like it's all been a theory and now it's actually going to happen. Well actually, it still feels a bit theoretical. Maybe I'm just in denial.

I know intellectually that I'm pregnant, but it just doesn't feel real. I can't tell by looking, and I don't suddenly feel like knitting bootees or protecting my offspring with the ferocity of a lioness. I have no more idea about raising a child than I did six weeks ago. No sudden illuminated shaft has split the heavens asunder, pierced the top of my noggin and said in a very deep voice, 'You are going to be a mother.' Just as well, really. I'd probably wet myself.

I am very grumpy indeed. Geoff has read somewhere that newborn babies look like their father so the father will stick around. I reply that all newborn babies look like Winston Churchill, and what's that got to do with anything? Geoff wonders why hormones would make you grumpy when surely nature intends you to keep the man happy, to protect you. I refrain from saying that being grumpy is a perfectly bloody natural reaction, and furthermore it is no doubt serving the important purpose of teaching you that if the bloke runs off with a sailor, or proves to be a complete flop at hunter-gathering, you can do it all yourself.

After all, most women with one child and a husband feel like they have two children and anyway why is there a mess in that corner and I believe you forgot to put the rubbish out again and WHERE'S MY BLOODY DINNER?

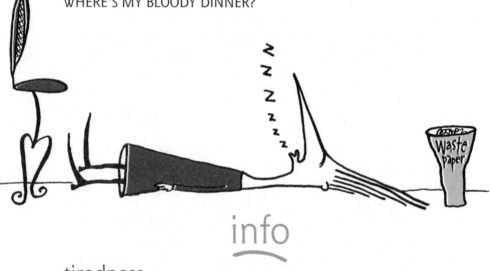

info

tiredness

One symptom of the first trimester can be an incredibly draining exhaustion – which you can't even complain about because most people don't know that you're pregnant.

Here's the weird thing: in the past, if you've been really tired, you have probably pushed through it. With first-trimester pregnancy tiredness, you find yourself following your feet up the hall and getting into bed. You have turned into a robot. Welcome to reality: your body is now running you, rather than the other way around.

A lot of women who go out to work full-time spend the first trimester coming home from their job, going straight to bed, waking up and demanding dinner from their partner or flatmate, or calling a takeaway pizza, and then going back to bed.

Most women start to feel perkier and less nauseated by week 14 (but the tiredness comes back in the third trimester).

Here are some of the reasons why you may be so tired:

⑥ The high levels of progesterone in the system during the first trimester can have a sedative effect.

⑥ Your metabolic rate increases 10–25 per cent to support the developing foetus, and a whole lot of other parts are working overtime, such as your heart.

⑥ Your body is putting the development of the foetus first – you are making eyelids and bones and sex organs and lungs and a placenta and stuff so for heaven's sake who WOULDN'T need to lie down with all that going on?

⑥ All that extra night-time weeing means you're not getting the deepest, most restful part of sleep.

⑥ Just being nauseated (see Nausea in 'Week 4') can make you feel exhausted.

Some ways to combat tiredness are:

⑥ Win the lottery; quit work; sleep all the time; get a cleaner, a masseur and, oh, hang the expense, a personal chef like Madonna's; live in a posh hotel.

⑥ Give in to it, don't fight it – your body will win this round anyway, so you may as well not start your life as a mother by being frazzled.

⑥ Let your doctor or midwife know the extent of your tiredness: a non-constipating iron supplement may work wonders.

⑥ Find a storeroom or sickroom where you can nap if work commitments mean long days at the office (and if all else fails you could always just Lie Down under your desk) – and don't forget to eat lunch at your desk if you use the lunch hour for a kip.

⑥ Nap when you get home if you work away from home.

⑥ Nap when you can if you work at home.

⑥ Meet friends for lunch or on the weekends rather than at night (smoky pubs and nightclubs, and alcohol are probably making you feel sick at the moment anyway) — you can always come back to daiquiris in a year or so.

⑥ Keep one day, or at least an afternoon on the weekend, completely free; and don't be ashamed in any way if you want to spend All Weekend in bed for the first three months.

⑥ If you have a partner or flatmate who has not been pulling their weight in the housework department, renegotiate so they see that doing the tasks/chores is about rights and responsibilities rather than about 'helping' you or doing you a favour; alternatively, get used to mess – or both.

⑥ If you already have little children, give them away to relatives. Sorry. No. Try to nap when (if) they do.

weeing all the time

Weeing all the time is a very common symptom of pregnancy in the first thirteen weeks or so. It's not that you're over-excited, it's just that your uterus is taking up more space, putting pressure on the neighbouring organs, including your bladder. Even more congestion is caused by the extra blood vessels and blood flow developing in the pelvis to sustain the placenta and carry the extra weight.

It may be less of a problem in the second trimester because the uterus 'pops' outwards at the front, making the pelvis temporarily

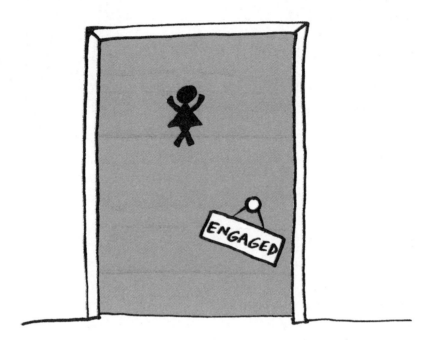

less crowded. But then constant weeing usually comes back in the third trimester when there's a serious space shortage – at which stage it can feel as if your baby is kicking your bladder, or grabbing it, or generally tossing it around and headbutting it.

You still need to drink lots of water during the day to avoid dehydration, but you can try drinking less in the evenings in an attempt to reduce the number of trips to the toilet during the night. (Experienced mums will grimly inform you that getting up to wee all night long is good training for the interrupted sleep caused by night feeding once the baby is born. I say try not to do it until you have to.)

If you get a burning or stinging sensation when you wee a lot, mention it to your doctor. You may have a bladder infection, which may need treating with antibiotics. Drinking cranberry juice can help relieve the stinging.

1
2
3
4
5
6
7
8
9
10
11
12
13
14
15
16
17
18
19
20
21
22

what's going on

You are continuing to wee more often because your bladder is being crowded by the uterus. A lot of fancy hormonal footwork is going on to keep building the placenta. You might feel nauseated AND constipated: jackpot! You may be starting to feel tired: your body has a lot to do that is normally not on the agenda. Your hair may be getting thicker, and downstairs there may be more vaginal mucus than normal.

Your embryo has become that classic curled shape, the big fat head with a tail (not a very attractive shape at this point, and similar to a prawn from space, sure, but we all have to start somewhere). It's still so tiny, but it's about a million times bigger than the fertilised cell that started moving and shaking six weeks ago. The external bits of the ears now start to be visible, and the tiny hands are webbed.

EEK 8

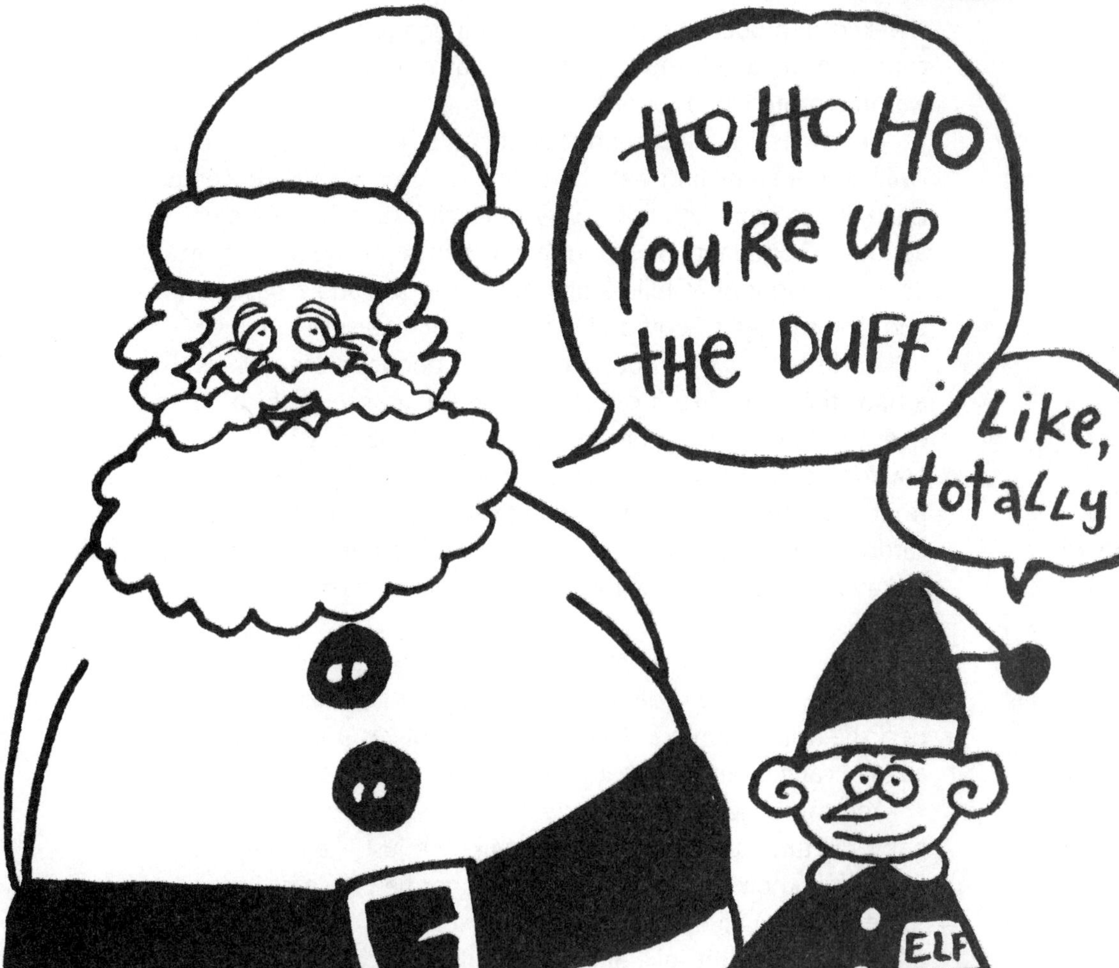

DIARY I am having strange, vivid dreams. Last night I dreamt that American author Gore Vidal came to afternoon tea and I gave him a Toffee Crisp on a silver plate and he said, 'How perfectly charming.' I was completely furious that Geoff woke me up at that precise moment to kiss me goodbye as he went to work.

'But I just gave Gore Vidal a Toffee Crisp!' I said accusingly.

'Yes, dear,' he replied, which was probably about the only thing he could have said.

I also dreamt I went to a funfair on the Isle of Wight with a well-known model who had too much luggage to fit in the helicopter. In the end it didn't matter as our turn on the Ferris wheel was interrupted by a tornado.

Christmas Day. We spend it pretty quietly, knowing that in the twinkling of an inkling we'll be agonising over whether to come clean about Santa and how to try to teach a rapacious toddler about the spirituality of giving rather than receiving. (Fat chance.)

I've bought Aunt Julie a pair of silk slippers and a flash handbag. She's bought Geoff and me a sandwich toaster.

Uncle Mike (we've got him a mobile phone) presents us with a book that looks like it came from the Oxfam shop, which he doesn't bother to wrap because wrapping paper destroys the environment. Instead he sticky-tapes a homemade card to the front of it. And when I say a homemade card, I mean a bit of cardboard from the inside of his girlfriend's packet of pantyhose. (Re-use, recycle, read my lips: my Uncle Mike has become a real eco-cheapskate.)

Uncle Mike's new girlfriend is twenty-five years younger than him and has purple dreadlocks and is a total fruitcake. I suspect she drinks hemlock. Her name, allegedly, is Aurelia. We are already calling her 'Oh Really' behind her back.

You can't choose your family, I guess. I wonder how our baby will turn out. Maybe just like Mike. Or just like Mum, but I wouldn't know because I can't remember her. At least I have some photos. Will I have more respect for what she went through, or for the way Aunt Julie and Uncle Mike raised me? Will our child inherit Aunt Julie's instinctive morbid dreads? Or copy

Aurelia's purple dreads? Or be influenced by Uncle Mike's habit of saving rubber bands, rolling them into balls and then trying to sell them to Jehovah's Witnesses who come to the door?

Bloody nausea. Queasy isn't the word for it. I am nauseous all the time and desperate for it to stop. Whoever called it 'morning sickness' was a complete maniac. (I keep involuntarily singing 'Get it in the morning, get it in the evening, get it at suppertime'.) Beck thinks it's just too much oestrogen in my system and my liver is having trouble clearing it out.

Aurelia would probably say if I was a Pisces I would accept my pregnancy and wouldn't get 'morning sick' and that it's all in my mind. At least I've got a mind, I could tell her.

'The HCG hormone almost certainly has something to do with morning sickness, but we don't really know what causes it,' Dr Fisher had said when I asked him about it during my first visit. Nor did he offer any fix, quick or otherwise.

Even my growing library of pregnancy books don't have much to suggest. 'Eat dry crackers before you get out of bed in the morning' doesn't seem much of a game plan. I mean, they might as well say: 'Sacrifice a chicken and study its entrails. An interestingly shaped spleen means you will continue to have nausea until the thirteenth week.'

Beck says, 'Don't worry, nausea means the baby is hanging on in there. If it stopped suddenly THAT would be a worry because it could mean a miscarriage.'

Nausea stops suddenly for a whole day. Oh my God.

Nausea starts again. Thank God.

Bloody nausea.

I'm also weeing all the time. In some circles this is regarded suspiciously, and one person even starts a rumour that I have such a severe cocaine problem I have to go to the toilet three times during a dinner party. In other circles you get smug looks from mothers who think they're onto you. And one of the girls at work asked if I was bulimic and suggested I try laxatives instead. Crikey.

Geoff and I take a long walk on the common and decide we don't want to have a Down's syndrome baby because it's not fair to have a child who might need constant medical intervention yet mightn't understand why. And we can't take care of our child forever: one day we'll be gone. We decide that we would terminate if we had to. Geoff says the decision is ultimately mine and he'll support it.

A part of me knows what he means, and I appreciate the sensitivity, but there's a part of me that gets really annoyed and thinks, 'I can't make this decision on my own – we'll both have to live with it.' Then I worry about whether I'm a selfish cow. It's all very tricky. Beck advises that if it comes to that, we could always say there was a miscarriage so other people who knew about the pregnancy didn't judge our decision to terminate. Sounds like a good idea. The result of all this is we decide I should have a test that estimates the risk of giving birth to a Down's syndrome baby.

We've chosen an interim name so we don't have to say 'it' all the time. Cellsie – as in bunch of cells – is what we're calling the embryo-baby-offspring-thingie inside me. We'll have to come up with something else before kindergarten but it'll do for the moment.

info

cravings

You know how you sometimes crave chocolate or pasta, or maybe red meat, when you're premenstrual? Pregnancy cravings (picas in medical talk) can be similar. Most pregnant women get brief crazes for one sort of food or another – usually ice-cream or things sugary. You can go through stages, craving steamed veggies, then chocolate, then tropical fruit. (You can also go right off a food that used to be a favourite. This can include strong-smelling foods and green leafy vegetables that are the slightest bit 'slimy'.) It's best to keep sugary snacks to a minimum as they don't provide real energy and can stack on extra weight you won't need.

You might also get a funny taste in your mouth that seems kind of metallic. This is thought to be due to the high level of various hormones in your blood, which can change the taste of your saliva.

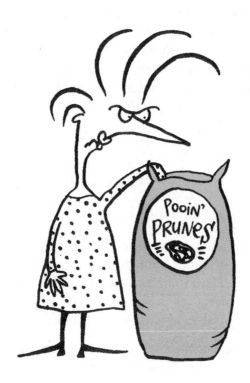

constipation

High progesterone levels are relaxing the muscles in your digestive tract, causing intestinal activity to slow down. This means your poo is going on a slower journey than usual, so it loses water and can become hard, causing constipation. (In the third trimester you can experience even worse constipation as your ginormous uterus squashes the bowel.)

Here are some ways to avoid constipation.

⑥ Drink at least 2 litres of water, spaced out across the day; try some warm water first thing in the morning if it doesn't make you feel nauseated.

⑥ Eat plenty of natural fibre – fresh and lightly cooked root vegetables, fruit, wholegrain breads, high-fibre cereals, such as porridge, and brown rice. Choose whole foods instead of processed foods and pre-prepared breakfast cereals whenever possible. If this is a bulkier load of fibre than your body is used to, have smaller meals more often while you adjust. Remember that the more fibre you eat, the more you need to drink.

⑥ Get plenty of exercise.

⑥ If chemical iron supplements are causing constipation, talk to your doctor or midwife about a herbal alternative (such as Floradix – see pp.27–28).

⑥ Constipation can also come with the added discomfort of bloating and farting. This should disappear when the constipation goes. Too much unprocessed bran, and sometimes too much raw food, which is hard to digest, can cause bloating. Lightly steamed veggies are easier to absorb than hard, completely raw ones.

⑥ Don't take any laxative preparation without discussing it first with your doctor – some laxatives, including those that contain senna, can produce violent expulsive actions, causing painful contractions of the bowel, which in turn can upset the uterus next door.

⑥ Don't have any kind of abdominal massage – a real no-no at this stage of pregnancy.

more info on constipation

A natural therapist or health-food shop adviser can help you with natural methods of dealing with constipation, especially after the birth.

WHO TO TELL? WHEN TO TELL?

Many people wait until the end of the first trimester (after thirteen weeks) to 'publicly' announce their pregnancy, when the greatest risk of miscarriage is over. This allows you time to adjust to the idea of being pregnant and to share feelings in private. It also delays the moment when relatives go berserk and can't shut up about it. Once they know, your whole family and in-laws (not to mention work colleagues, acquaintances and complete strangers) will descend with advice, horror stories, theories and judgements about your plans to return to work or not return to work. Even expressions of joy from your extended family can be overwhelming. Maybe you'll want to pick a weekend to break the news so everyone can celebrate together.

Parents often choose not to tell their toddler until the pregnancy is visible because for a littlun it seems like an eternity until something interesting happens. (Well, actually, you don't have to be a toddler.)

Work Exactly when you want to tell your employer will depend on your relationship with them and your position within the organisation, but they should hear the news from you and not on the office grapevine. Your employer should be advised in writing that you are pregnant and when you plan to start your maternity leave. You will need to give your employer the MAT B1 form which states the date when your baby is due. You get given this form by your doctor or midwife when you are 20 weeks pregnant. Legally, you don't need to tell your employer until ten weeks before you plan to stop work, but it's hard to imagine that nobody would have noticed by then, and you might want to give as much notice as possible so your employer can plan how to best cover your job while you are on leave ... and give it back to you if you want it. Before you tell your employer, find out your leave rights (see Getting Ready for Pregnancy in 'Week 1').

▶

Friends with pregnancy troubles You may have a friend who wants to be pregnant but it's not possible for them right now. They may be having trouble conceiving, have had a miscarriage or several miscarriages, or they may be on the in vitro fertilisation (IVF) program. You may even have a friend whose baby died. The news that you are pregnant will be bittersweet for them. Here are a few hints that might make it easier.

● Tell your friend about your pregnancy privately, perhaps in her home when nobody else is around. Although she will be happy for you, she may have a cry because your pregnancy reminds her so much of what she wants for herself. Don't tell other friends about her situation if she wants to maintain privacy.

● Let your friend know that you will answer any questions about your pregnancy, but that you'll try not to talk to her about it all the time, and she has your full permission to tell you to shut right up if you get obsessed with baby business.

● It might be a good idea to arrange that your friend first visits you and your new baby at home, away from the hospital, when you won't have other visitors. Don't insist that she hold the baby, or discourage her. Don't be alarmed if she cries when holding the baby. She will find her own way to deal with it in her own time.

● Don't for heaven's sake tell her to 'just relax' and she'll get pregnant, or insist she try some folk remedy you've read about, or suggest that she do whatever you did. She may already know about an infertility support group or counsellor. Often available in both city and rural areas, these services can usually be contacted through GPs, family planning centres and hospitals.

your record

✳ Are you feeling queasy? When?

✳ What smells and/or foods make you feel sick?

✳ What are you doing to combat queasiness?

✳ How have you changed your eating habits during pregnancy?

✳ If you're taking supplements, record them.

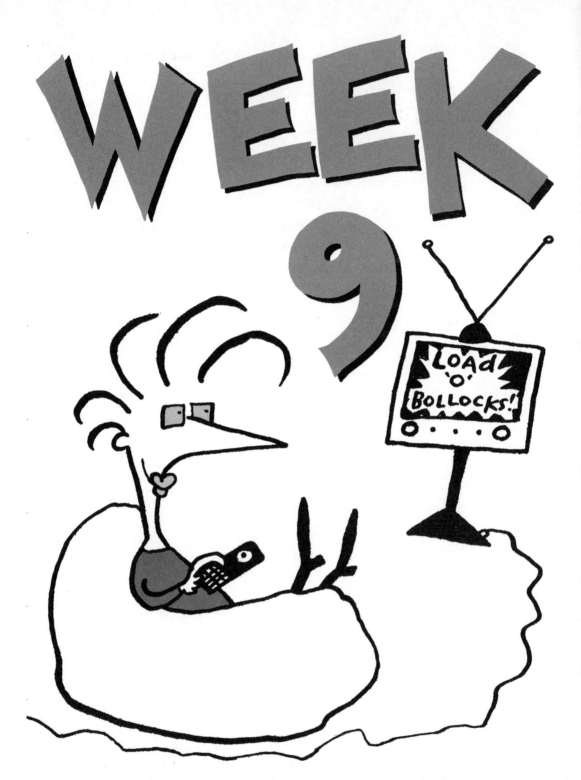

INTELLECTUAL at WORK

what's going on

Your stomach may not be at all preggie-looking yet – after all, the embryo is yet to hit the 2cm ($^3/_4$ inch) mark. But as it grows, your centre of gravity will change and you will become, well, a person with the grace of a hippopotamus rather than a fruit bat. So this is the time to attend to any handy-type problems around the house – loose carpeting, tricky steps, bits of bathroom that get slippery or dangerous or awkward to manoeuvre around. And if there's something you need to get at regularly that involves standing on stepladders or a chair, lower it for the duration.

The embryo's eyelids appear and its body elongates. The internal sex organs are starting to develop into boy and girl bits, but you can't tell the sex from the outside yet. An ultrasound will be able to show the embryo's early movements. The ends of the limbs are looking a bit more like hands and feet but you still couldn't play 'This little piggy goes to market' unless you changed the words to 'This little webby bit . . . ' Birth guru Sheila Kitzinger's fruit alert says the embryo weighs as much as a grape.

DiARY Picked up a leaflet on child benefit from the post office and did a double take when I saw the figure. £15. Now what exactly does that get you? A round of drinks in Clapham, if you're lucky. And to think that *Daily Mail* readers are forever going on about how single mothers have Never Had It So Good scrounging off us all. I read somewhere that it costs £100,000 to raise a child from nappies to university. Not entirely sure where that's going to come from. Even Geoff the breezy optimist paled when I told him, temporarily adopting a look of Hitchcock horror before rallying with 'We could always live in Spain.' So there we go, only nine weeks gone and we're looking at emigration.

But where was I? Oh yes. Even though it still seems miles off, I have to make plans for the actual (it's hard to say this out loud), um, you know . . . birth. I went for a checking-in appointment with the midwife team at the hospital and we discussed my options for antenatal care, the tests available, and the delivery options – which basically came down to hospital or home birth. I'd heard about places called birth centres, which seem a bit like Wendy-house hospital extensions, with subdued lighting, and a midwife-only team looking after your needs. However, the nearest one to us could be a white-knuckle ride in bad traffic, so I've plumped for a regular delivery in the local hospital.

DIY home delivery seemed attractive for a brief moment of fantasy, but even with a couple of midwives in attendance – well, I'm just too neurotic. I'll take the twenty-first-century technology, I said to the midwives. It's still twentieth century round here, they replied. But there you go. The midwives also asked if I had private health insurance (no luck). Seems like you sometimes get a few options thrown in if you do, like a private room and executivey food after the delivery. Oh well.

Beck had sent me a pamphlet advertising the services of independent midwives, who for a rather hefty consideration will look after you through pregnancy and into babyhood. That sounded a nice deal, if you had the money, and very modern: the mother on the front cover, holding her minutes-old baby in a birthing pool, had a very charming tattoo on her arm. I have

informed Beck that in the absence of funds for such luxury, she
will have to be my private midwife, but I refuse to get a tattoo.
Beck agreed and now I just have to square it with the midwives
that I can have her as an extra birthing partner at the delivery. It
feels like being a kid and asking if a friend can stay over: a real
sense of the authorities already being in charge (they'll be taking
Cellsie off to school soon). Still, best to check. You don't want any
punch-ups on the day.

On my admittance form booking a hospital delivery it said
'Diagnosis: confinement'. A word out of a Jane Austen novel, or
some 1950s sitcom, when pregnant bellies were hidden indoors
for the last few months so nobody had to be reminded that
pregnant women HAVE HAD SEX. Confined, for Christ's sake. It's a
wonder the form doesn't say 'BYO handcuffs'.

The list of things we're instructed to bring to the hospital
on Cellsie's birth day is more mystifying the longer I look at it.
'Underclothes including underpants and maternity bras.' Well,
what other kinds of underclothes are there? Do people usually take
their own bondage gear? 'One to two packets of nursing pads.' Oh
dear. Not a clue what they are. Surely nurses can look after their
own needs?

Then there's a whole list of baby stuff, for which we'll need to
use Geoff's van. 'Four babygros.' These are the all-in-one costumes
babies like to adopt, apparently. But four? What's going to happen
to the other three? Does the baby shred them during post-birth
tantrums? Do they all go on at once? How cold can the kid get?
'Baby hat, and bootees or socks, and mittens (optional).' Well, I'm
glad it's all optional. Because to be honest it hadn't previously
occurred to me that a person less than a week old should have
a hat and gloves. Stockings, maybe, but let's not go overboard.
The kid can develop its own sense of elegant matching accessories
when it leaves home and can afford to buy its own formal wear.

Under 'What to bring for partner' there is a most unsatisfactorily
short list. 'Men's night attire please if staying overnight eg
tracksuit, pyjamas, dressing-gown.' (I asked about this, and
apparently most of the midwives have seen willies before, but
an elderly cleaner at the hospital copped an eyeful of a bloke's

leopard-skin posing pouch early one morning and took early retirement.) As Geoff has none of the recommended items except track bottoms this could be a bit of a problem. And anyway, why assume the partner is male? Why should a lesbian partner be forcibly levered into 'men's night attire'? Plus the list of what a partner really should bring to the hospital might more imaginatively include: enormous boxes of chocolates, current copy of *Hello* magazine, new and attractive clothes, tickets to Paris (springtime) etc. Diamonds would be acceptable or a modest-sized yacht with a bowling alley.

The upshot of reading all this material from the hospital is that you get wildly ahead of yourself. You've still got months and months to go and you're wondering what to pack. Not to mention a few decisions about ambience. For delivery, the hospital suggests 'relaxation music'. Not a good start. Relaxation music always makes me very tense. I remember some stand-up making a joke about how it sounded like dolphins playing the piano. Besides, if you gave birth to an Enya album, the quietly contemplative ambience might be somewhat offset by the fact that you are screaming the place down and something huge is coming out of your vagina and at least two people you don't even know are watching. And anyway, if we can subliminally remember birth, why would you want the poor child to recall Enya's latest hits?

Further suggestions include 'camera, essential oils, glucose lollies, large T-shirt or old nightie, socks, toiletries, book or magazine, etc, T-shirts and shorts or swimwear for partner if desired'. This must refer to the mysterious birthing pools everyone mentions before the birth but which apparently are never available at the time. Still, I wasn't imagining labour as a scenario in which I am lying back reading while Geoff does a few laps. And at what exact point during labour would one read a book? 'The baby's head is crowning!' 'Don't bother me now, Mr Darcy's just going for a swim in the pond.'

info

choosing your birth place and team

Even though it seems such a long way off, it's time to start asking around and thinking about what sort of birth you'd like, generally, and who you would like to help you through it. And so begins the search for your 'place of birth' and a decision on 'birth alternatives'. Remember that the choice you have about where to have your baby and how you are cared for will depend to some extent on where you live and what is available in your area. But it is still a choice – your's. There are various options so it's worth getting informed and thinking through what you want.

fig (A): OBSTetRiciaNS to Avoid

hello fatty

Birth choices are contentious terrain. Some people argue that because birth can become a medical emergency very quickly, it is crucial to have your baby in a hospital – ideally one that can provide an atmosphere you'll feel comfy in, but with specialists and equipment on call. Meanwhile, home birth advocates say that most medical emergencies develop with plenty of warning, and home is a much better (and healthier) place to give birth if you have an uncomplicated pregnancy.

Most women look for a safe balance between a comfortable environment and the best care available. Giving birth on the kitchen floor is a much safer proposition if there's an ambulance minutes away than if you're in the middle of nowhere with only a confused sheep and a potato peeler instead of an experienced midwife.

Additionally, some birth options are only available if you have what is called a 'low-risk' pregnancy. Your pregnancy is considered 'high-risk' if, for example, you're going to have a multiple birth, or you have chronic high blood pressure, a family history of thrombosis, or a pre-existing condition such as diabetes, or you develop a complication during pregnancy – most commonly a baby in the 'breech' position, with its head pointing up (under your ribs), instead of down (towards your pelvis).

Before you make your choice, have a good read of this section, discuss the local options with your GP or midwife, and try to talk to other mothers who have had a baby recently, or to your local branch of the NCT (see 'Week 5').

medical insurance

If you have private medical insurance, it is worth checking out, at this stage of your pregnancy, what if anything is covered. Most regular policies will expect you to use regular NHS services unless you have particular complications, in which case they may cover you for private consultations and care. Only the real Rolls Royce policies offer anything of much use in a 'normal' pregnancy, other than, possibly, the cost of a private room in an NHS hospital. Still, that could be worth a lot. Make that call . . .

hospital, birth centre or home birth?

What you decide will have a bearing not just on the birth, but also on your antenatal care, and often your postnatal care as well. First you need to decide where you want to have your baby. There are three main options – hospital, birth centre, or home.

hospital births

If you have decided to have a hospital birth there may be several choices in your area and it might be possible to visit them before making your mind up. Many hospitals have tours especially for parents who are in the early part of pregnancy and wish to look around. Speak to either the antenatal sister at the hospital or write to the Director of Midwifery to see what is available.

When you see the hospital do not be put off by the surroundings and interior decorations. Don't look for the en suite bathroom and private room, but remember it is the people who make the hospital what it is. The attitude of the obstetric doctors (obstetricians) and the midwives towards you and your baby's birth an important factor in making the experience a rewarding one.

Once you have decided on the hospital, your GP has to write a letter of referral. Your GP will refer you to one of the following: a midwife, a midwifery team or an obstetric consultant depending on your health needs for the pregnancy and the nature of the local organised care plan. Do mention if you would prefer a particular midwife or obstetrician, who has been recommended to you.

Realistically, you will probably only see an obstetric consultant if you need their specialist care in your pregnancy. The majority of antenatal care is carried out by midwives as they are the specialists in normal pregnancy. Should a complication arise you would be referred to the consultant.

If you can afford it, or you have an insurance policy that covers it, you could book for private obstetric care and see the consultant throughout your pregnancy; they would agree to be present at the birth and may even deliver the baby. Or you could go for broke and book into a private maternity hospital, if there is one in your area. However, it's important to know that few obstetricians are able to attend an entire birth. They usually pop in and out during labour and are really present only at the end, for the birth, unless something unusual is happening. So your other support people and in particular the midwife team (remember that they operate in shifts) are likely to be just as important.

hospital midwife care

The majority of NHS maternity care is well organised, in defiance of threadbare surroundings and occasionally alarming shortages of staff. Hospital midwife departments all strive to provide continuity of care throughout your pregnancy, birth and postnatal period. But there is quite a variation in the styles of how they do it. Here are the main ones:

Shared care Shared care is the most common style of hospital care. You see the local community midwife and your GP during your pregnancy and have a hospital midwife attending you at the birth. You may have one or two visits to the hospital obstetrician during your pregnancy, with the first generally at 12 weeks (when you have your first scan) and the second towards the end (at around 36 weeks). After the birth the same local community midwife would visit you at your home – NHS midwifery care continues for 10 to 28 days after the birth. This system aims for you to see a familiar face throughout your pregnancy and in the first few weeks after the birth.

Team midwifery, Case holding and Domino schemes Some hospitals have gone a step further and introduced Team Midwifery. This is where you are offered care from a team or group of midwives throughout your pregnancy and during your labour including the home visits in the postnatal period. The team of familiar faces should be able to offer you more personalised care and make the whole experience around the time of birth more rewarding.

The two other schemes that aim to offer continuity of care are referred to as 'Case holding' or 'Domino care'. There are regional variations and these may not be offered in all hospitals. The idea is that the midwife who you have been seeing during your antenatal period attends you at the birth. She may visit you at home during labour, go to hospital with you for the birth, and then see you at home in those first postnatal weeks.

High risk care If you are having a pregnancy that is described as 'high-risk' it will mean that you and your baby/babies will need extra attention throughout your pregnancy and during your hospital stay. It may mean that you need to see your consultant obstetrician on a more regular basis and possibly other specialists within the hospital. You may still receive Shared Care and get to know your local midwife but it is unlikely that you will be offered midwifery-only care. If your health or that of the baby is being compromised

INDEPENDENT MIDWIVES

You can choose (at upwards of £1000) to hire an independent, 'freelance' midwife – not a hospital employee – who advises you before the birth, stays with you during the birth, and helps you afterwards with breastfeeding and other issues. Having a private midwife gives you the comfort of a chosen and familiar adviser through your pregnancy (including any consultations with an obstetrician) and they will (if all goes well) personally deliver your baby. However, births being the unpredictable things that they are, there is no absolute guarantee of your midwife being available when you go into labour: private midwives tend to work in small groups and provide back-up for each other, so be sure you are comfortable with all members of the team.

Independent midwives can attend home or hospital births. If you are planning on a hospital birth, make sure that the hospital will accept your midwife as your primary carer during the labour (ie the person who delivers your baby, with the doctor). For legal reasons, all hospitals will insist on the independent midwife having an honorary contract with them. If the hospital does accept the private midwife, then they will be part of a 'shared care' team with your GP and obstetrician, or your hospital.

For contact numbers, see under Midwives in 'Help' (p.408).

during pregnancy a hospital setting for the birth is probably the safest place.

Students If you are having your baby in a hospital you should be prepared for students during your pregnancy visits. These can be either medical or midwifery students in training and they follow around in the wake of a mentor to learn how to communicate well and provide care. Thankfully an audience of eager students peering up your girly bits at the time of birth is now considered an old-fashioned training method. Your privacy is a right, so feel free to say you don't want students to attend any consultations or procedures. Just don't say it's okay and then try to bite them.

birth centres

Birth centres (often called GP or midwife units) aim to be more 'homey' places to give birth in than a surgical-looking hospital room. They are often seen as the result of hospitals responding to public demand – a safer option than giving birth on a couch at home and a more pleasant and natural option than giving birth on a trolley under bright lights in a room that smells of industrial-strength Dettol. But there's much more to a birth room than a double bed and a potted plant and you can't assume that an inviting-looking birth centre necessarily means an absence of hospital attitudes. If you are looking at a birth centre with a view to having a more 'natural' birth you should ask (just as much as of a hospital) the rates of caesarean deliveries and inductions, and how many women are transferred from the birth centre to the main maternity unit during their labour – and the reasons why.

Birth centres may be part of a regular maternity hospital or a separate unit a few miles from the main hospital. These units are for low-risk care where it looks as if everything is going to be straightforward. In the event of an emergency during labour you may need to be transferred to the main hospital. If the unit is part of the main hospital, then emergency facilities are close at hand.

Your baby can be delivered at a birth centre by your community midwife, who has been involved in your antenatal care, by your GP, or by a hospital midwife. The care in the unit tends to be more personal since you will usually be looked after by people you know. The length of time you will remain in the unit after the birth depends on how well you and your baby are. If you were transferred in labour to the main maternity unit you may find yourself back at the birth centre for a period of rest and recuperation with all the familiar faces around you again.

Private birth centres A few independent midwife practices maintain their own birth centres – sometimes close by a maternity hopital in case emergency care is required. A stay at a birth centre will generally be charged on top of the regular fee for having a midwife care for you through your pregnancy.

home births

A birth at home is an option for all women with a normal uncomplicated pregnancy who fancy the idea of having their baby at home – and, of course, it is sometimes an option that happens by default if birth time arrives without time to move to hospital (this is unlikely to happen with a first baby).

If you are considering a home birth, it is advisable to talk it through with the midwives, or the Head of Midwifery, at your local hospital so they can tell you about the home birth services that are provided in your area. You are usually cared for by a midwife, who provides all the antenatal care and becomes a familiar face. At the time of birth, the midwife will bring all the necessary equipment to your home and another midwife will accompany her to assist in the birth.

Many women who choose to give birth at home relish the opportunity to be in a familiar, comfortable and non-medical environment. They want to be able to choose who will accompany them during the birth – grandma, siblings, partner, neighbours, milkman and the lady who lives down the road – and exactly how and where it will take place. (Keep in mind that a home birth can be a difficult experience for little children, who may not understand what mummy is going through. Many mums decide to have only grown-ups in the gallery.)

You may encounter negative reactions to your decision to give birth at home – including occasionally, from your GP, who may try to talk you out of it. If this is the case, talk to the local Supervisor of Midwives who has a responsibility to ensure that the care being provided is of the highest standard and will act as an advocate for you.

It's also possible to hire the services of an independent midwife to attend you at home (see box on p.97).

any questions?

Some questions you might like to ask when choosing your place of birth and type of care include:

ⓖ Would I go to the hospital antenatal clinic for all or just some of my antenantal care appointments?

⑥ Does the hospital run antenatal classes?

⑥ Does the hospital offer Team Midwifery, Domino Care or Case-Holding schemes?

⑥ What are my chances of knowing the midwife when I am in labour?

⑥ What are the policies on pain relief, different labour positions, electronic foetal monitoring, episiotomy and forceps delivery?

⑥ Are fathers, relatives or friends welcome in the delivery room?

⑥ Does the hospital encourage women to move around in labour and find their own position for the birth?

⑥ What services are provided for sick babies?

⑥ What is the normal length of stay?

⑥ How do you feel about following my special wishes for the labour? (We'll get into the birth plans later . . .).

relationships and support

The relationship with your GP, obstetrician and a midwife who goes with you through pregnancy and beyond is intimate and dependent on trust, mutual respect and free communication. You'll come to depend on the midwife (or midwives), in particular, over a number of months. You will be entrusting them with your life and your child's life. In an ideal situation, they will be equal partners with you in the process.

Tell the obstetrician and your midwife what sort of birth experience you are hoping for and what sort of patient you are. Say, for example, that you like to have clear explanations given to you about why things are done, or that you will be needing extra reassurance because your last pregnancy ended in a miscarriage, or that you are terrified of the whole idea and thinking of a general anaesthetic or hiding under a rock.

choosing a birth partner

If you have a partner, you'll probably want to have them at the birth. But if your partner isn't keen, it's probably better to choose a birth partner who'll be more useful and supportive at the time. Many women opt for sisters and friends, or occasionally mothers. You might also want to consider employing a doula – an experienced birth partner who can offer emotional support and encouragement during your labour, and practical support during your first days at home, with breastfeeding and babycare. Some antenatal teachers offer this service in addition to their classes.

Don't forget that if you have a long labour, it's better for everyone if your support person gets rest breaks or even a bit of shut-eye. They won't have your endorphins, and you don't want them fainting at the wrong moment. (Whatever a right moment is.) Many people want a record of the event in photos or on video: some even want it shown live on the Internet. It can be hard for somebody to be in charge of support, lollies and multimedia at the same time. When in doubt, ditch the Internet.

Some people invite a cast of thousands, only to regret it later. Don't forget the people who are actively involved need room to do their work. Some midwives and doctors believe that the more people in the room, the longer the birth. Most women don't want to be distracted by visitors or worried about how their children are coping with what for them can be quite a traumatic scenario.

your record

✴ What kind of prenatal and birth care have you chosen?

✴ How did you find your midwife?

✴ Who else will be on your support team and why?

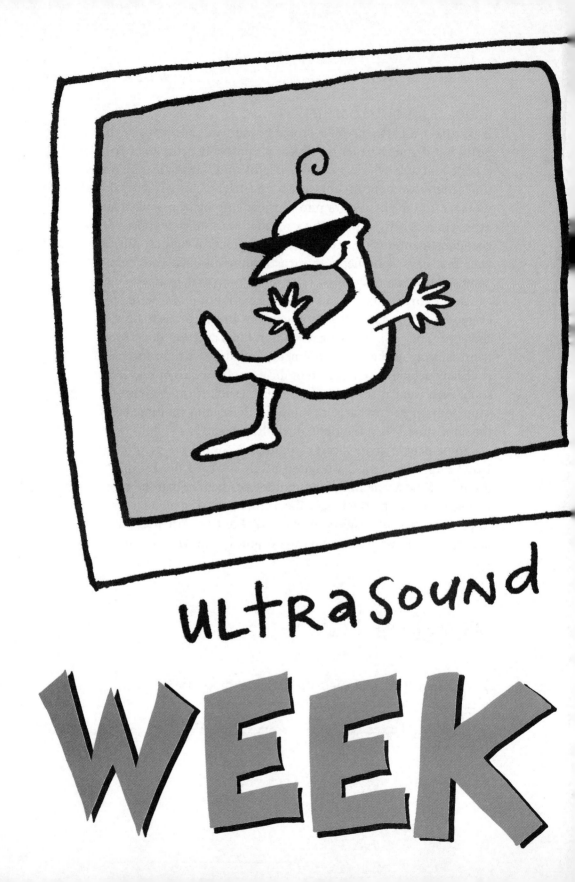

ultrasound

WEEK

cm
1
2
3
4
5
6
7
8
9
10
11
12
13
14
15
16
17
18
19
20
21
22

what's going on You're hungry. Eat. Your

body is doing a lot of work and you need more fuel than usual.

The embryo officially becomes a foetus this week. Very

few organs are actually working yet, but they're in the right spot.

The head is still big in proportion to the rest of the foetus. The

nostrils and tear ducts are finished off. (If anybody asks why

you're tired, just say you've been making eyebrows all night

long.) Around about now the little tail will 'disappear' as the

rest of the foetus grows. The limbs get longer; the arms can

bend; hands and feet can touch each other; and toes and

fingers lose their webbing and become fully separated. Sheila

Kitzinger's never-ending supply of fruit comparisons says

your uterus is now the size of an orange.

Foetus weight: about 8 grams ($^1/4$ oz).

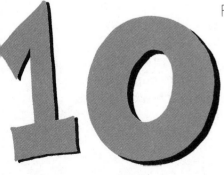

DiARY

I'm not sure but I think some of my wrinkles – sorry, I mean character lines – are less obvious. This is because my body is making extra collagen and all that stuff the cosmetics companies would probably kill us pregnant women for if they knew how to get it out of us. Most of my daily thoughts consist only of the following mantra: 'I have no interest in food, I cannot cook, I must lie down, I need to watch soaps on television.' It's all just too exhausting. If only I was the sort of person with four servants and a heart-shaped box of chocolates and a four-poster bed with a satin quilt and siamese cats, it would probably all look quite glamorous.

I go for the nuchal fold ultrasound. This is an ultrasound that looks for a thickening at the back of the baby's neck, which is an indicator of Down's syndrome. For some reason everyone thought I might be eleven weeks pregnant but it's actually only about ten according to the ultrasound operator (a woman, this time – not the sweet man who talked wastage four long weeks ago). This meant it was too early to do any sums and I'll have to come back.

It was disappointing not to get a definitive answer about the nuchal fold thing, but I'm happy that somebody else is as bad at maths as me, and we got to see Cellsie again on the small screen.

'There's your baby,' said the operator, pointing to an insecty shape wiggling a lot of little legs in the air. 'Look, it's waving,' she added, pointing out a head, two arms and two legs.

The head seemed to turn towards us, like something out of an alien movie. 'Oh fuck, that's too weird,' I say and nobody answers. It occurs to me that you're not supposed to say fuck during an ultrasound. Repeat after me: Mummies ought not to say fuck. Sigh. So much to learn.

The creature is only about 3.5 centimetres (1^1/$_3$ in) long, but on the screen it looks as long as an adult hand. This is very disconcerting. Makes it seem more advanced and less human at the same time. Suddenly the heartbeat monitor at the bottom of the screen shows an up-and-downie, mountain-shaped graph running along like something out of 'ER' – and the sound! Like a Latin techno beat! The fastest heartbeat I have ever heard. Looking closer, we can see the heart actually beating.

'That's not my heartbeat is it?' I ask. 'Because if it is, I think I'm having a heart attack.'

The operator, Tania (we get quite chummy in the warm wash of good news), doesn't know why foetal heartbeats are so fast, but she says it's quite normal. Everything is normal. Size, normal. Shape, normal. All bits present so far. Tania then gives us her take on tests, which is basically do the nuchal fold ultrasound and, so long as that doesn't show a problem, leave it at that. However, if the nuchal fold suggests a high risk of Down's syndrome, then we should do an amniocentesis, which will give us a conclusive result. She says an amniocentesis (or 'amnio') is not something you should consider unless it's absolutely necessary, as there's a one in 100 chance of the test causing a miscarriage.

After Tania has finished completing the forms, we go on to another consultation with one of the midwives, an enthusiastic man (yes, a male midwife) called Richard, clutching the normalnormalnormal ultrasound report. There I produce a jar of wee, and trot onto the scales to have my weight jotted down. It seems a lot more than I declared. Must be the hiking socks. I then distinguish myself in the midwife's consulting room by whipping off my trousers and undies when he actually just wanted my blood pressure and a chat.

Richard obviously thinks I'm some kind of crazed exhibitionist who enjoys lying on couches naked from the waist down except for boots, with her ankles somewhere near the light fittings, while her boyfriend sits in the corner reading a pamphlet. Well, maybe I am. What's it to ya? I suddenly wonder in my scatterbrained way, why is there a poster of a skeleton in here? Doctors can't do décor.

Richard expands on the statistics the ultrasound operator had outlined, talking about various possible but unlikely risks. It leaves my brain in a whirl of confusing maths, so it seems best to just wait and see what's on the next ultrasound.

I have started to wrestle with constipation: I decide to adopt Beck's secret seed-breakfast method. Every time I get constipated I get at least one pimple, probably two. But after a day or two of crushed mixed seeds on my muesli, I'm running like a train again and zit-free.

info

chromosomes and genes

At conception the egg and sperm join to make a single cell. This one cell, combining twenty-three chromosomes supplied by the egg and twenty-three from the sperm, contains the entire genetic blueprint for your child. At that moment, your baby's destiny is decided: what sex it will be, how tall it will be, how much natural musical or sporting talent it will have, what colour skin, hair and eyes, what shape it will become after puberty, and maybe what kind of illnesses it will be prone to.

Even though its genetic inheritance comes from both parents, a baby will not be an exact 50:50 mix of both parents' characteristics. It may end up with red hair that has 'skipped' a generation, or with a skin colour that is far more Dad than Mum, or vice versa. Your child may look not much like either parent, but more like long-lost Great-Aunt Agatha. Some families have genes that always seem to win out, such as a family nose or a build.

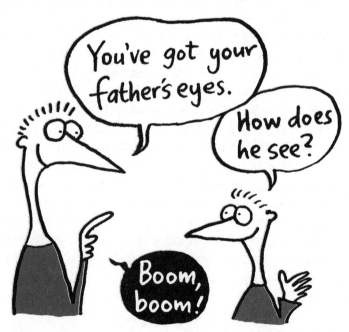

Your baby will eventually have millions of cells. The forty-six chromosomes inside the nucleus of each cell are made up of two chains of your genetic code, called DNA (deoxyribonucleic acid), which control growth and functioning of the baby. The chromosomes contain thousands of genes, which determine the physical and intellectual characteristics.

problems with chromosomes and genes

The term 'genetic disorder' refers to changes in the genetic code – like a typing error – that occurred in the formation of the genes and chromosomes in a particular baby, as well as to medical conditions or health problems, often also called genetic, which are inherited through the family.

Some inherited genetic diseases such as cystic fibrosis happen when both parents carry a recessive problem gene. This gene doesn't affect either of the parents, but when the two potential problem genes are combined the foetus is affected. Other problems such as haemophilia may be 'activated' only if the baby is of a certain sex. Some genetic disorders are linked to geographic regions or ethnic groups. Sickle-cell anaemia is the most common genetic disease in people of African descent, for example.

down's syndrome

Down's syndrome is a genetic condition with a high profile. The most common cause of intellectual disability, it affects about one in 800 to 1,000 pregnancies. It is also known as trisomy 21. Because of an accident during the division of cells when still an embryo, the foetus has three copies of chromosome 21 instead of the usual two. A Down's syndrome baby (and adult) will have learning disabilities, will have characteristic facial differences (especially a distinctive eyelid shape), a stocky stature and loose muscle tone, and may also suffer from medical problems, such as heart abnormalities, that need corrective surgery.

The incidence of Down's syndrome increases dramatically in the foetuses of older women. The ratios are:

21-year-old women – one in 1,520 pregnancies

35-year-old women – one in 355 pregnancies

40-year-old women – one in 95 pregnancies
43-year-old women – one in 40 pregnancies

You can get routine, non-invasive testing which establishes a more accurate risk of your embryo developing Down's, and if you are judged 'high risk' you may decided to have a diagnostic test called amniocentesis. As the statistics show, even among older women, the vast majority of tests are negative. For more on this and other tests, see 'Week 11' – p.114.

genetic counselling

Your hospital or your obstetrician can refer you to a genetic counsellor for any of the following reasons, but it is not automatic. If you have any worries you may need to bring up the subject.

⑥ You've had a diagnostic test confirming a chromosomal abnormality.

⑥ You've had miscarriages.

⑥ You or your partner has a family history of inherited physical or psychiatric disease.

⑥ Blood tests have indicated a partner carries a genetic disorder.

⑥ You've already had a baby with a chromosomal or genetic abnormality.

⑥ You or your partner or a member of either family was born with an abnormality caused by a genetic problem that was not inherited through the family – this is known as a 'congenital abnormality'.

⑥ You and your partner are related (cousins, for example).

⑥ Genetic counsellors can accurately assess your risk of having a baby with a hereditary disorder. If you have already had a child with a disorder, they may be able to predict your chances of it happening again. They can tell you if you carry genes that cause certain disorders, and very often reassure you that the chances of a problem are very low. The techniques used to arrive at this information can include blood tests, genetic analysis and examination of both families' medical history. So of course it will always be a bonus if you have access to family histories on both sides. If you don't have access because you don't know who the father is or he is unco-operative, you probably don't need to worry at all. Genetic problems are very rare.

more info on gene and chromosome problems

There are support and info groups for various genetic disorders. Check phone listings for your area or go through the counsellor at the biggest local hospital. Also see 'Screening and Blood Tests' in 'Help', p.410).

Antenatal Tests (National Childbirth Trust Guides) by Mary Nolan, HarperCollins, UK, 1998.
For anyone facing difficult choices, this is a compassionate and informative book that explains risks, tests, results and the decision-making process during what could be your most confusing moments.

1

2

3

4

5

6

7

8

9

10

11

12

13

14

15

16

17

18

19

20

21

22

what's going on
Nausea should start to settle down from now on. Hurrah. Outside influences, such as certain drugs and chemicals, could have damaged the foetus while it was still forming; the dangers are still there after week 10, but are no longer so acute. (This does not mean you can get on the vodka.). The placenta is continuing to get bigger, keeping pace with what the foetus needs. The heart is completely formed and pumping away. The ear and hearing structures are nearly finished and ready to grow. Your foetus is looking a lot more like a tiny human with a big head, short limbs and not much clothes sense. (In fact, about now the head is almost half the size of the whole foetus.)

Weight: about 10 grams (1/3 oz).

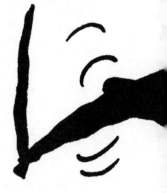

oops

WEEK 11

iNADViSABLE ACROBATiC DANCiNG

DiARY I've been lent a lot of baby-care books for the
duration. One is Aunt Julie's decrepit second-hand
copy of Dr Spock from approximately the Jurassic
Period, which she immediately borrowed after
Mum died to work out what she and Uncle Mike should do with
this small creature (me) suddenly on their doorstep.

I fancied a look at the modern pregnancy and child-care
books, but I discovered most of them are absolutely shocking.
For one thing, they're always banging on about husbands as if
every pregnant woman had to have one. Mind you it's not just
insulting to the single mother-to-be. The blokes don't come out of
it well either. One book actually recommends that you teach 'your
husband' to make his own breakfast before you go to hospital, say
by week 32 to be sure. If a bloke doesn't know how to make his
own breakfast, I say you're better off without him.

The books also seem to disagree on lots of points, which is
kind of comforting – it means you don't have to get worried if
you're not at exactly the stage a book reckons you should be. On
almost every major yardstick I'm not.

Even some of the good books have the most absurd
photographs to enliven their pages. Under the section on nutrition
or appetite there is usually a photograph of a woman with a plate
of food, in case you have forgotten what a plate of food looks like.

And I don't wish to be rude, but I'd like all the people who
have done illustrations for pregnancy books rounded up. Who
ARE all these women in the illustrations, pale-as-pastry, frumpy,
with disgusting haircuts, wearing duvet covers? And who are
these husbands looking manfully into the distance with gigantic
sideburns? One book has four filthy drawings of bright pink
couples 'making love' during pregnancy, in different positions.
In the first position they look bored. In the second they look like
they've had a lobotomy. In the third they look really smug, and
in number four, I don't know how this is quite conveyed, but I'm
pretty sure they were singing 'Michael Row the Boat Ashore'. (This
could be dangerous. If you don't know by now that it's possible to
have sex from behind, a line drawing is going to send you into a
state of shock.)

Another book, called *A Child Is Born*, has extraordinary photos of the foetus in the uterus. It's disgusting. Geoff reads it every night. He's fascinated by the pictures. They make me want to projectile vomit. 'Look, that's what Cellsie looks like now.' I scream and hide under the sheets. 'That looks like a prawn made of snot!' 'But it's amazing. Look at this one – this is what it'll look like next week.' Great. A portion of especially dumb plankton, with eyes like ball bearings. I cannot relate to this. Nobody could love a snot prawn. How can I bond with a crustacean?

There really is too much information in these books, and yet not enough. For example, 'Acrobatic dancing is, of course, unwise at any stage during pregnancy'. How acrobatic? Are we talking those circus girls who can put their head up their own bum? Do we refer here to the sort of wafty crap, Stevie-Nicks-type hippie dancing while waving shawls? Which is surely ultimately more offensive and therefore more dangerous than the lesser known acrobatic dancing. Perhaps it means chandelier work.

One of the books, by Miriam Stoppard, has an entire section devoted to how to wear make-up during pregnancy, with handy hints such as how to cover up dark circles under the eyes; and camouflage puffiness by shading a little brown blusher subtly beneath the jawbone and on either side of the neck. Look, this might work if you are standing still, being professionally lit and photographed, but if you're walking around like a normal human being no amount of brown blusher on your neck is going to disguise the fact that you're a bit puffy.

You would be better off constantly introducing yourself to people by saying, 'Hello, I'm a bit puffy. It's because I'm up the duff and a big fat baby is going to come out of my vagina', and getting on with things. I can guarantee nobody will mention any puffiness after that. Not to your face, anyway.

info

screening and diagnostic tests

There are a range of screening and diagnostic tests that will give you an idea of how your baby is developing, and which can pick up on possible problems.

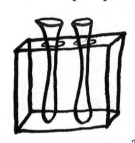

A screening test, such as an ultrasound scan or blood test, looks for pointers for certain conditions and assesses your risk against the average risk of having a baby with certain abnormalities. This is a more accurate risk assessment than using your age alone though a 'positive' screening-test does NOT mean the baby has an abnormality – in fact, chances are very much in your favour that the baby is perfectly fine. But the result means that a further test is offered to you – a diagnostic test.

The two main diagnostic tests are amniocentesis and CVS. These tests can provide you with a definite answer about whether your baby has a specific abnormality. However, they are both invasive tests that increase your existing risk of miscarriage – commonly a risk figure of 1 in 100 is quoted.

The vast majority of women having screening or diagnostic tests will have no abnormality at all, and ultrasound is now very much part of routine pregnancy care, a first and reassuring step to feeling your baby is real and developing as it should.

routine ultrasound

An ultrasound examination bounces high-frequency soundwaves into your body to create an image of the foetus and your internal organs on a computer screen. You lie on your back while an ultrasound technician or obstetrician performs the test. A small object a bit like a computer mouse will be run over the top of your tummy, after some gel has been spread on it; or, if the test is done before twelve weeks of pregnancy, a 'probe' is put into your vagina. Luckily the probe is only about the size of a large pen. Ultrasounds don't hurt. Unless you hospital has very new equipment, you'll need to have a full bladder in order for the examination to be performed; this means drinking at least a pint and a half of water an hour before your scan.

Hospitals differ in the way they offer screening tests but most will offer you an ultrasound at eleven to fourteen weeks – and a second one at twenty to twenty-three weeks. An ultrasound is a great chance to see your baby on screen for the first time – so bring your partner, or a friend who might get a kick out of it. If you're lucky, the baby will give you a wave. It can be an emotional moment seeing your baby for the first time; be prepared to get misty eyed.

An ultrasound after 18 weeks can confirm an estimation of how advanced your pregnancy is (give or take a few days); catch sight of twins or other multiple births; and locate the position of your placenta (if it's low lying, another ultrasound will be done later in the pregnancy to see if placenta praevia has developed – that's when the placenta grows over or very close to the cervix). The ultrasound will show any uterine growths, such as fibroids. Most fibroids are harmless and you wouldn't even know you had them unless you'd had the ultrasound.

An ultrasound allows the operator to measure and observe limbs and organs; it also shows the baby's sex (it's about 98 per cent accurate, but sometimes the position of the foetus can make identification difficult). If you don't want to know the sex of the baby you should let the operator know, otherwise they're likely to blurt out something like 'Look out, there's a big willy.' (Conversely, some hospitals actually have a non-disclosure policy on sex).

A specialist ultrasound operator can usually identify certain foetal abnormalities such as spina bifida, cleft palate and mis-shapen feet by using measurements and observation.

Digital technology has made it possible now to have a three-dimensional ultrasound. Distributors of this technology say it is better than the routine ultrasound at picking up some abnormalities early on. It is still too expensive (about double the price of the standard machines) for routine use in the UK.

nuchal fold ultrasound

You may be offered, or you can request, an ultrasound at eleven to fourteen weeks that is sometimes called the nuchal fold, or nuchal translucency, test. This is a screening test for Down's syndrome which has all but replaced the blood tests previously offered as it appears to be more accurate (it picks up about 80 per cent of Down's syndrome cases). However, it is not yet routine in the UK and you may need to be referred to a different hospital or centre – and may possibly have to pay for the test.

The procedure is as for a routine ultrasound but the operator concentrates on getting a good image of your foetus's neck on the screen and measures a layer of fluid at the back of the neck. The thicker this layer is, the greater the chance the baby will have Down's syndrome.

You will be given an indication of any problems while the operator is doing the measurements, and then a more accurate result to take away with you. This is expressed as a probability (a one in 10,000 chance, one in 100 chance, and so on) of Down's. It may also be expressed in terms of age-risk – a 40-year-old may be told she has the same (very low) risk as a 20-year-old, for example. If your risk is high (one in 100), and the neck swelling is there, you will be offered a diagnostic test – amniocentesis or CVS (see opposite) – which can tell you whether or not your baby has Down's syndrome.

blood tests

If you are not offered the nuchal fold ultrasound you may be offered a blood test called an alpha-fetoprotein test. This is a protein made by the baby and passed into your blood during pregnancy. High levels are associated with spina bifida and low levels with Down's syndrome. Further blood tests such as the 'double' or the 'triple plus' may also be carried out to measure other blood chemicals and the results of these tests are combined to give an estimated risk of Down's syndrome. (These tests are not suitable for diagnosis for women expecting twins or multiple births because of the extra proteins being produced naturally by the babies.)

When you have the test, a small amount of blood is taken from your arm and sent off to a laboratory. The result comes back within a week as either 'screen positive' or 'screen negative', often, as with the nuchal fold test, expressed as a statistic (a one in 10,000 chance, one in 100, and so on). Nineteen out of twenty women tested will have a 'screen negative' result.

A 'screen-positive' (one in 100) result does NOT automatically mean your baby has the conditions tested for – most 'increased risk' women will be found to be carrying a healthy baby – but you'll be advised to take a further diagnostic test: an ultrasound, CVS or amniocentesis. So you will need to prepare yourself for a drawn-out two or three weeks' further wait for results.

amniocentesis and CVS

Diagnostic tests such as amniocentesis and CVS are usually offered if you're over 35, you have a family history of Down's syndrome, you've had an 'increased risk' blood-test result, or you've had an inkling from the nuchal fold test that your foetus may be at greater risk.

As mentioned, both amnio and CVS are invasive tests that slightly increase your existing risk of miscarriage: one in a hundred women miscarry following the operation. It is this risk that makes the tests an option rather than a routine for every pregnancy. You will be weighing up a statistical risk – the chance of discovering a defect versus the chance of causing the miscarriage of a healthy foetus. Help in making that decision is available from your obstetrician, and from your midwife or hospital antenatal clinic.

Amniocentesis is used to test for Down's syndrome and other chromosomal disorders. The test is carried out at about 15 weeks. It involves you lying very still while the obstetrician uses an ultrasound to see exactly where the baby is inside the amniotic sac. The obstetrician will then insert a needle through your abdomen and into the uterus (but not near the baby) to draw in a small amount of amniotic fluid. This contains cells from the baby which give a definitive answer to questions about chromosomes.

CVS is used to test for most of the same conditions as amnio. The test is often done earlier than amnio and can be done at any time after about eleven weeks. Some studies have shown that if the test is done before ten weeks there is an increased risk of the baby having abnormal fingers and toes. The technician operates in much the same way as for amnio, but takes a needle sample of tissue from the chorion – the name for the placenta in its early, growing phase. The needle can go in either through the abdomen or through the vagina.

Either test takes around 10 to 20 minutes and it is usually considered to be uncomfortable rather than painful. But it's no fun having a big needle put into you near your baby, nor dealing with anxiety about the result. It's good to have someone come with you to the procedure, who can then take you home, where you should lie down for the day, or even two days, depending on the advice of your obstetrician.

Results for amniocentesis tests take up to three weeks; CVS gives a preliminary result in about four days, with confirmation in two weeks. Because CVS can give a result earlier in the pregnancy than amnio, it's often helpful if you have to decide whether to discontinue a pregnancy involving a baby with an abnormality. It is easier emotionally and physically to terminate a pregnancy as early as possible. Most people do decide to terminate a baby with a severe abnormality, but some would not do this whatever the circumstances.

Decisions about terminations are always difficult, even if you're sure you've made the right choice. Take as much time as possible to work through the decision. Non-directive counselling is available to help you to understand and process the issues, without any urging in a particular direction; it can also be useful in resolving any differences of opinion between you and your partner. Some elements to consider are the nature and severity of the diagnosed condition, the likely survival or quality of life of the baby after birth, any ethical and religious aspects, your willingness or ability to deal with the baby's condition, and the likely impact on members of your family such as other children.

Even if for religious or ethical reasons you would not consider terminating your pregnancy, these tests can help you and your family to prepare both emotionally and in a practical sense for the birth requirements and care of a special needs baby, or for the possibility of a miscarriage.

more info on tests and beyond

 Your nearest family planning clinic, maternity hospital or obstetrician will have staff and counsellors to help you, and pamphlets or booklets you can read on specific issues, relating to abnormalities highlighted by tests. There are support groups for parents of babies and children with special needs. Your doctor or nearest hospital should be able to help you get in touch. Grief counsellors can help with anything from a decision to terminate or miscarriage, to dealing with a special needs baby.

See also the book on Screening Tests recommended in Week 10 (p.109), and the sections in 'Help' on Grief and loss (p.406) and Babies' health problems (p.402).

your record

✳ What tests have you decided to have?
✳ If you had an ultrasound, what could you see?

1

2

3

4

5

6

7

8

9

10

11

12

13

14

15

16

17

18

19

20

21

22

what's going on This is often the first time

you'll visit the obstetrician. Don't forget beforehand to write

down any questions that you may want to ask. You may be

feeling very tired – after all, you're not just a fascinating,

sophisticated minx any more, you're a walking host organ.

Inside, your foetus looks more like a baby but with the

head still bent forward. The face has a human profile and

the jaw hides twenty developing tooth buds. Muscles are

growing and increasing the movement of the foetus, but you

still can't feel it because it has plenty of room to slosh about in

the amniotic fluid without touching the sides. As the placenta

has been doing since week 5, it is routinely sending oxygen

and nutrients down the vein of the umbilical cord, and taking

away waste such as foetal wee, which travels back up

the two arteries in the cord. Weight: about 18 grams ($^2/_3$ oz).

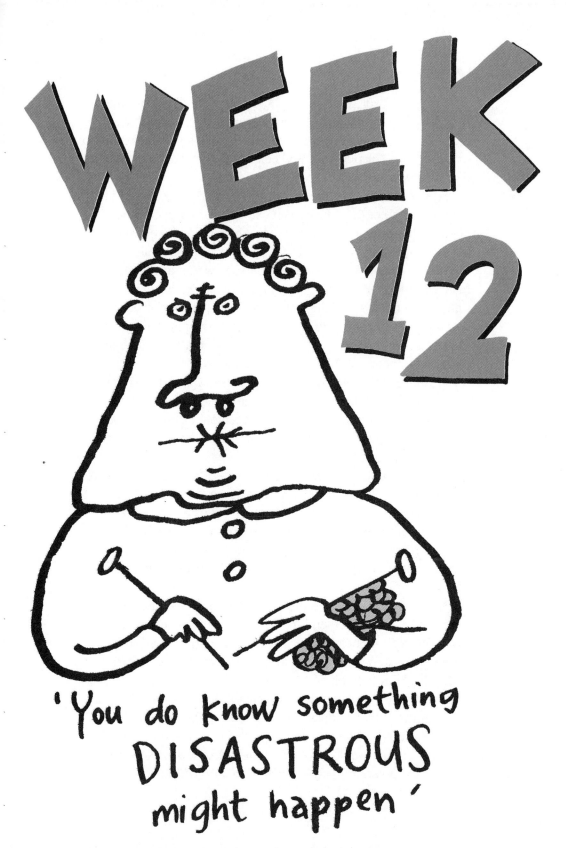

DiARy

For some reason my sense of smell has become really acute. I can only wear men's aftershaves. Any even slightly girlie, florally scents make me go bleuuuergh. God help me if I get stuck in a lift at a department store.

Finally I get to have the proper nuchal fold ultrasound. This time the operator (it's Tania again, which seems a good omen) pokes Cellsie around to get it in the right position by pushing hard on my tummy. I really don't feel so good about this but all the measurements are fine, she says, so she would advise against me having further, invasive tests. Again we are at the whim of statistics, reminded that the test picks up 80 per cent of Down's syndrome cases. For a wild maths-phobic moment I think this means we have a 20 per cent chance of having a Down's syndrome baby, but of course it doesn't mean that at all.

We leave, and I surprise myself by bursting into tears. For some reason I feel great indignation at Cellsie being unceremoniously poked to get him or her into a better position. I guess the baby must be starting to feel more real. I didn't expect to feel protective of my little space prawn.

We're close to the magic, don't-have-to-be-so-scared-about-miscarriages point, and we decide to tell everybody we haven't told. Geoff's parents are thrilled, and send us a lovely fax from Pembrokeshire, where they are on assignment investigating a rare fungus up some mountain. Aunt Julie is very happy, I think, but it's hard to tell. Aunt Julie cries no matter what happens.

Uncle Mike seems seriously avuncular about the idea of a grand-niece or -nephew and makes the same joke he does every two months about being glad we're not getting married so he doesn't have to pay for the wedding. 'Oh, we've been thinking about that,' Geoff deadpans, which gives him a quick jolt. Mike's girlfriend Aurelia, meantime, is shrieking, throwing herself onto Geoff, getting coral-coloured lipstick in his eyebrows and his ears. She's thorough, I have to admit.

'Your mother would have loved this,' Mike whispers to me while this is going on, and I suddenly well up with tears. I've always missed my mother, but I think I'll feel it more when the baby comes.

Geoff's cousin Annie, mother of six, which is a truly appalling prospect, the one who spent years before the pregnancy asking when I was going to get pregnant and then, when told to knock it off, asked everyone else in the family every time she saw them, is continuing to be insufferable. She announces loudly and frequently, 'I *knew* you were pregnant!', and has taken to poking me in the stomach and squeezing me on the arm as if she's about to buy me as a Shetland pony for one of her children. 'Mmm,' she says each time. 'Yes, you're definitely pregnant!'

Other immediate reactions to 'I'm pregnant' have included:

'You'll never get rid of them!' (60-year-old woman)

'That's wonderful!' (all the nice people I know)

'Your life is over!' (Francine, my beauty therapist)

Complete silence and choking sound. (my boss)

One of my clients buying the latest range wants me to commit to a fashion conference in Cannes, in September. Cellsie will be four weeks old. 'It will only be for a day and a half,' he says. 'You'll be dying to get out and about by then, and reclaim your identity. When we had kids it satisfied my creative urges for a while, but then you really need to reclaim your own space.' What a dork.

Another visit to Dr Fisher so he can check out the ultrasound results, and me. In the waiting room the woman next to me has a small boy she speaks to in a Very Loud Voice. She is Extremely Annoying. The toddler looks at pictures in a book.

'Here's Daddy,' he says, pointing to a man.

'That's not *our* daddy,' she bellows, cheerfully.

Our daddy! 'Madam,' I feel like saying, 'he is the child's daddy. He is not your daddy.' I ponder the whole spooky idea of calling your sexual partner mummy or daddy.

Finally I get to see Dr Fisher. He gives the old tummy a bit of a poke and a feel (this is called 'palpation' apparently) and seems pleased with the progress.

'It's definitely growing.'

Despite the obviousness of this banality I am absurdly pleased. He smiles. 'Everything's going as well as could be expected.

Couldn't be better.' I beam. Oh hurrah. I feel like I've received a gold star and an elephant stamp on my homework.

'You'll be having most of your pregnancy care, from now on, with the hospital midwives,' Dr Fisher goes on. 'But I'm on hand if any worries come up along the way.'

This is the opening I need to 'fess up about the booze. I've been brooding about it ever since reading the first of those pregnancy manuals. 'Well, there is something,' I stumble. 'I had some seriously alcoholic punch at a party when I was already pregnant.'

'How much?' asks Dr Fisher.

'About two glasses. Erm. Maybe three. Four, tops.'

'It's very unlikely to do any harm at all.'

Phew.

I have written down three questions: can Beck be an extra birth partner? (Yes – Dr Fisher says it's very trendy to have an experienced birthing partner along – in fact there's even a name for these women – doulas. Beck is now my official, unpaid doula). Is the hospital set up for any emergency and will it be equipped to perform a caesarean if needed? (Yes and Yes.) And what books does he recommend? (Janet Balaskas's *New Active Birth*. He's a bit of a New Man, my Dr Fisher).

Talking of worries, Aunt Julie is driving me insane. She has been depressed since 1957, but carries about her the air of a wounded martyr delivering vital messages to the front. Unfortunately now she knows I'm pregnant, she has decided the front is me and the messages must be as tragic as possible. She always has a horrendous story to tell, usually about some dreadful thing that has happened to a small child: left in the wilderness, flung from a train, attacked by feral guinea pigs – you name it, Aunt Julie can tell you the long version.

'I'm not congratulating Geoff yet, dear,' she announces on the doorstep instead of saying hello, 'in case something goes wrong.'

Tact and optimism are strangers to our Julie. After a few other pleasantries (babies who have been abused, small children murdered by their estranged parents, the children of women who drink too much in pregnancy), she bursts into tears and tells me all about some friend's daughter who miscarried after carrying a toddler in a buggy up the stairs in the tube, when the escalators had broken down. 'Promise me,' she sobs, looking at me accusingly. 'You're not lifting anything, are you?'

Aunt Julie eventually leaves, temporarily reassured, after pressing some packets of herbs into my hands, neatly labelled with their names. 'Make yourself some tea with these, dear, they're very natural,' she confides.

Not bloody likely. After she goes I ring Beck for the herb inside story, and sure enough, one of the herbs is an abortifacient, which means it could abort or deform a developing foetus. Now I have to ring Aunt Julie and tell her to stop being an amateur herbalist around the joint before somebody comes out in hives, loses their hair or carks it. (What is it about pregnancy that brings out the amateur doctor or herbalist in people?)

'Your Aunt Julie,' says Geoff that night, 'is mad. It probably runs in the family.'

info

pregnancy hormones

Every time you mention a symptom of pregnancy – from bigger breasts, to wanting an ice-cream, to feeling unspecific morbid dread – somebody will say in tones of enormously ponderous knowledge, 'It's the pregnancy hormones.' Well, what exactly are the pregnancy hormones, and which ones do what?

⑥ Many of these pregnancy hormones are produced by the placenta, the organ inside the uterus that sustains the developing baby through the umbilical cord. This is kind of a neat trick as the placenta comes out just after your baby does, right when you won't need those hormones any more.

⑥ The 'thin blue line' hormone is called human chorionic gonadotrophin (HCG). HCG in urine triggers a 'positive' result in pregnancy tests. A high level during the first three months is one of the suspected reasons for nausea. HCG stimulates the ovaries to produce more progesterone, which in turn shuts down the monthly period department for the duration of the pregnancy.

⑥ The 'Oh my God, look at these bazoombas' hormones needed for milk production are the human placental lactogen (HPL), prolactin, oestrogen and progesterone. HPL is responsible for enlarging the breasts and the secretion of colostrum, the 'pre-milk' or 'practising milk', which may leak from your nipples from about the fifth month (or not) and is produced for the first few days after the birth.

⑥ Relaxin, the 'hang loose' pregnancy hormone, makes ligaments and tissues soften up and become more elastic, which provides the increased flexibility in the joints of the pelvis and back needed for labour. It may also contribute to the 'waddle' and aches and pains of later pregnancy. (The other contributing factor being that you've turned into a giant wombat.)

⑥ Oxytocin is the squeezer hormone: it stimulates the practice (Braxton Hicks) contractions of the uterus and the contractions during childbirth. Injections of this hormone are often used to induce labour and to expel the placenta.

⑥ The 'colouring-in' hormone is melanocyte-stimulating hormone (MSH). In the later months of pregnancy, high levels of MSH can make your nipples darken, and can cause dark patches on your face and a dark vertical line down the middle of your tummy called the linea nigra ('black line').

⑥ One of the big two girlie hormones, progesterone affects every aspect of pregnancy. It's produced by the ovaries when you're not pregnant, but eventually the placenta takes over the task during pregnancy. It relaxes smooth muscle: in the uterus so it's less likely to contract and cause miscarriage, and in the bladder, intestines, bowel and veins so they're more flexible as they're squashed by the growing uterus. It increases your body temperature and breathing rate, causes dilated blood vessels, which can reduce blood pressure and make you feel faint and nauseated, and helps produce breast milk. Immediately after the birth, the level drops and continues to drop for a number of days.

⑥ The other major girlie hormone, oestrogen (or more correctly group of oestrogens), is also produced by the ovaries and then the placenta during pregnancy. Oestrogens help make everything in the reproductive department behave as it should throughout the pregnancy, including the breasts (enlarging nipples and developing milk glands), the uterus (strengthening) and body tissue (softening). Many believe that excess oestrogens cause nausea in the first three months. As with progesterone, the relatively high level of oestrogen drops immediately after the birth, and continues to drop in the days that follow.

⑥ Endorphins, which mimic the effects of morphine and help blunt perceptions of pain and stress, are hormones produced by the brain up until and during childbirth. After the birth the levels drop sharply. This has been implicated in the temporary 'baby blues' most new mothers experience, and the more lasting feelings of depression that sometimes follow as your 'happy hormones' are switched off.

your record

✳ What are your fears and hopes for the pregnancy?

WEEK 13

what's going on

Your tummy is probably starting to stick out. Soon it will seem to 'pop' and everyone will begin noticing (scan done, you may want to go public soon). Any nausea will probably stop or trail off about now.

Down in foetusland, reflexes for sucking, swallowing and breathing have begun. The amniotic sac surrounding the foetus contains 100 millilitres of amniotic fluid, a fully appointed unit still with lots of room to bob around in. The ears are finished but can't hear yet. The lungs, liver, kidneys and digestive bits are still maturing. The head has been growing more slowly than the body since week 11. By the end of this week almost everything should be formed and ready to grow. But the foetus almost certainly wouldn't survive on its own because the organs wouldn't function well enough. Weight: about 30 grams (1oz).

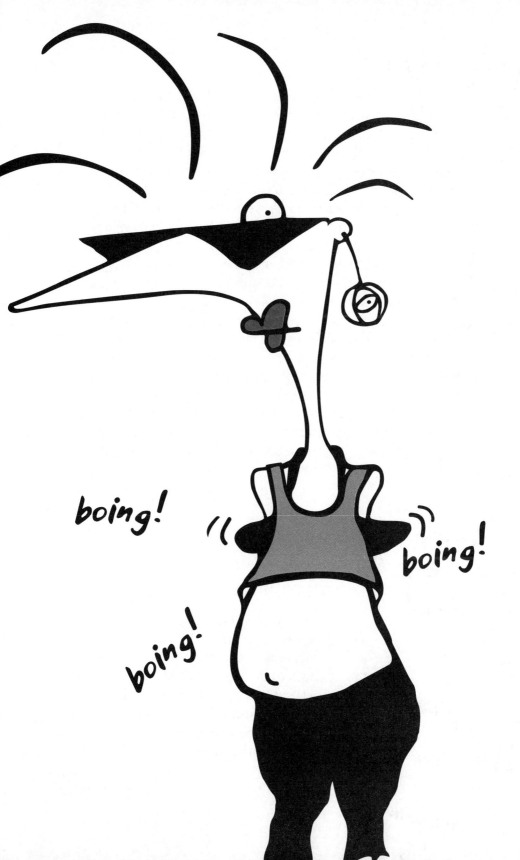

DiARY

I am so grumpy. All I want is an extensive personal staff to clean the house, fluff the pillows, cook my dinner and suck up to me. I have injured myself by sneezing in the middle of a yoga stretch. It felt like I tore through muscles or ligaments on each side of my tummy, down low near the hip bones. Bloody exercise: it's bad for you.

And there is far too much palaver written these days about balanced meals for the pregnant woman. A perfectly nutritious and attractive meal can be had by eating three pieces of marmite toast and half a carton of chocolate milk in 7 seconds flat. Although it is true that I'd probably be dead if I wasn't taking all those vitamins, come to think of it.

It's the weirdest thing being nauseous and getting no fun out of food, but still feeding your face relentlessly.

My gums keep bleeding. This is obviously some sort of design fault. Again, many of the pregnancy books are hopeless, presuming the 'mother-to-be' has the brain of the average anteater: 'The baby hormones may be making your gums bleed. Take special care with dental hygiene.' I always lose consciousness at about the word 'hygiene'. I phone my midwife who suggests more vitamin C, which seems to help. Maybe I just had scurvy.

weepiness

At times during pregnancy you can feel ecstatic, elated, like a fertile winged mythical love goddess (well, okay, maybe not), contented, confident, optimistic and relaxed. But you can also feel depressed, terrified, worried, tense, crabby, moody and like a blundering water buffalo. Tears are almost inevitable.

Sometimes it can seem that you're on a hair-trigger. Anything can suddenly set you off: sad movies or the news stories about bad things that happen to babies or mothers. The rest of the world goes on despite your pregnancy, and with a bit of bad luck yours might coincide with a relationship break-up, other personal complications, or a death in the family.

Even without extra stress, you can feel miserable, especially during the first trimester when your hormones seem to be stuck on the spin-cycle. Maybe you recognise some of the symptoms from PMS (premenstrual syndrome). About 10 per cent of women have mild to moderate depression while pregnant.

Your moodiness might be manifested by you being cranky and overcritical; or flying into rage or panic about something that isn't really so important; or crying for no specific reason. Thinking about pregnancy and becoming a parent can also bring up unresolved issues you may have with your own mother and father, or feelings of sadness or anger about your own childhood. And it's natural to feel ambivalent about being pregnant, and worried about many aspects of pregnancy and parenting, and grief for a lifestyle lost.

Your more pressing and immediate pregnancy worries might include the following.

Will my baby be born healthy and 'normal'? (Very probably.)

Do I deserve a healthy baby? (Oooh, yes.)

How will I juggle parenting and career? (You won't know until you get there, but you can talk to people who do it and see if any of their strategies might suit you.)

How will I cope with childbirth? (The best way you can.)

Sleep deprivation? (Get all the sleep you can now.)

Breastfeeding? (There's lots of help available, and in the end it isn't compulsory.)

Curtailed freedom? (There are compensations. But yes. Life ain't perfect. Prepare to be curtailed.)

And loss of autonomy? (It will pass to some extent in about twenty years or so.)

Will I have 'maternal instincts'? (Being a good parent is about being kind, patient and ready to learn, not about 'instincts'.)

Will I bond with my baby? (Probably, and if you don't there is help available.)

How will my relationship with my partner be affected? (You'll probably both be sleep-deprived and grumpy for a while. Express your fears and keep talking.)

How will my partner cope with the demands of parenting? (Don't know, but again there's help available.)

Will my baby suffer from me being a single parent? (Children need a stable, loving environment. You can do that.)

Will I ever recognise my body again? (Yes, and you should stop looking at photos of famous actresses and models who have had children. They also have forty-seven nannies, personal trainers and teeming hordes of hair and make-up artists.)

How will I/we cope with a reduced income and increasing expenses? (Have a strategy.)

Why wouldn't you have the occasional wave of panic when you remember any or all of the above, plus the fact that your life is about to be transformed, and there's no going back?

Maybe you just need a good cry every now and then or to share your feelings with your partner or a friend. If a particular issue is really getting you down, or if you feel depressed most of the time, it might help to get some professional counselling. It's better to sort things out now than when you have a real, live, non-theoretical baby on your hands.

Here's the bit everyone bangs on about, but only because it's true: if you're feeling shocking, don't guzzle alcohol and caffeine and stuff your face with junk food. Eat a healthy diet, and get yourself some exercise, fresh air and plenty of rest.

Partners and friends, who are always on the lookout for a way to help you, should be ordered to cheer you up. And you need to hang out with some cheerful parents.

the way people react to the news

When people react to your pregnancy, it's not about you, it's about them. If they say negative or rude things, it comes from their own experience or their own personality, their own fears or their own problems with body image, babies, their mother, whatever. Every time you hear something discouraging ('Your life is over') or ludicrous ('Childbirth doesn't hurt at all'), just say to yourself, 'It's not about me, it's about them.'

your record

✳ Who have you told about your pregnancy?

✳ How have they reacted?

✳ What's the maddest advice you've been offered?

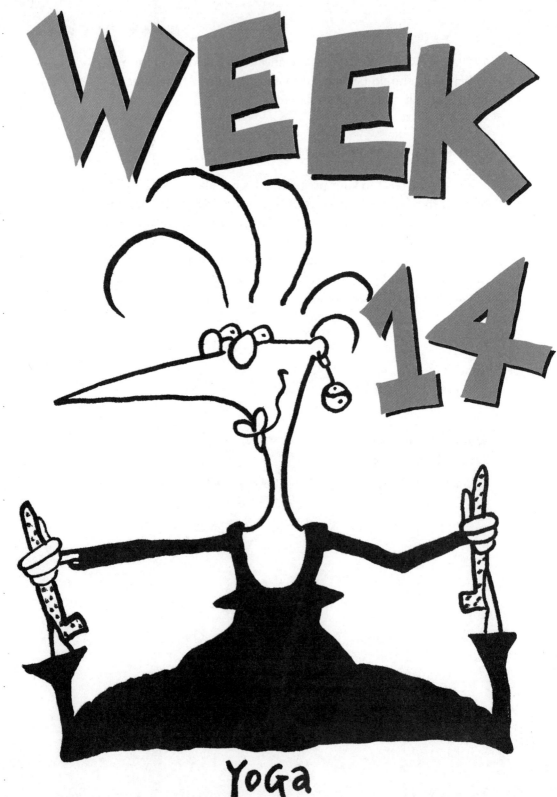

what's going on The second trimester

kicks off this week. You'll probably start to feel a bit more

energetic. With a bit of luck the nausea should be gone or

almost gone. You may get a dark line from your navel to your

pubic hair. This is called the linea nigra because doctors

can't resist Latin. In fact the 'black line' is not a black line

if you have white skin: it varies from a pale, shadowy pink to a

browny colour. On dark skin it can look darker, or not be visible

at all. You will almost certainly be 'showing' – meaning

that you have a pronounced bump in your tummy. According

to the fruit-metaphor brigade your uterus has attained the

size of a large grapefruit.

By now an expert ultrasound operator can usually

see whether the foetus is a boy or a girl, by the presence

or absence of a suspiciously willy-like object. The bones are

forming in the arms, legs, rib cage and skull. It's the start of

your baby's skeleton. Weight: about 45 grams (1^1/2 oz).

Average approximate foetus length this week from head to bum

cm
1
2
3
4
5
6
7
8
9
10
11
12
13
14
15
16
17
18
19
20
21
22

DiARY I've stopped being grumpy and started being weepy. I'm trying to regard this as progress. I'm getting more forgetful: this might be pregnancy hormones, or just having more to think about. So much for the alleged energy surge of the second trimester that everyone goes on about . . . I feel a little better by the end of the week. At least the nausea's gone and only pays a surprise visit now and again.

I investigate my sneezing/yoga injury. There is a muscle called the psoas that extends from the lower back to the front groin and I have injured mine waving my legs in the air. My chiropractor, a reassuringly sensible woman of the world, gives me an extremely gentle exercise to do three times a day and says a walk of ten minutes or so at a time is plenty until it gets better. She can't feel around because the foetus is in the way, and she says since everything is changing in the pelvis, healing the muscle isn't going to be top priority for my body.

I decide that my ill-fated attempts at yoga are simply folly. If you're not already a yoga enthusiast you can end up injuring yourself. On the other hand, if you are the sort of person who ties themself up into a pretzel every Wednesday night, if you stretch every day and can climb up your own left leg, well, there's no problem. But if you start yoga cold in pregnancy, you can do more harm than good. I should have taken instruction from an exercise person who is trained in pregnancy – I suspect that a lot of people who work in gyms or conduct yoga classes say they know about pregnancy exercise, but don't really.

Beck asks whether I've had any puffiness. Nobody mentioned puffiness. There had better not be any puffiness. I'm against it. I've got enough to deal with, thank you very much.

The fact that I feel like I weigh about 56,795 kilos is beginning to depress me. Beck says I will have to exercise from week 20 on, but I shouldn't do too much exercise before then because my system would be not so much shocked as horrified.

'But what about the people who swim five kilometres a day and hike around Borneo when they're pregnant?' I ask.

'They are not your type,' she replies.

She's right.

Feeling a bit fixated, I buy a pile of pregnancy magazines at the newsagent, call in sick, and take to the couch. Some of these magazines seem to belong to an alternative universe. Most seem very keen on giveaways. I remind myself that a whizzbang product being given away is probably not in the magazine because it's necessarily the best or safest thing. It's there because its manufacturers get a free plug and a picture of their stuff in the mag. Pregnancy is clearly big business.

Fitness is a big theme of all the magazines. One of them that seems especially focused on body image (honestly, is this the time?) actually talks of 'training' instead of exercise and has pages of suggested menus so you don't put on weight in the wrong places. All the models in the pictures seem to go through pregnancy a size eight with a cantaloupe up their micro-mini frock. How appalling of me not to look like a whippet in a wig and cook up some Tuscan, three-course, delicious, low-fat, gourmet meal every two minutes.

One mag claims to have 'Amazing facts about pregnancy and birth'. And they're right. They *are* amazing. 'A child born feet first will have the power of healing later in life.' This is such amazing bollocks it makes you doubt some of the rest such as 'The heaviest baby born to a healthy mother weighed 10.2 kilograms (more than 22 pounds)'.

Nonetheless, that is a pretty scary idea.

info

second-trimester hassles

This is often the most comfortable trimester of the pregnancy. For most women, nausea stops or decreases, energy levels are up and mood swings moderate. However, in this trimester, you may need to deal with one or more of the following.

sore, bleeding gums

Your gums may develop gingivitis, becoming sore, puffy, inflamed, and prone to bleeding, especially when you brush your teeth. This is caused by the increased progesterone and oestrogen in your blood, which makes gums softer and increases the blood pressure in the capillaries at the point where gums and teeth meet. This makes gums more susceptible to damage from food and being bumped by your toothbrush.

Try daily flossing, frequent brushing with a soft toothbrush (after each snack or meal if possible) and at least one dental visit during pregnancy for a professional cleaning job. (Make sure the dentist knows you're pregnant so you're not given an X-ray or medication. Many dentists say local anaesthetics are safe during pregnancy, but if you wait until you're not pregnant any more there will definitely be no risk.)

Proper levels of calcium, vitamin C and other nutrients will also help. As well, avoid eating toffeelike stuff or sticky date puddingy things that can get stuck in all the nooks and crannies and encourage infection.

congested nose

Something else you may share with the pregnancy sisterhood is a blocked, congested nose or one that is runnier than usual. You may also get nosebleeds. These schnoz problems are the result of the same hormonal effect that creates gum problems, which causes an increased blood supply, softening and swelling of the mucous membranes inside the nostrils, increased mucus production and easier bleeding. This means colds and upper respiratory tract infections can take longer than usual to clear up.

Bleeding can be triggered by unrestrained honking (over-strenuous nose blowing) or even by a dry atmosphere, which can harden mucus and make it more likely to cause damage to mucous membranes when you blow your nose. Try to avoid allergens. Humidifying the atmosphere and making yourself steam inhalations can help relieve the symptoms. You can also rub some emollient cream inside each nostril at bedtime.

STIR CRAZY? TIME TO TRAVEL

For many women, the middle trimester – Week 13 to Week 26 – is the prime time for a last spot of pre-baby travelling ... or, let's be honest about this, taking a holiday. There are women who keep going with plans for a trip to India or Peru late into their pregnancy, but the appeal of such trips tends to fade as you grow. Nonetheless, if you can afford it, you will almost certainly want to get away some time soon. For some ideas and advice on holiday and work trips, read through the section on travel in 'Week 23'.

To stop your nose bleeding apply gentle pressure on the affected side of the nose while leaning your head forward. Frequent or heavy nose bleeding should be mentioned to your doctor. Don't use any nose drops or sprays without checking first with your doctor. And . . . er . . . hate to sound like your granny, but don't pick your nose.

vaginal secretions

I realise this is hardly dinner-party conversation, but you'll be pleased to know that all those extra-wet knickers are actually normal. Your vagina is producing more mucus and I think it's time we had a better term. Like lady's lotion. God. Sorry. Maybe not.

It's caused by the combined effect again of progesterone and oestrogen: the softer, more swollen mucous membranes of pregnancy produce more secretions. (Unpoetically, the medical description is 'an increase of normal mucoid discharge', which sounds like something a special-effects technician would say on the set of a critter movie.)

This normal discharge, called leucorrhoea if you want to get technical, should be clear or milky white. There can be rather a lot of it, and it's likely to increase as the pregnancy progresses.

To help with the hassle of vaginal secretions in overdrive:

⑥ Avoid tight undies or trousers.

⑥ Wear undies and trousers made from natural fabrics such as cotton or wool – avoid nylon and polyester.

⑥ Wear panty-liners and change them frequently during the day.

⑥ Don't use tampons when you're pregnant because there is a higher risk of vaginal infection.

⑥ If it's easy, take a couple of changes of underpants with you in your handbag (and if you think you need a bigger handbag to leave the house now, just wait until you have a baby!).

Increased blood flow to the genitals can mean a more sensitive than usual clitoris – another reason to stay away from tight undies or trousers. (Or not.)

infections

If your vaginal discharge is yellowish or greenish or has an unhealthy smell, you have probably got an infection, which will need to be treated. An imbalance of friendly and unfriendly bacteria and high oestrogen levels in the vagina can make you more prone than usual to thrush, also known as candida, which may need to be treated by a doctor who knows you're pregnant. Symptoms include a curdlike white discharge and an itching and burning feeling.

If you are having thrush problems, remember to be careful to wipe front to back after going to the toilet. This is because thrush can hang out in the bowel and be transferred to your vagina. Thrush is linked to a high yeast diet, so try avoiding refined sugars, and eat lots of yoghurt with live Lactobacillus acidophilus cultures. Yoghurt can also be applied inside the vagina.

Air the nether regions when possible. You may do this by running around in the nude and waving your legs in the air, or by doing things like wearing no clothes or a nightie to bed instead of pyjamas. If you're lucky enough to have warm weather, wear a sarong or skirt with no undies when you can.

your record

✳ How are you feeling now you're in the second trimester?
- ❐ better
- ❐ happy as a clam
- ❐ get out of my way, I'm going to throw up
- ❐ excited about my changing body
- ❐ like my wardrobe just shrank to one ensemble and a queen-sized duvet
- ❐ full of beans
- ❐ completely exhausted, now that you mention it

1

2

3

4

5

6

7

8

9

10

11

12

13

14

15

16

17

18

19

20

21

22

what's going on

Your heart is doing a lot more than it used to and has a lot more blood to pump. (Contrary to old ludicrous persons' tales, your heart doesn't actually get bigger.) Nausea might come back if you let yourself get too tired or hungry. You may be looking even more divine than usual as your hair isn't falling out at the rate it normally does, so it looks thicker, your skin looks plumped out and the extra blood in your system is giving you what they call the 'glow'.

The foetal fingernails are developing, and the facial features are clearly defined. The foetus may suck its thumb. (All together now: awwwwww!) The skin formed is still very thin, so if there was a tiny camera in there transmitting pictures you could see blood vessels underneath. The foetus begins to put on weight more rapidly about this time. Starting soon the arms and legs will begin to be more co-ordinated when moving – imagine languid foetal aerobics. Weight: about 80 grams (2³/₄oz).

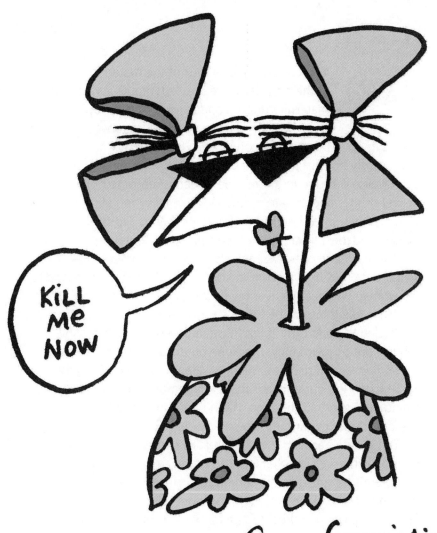

DiARY Geoff and I go for a tour of the maternity ward at the hospital we're booked into. Our visit to the maternity unit is conducted by a very capable midwife called Helen. In the nursery we look at babies in open plastic boxes on wheels, tethered next to their otherwordly but distinctly knackered-looking mothers.

Because they are in the middle of being renovated, the delivery suites and private rooms look like tacky motel rooms after being trashed by a desultory heavy metal band. Except that they all have hideous, floral, flouncy bedspreads. I couldn't possibly give birth on one of those, I tell Helen, wondering even as the words come out how it is I'm talking *World of Interiors* magazine to the woman who may deliver my baby.

'They like things to be feminine,' she says.

'Helen,' I point out, 'if you're squatting down with a baby coming out of your fanny, I reckon you'd know you're a woman.'

Some random realities: Sunday. Valentine's Day. We realise we've forgotten our anniversary nearly a month before. Start eating Refreshers all the time. Hadn't had one since I was about eight but I'm a confirmed two-packs-a-day woman now.

Drag myself around. Leg hurting. The bottom half of me is a milk-white sea of cellulite. I'm starting to have the feeling that there's no going back. Getting to bed far too late, then not sleeping, then waking early and can't get back to sleep, then finally sleeping in and being late for work. I think I may have jet lag, without any jetting.

Nausea, at least, seems to have gone except when I allow myself to get tired and hungry. Weeing all night long. The idea of wearing my normal clothes – eg anything with a ZIP or WAIST – is totally laughable. And the books say, 'You won't be showing yet'. Showing? I'm not just showing! I'm showing OFF!

Searching for maternity clothes in the shops is like wading through the rejects of every other season. A few years ago it was orange and lime-green clothes for women – so now it must be orange and lime-green maternity wear. P-lease!

As a clothes designer I know people try to reduce costs by cutting things thinner rather than wider, and shorter rather than longer, but in this case it seems pretty damn mingy. You don't want to be in a hobble skirt when you're already going to be waddling, surely? And why is there nothing between mini- and maxi-length? It's as if only Queen Victoria and one of Rod Stewart's girlfriends buy maternity clothes.

I end up buying sensible items in black – two pairs of trousers, one T-shirt, one jumper, a frock, two pairs of tights – and hand over the equivalent of the Mexican national debt. You'd think they had emeralds sewn into the hems. And that's in the normal maternity shop. The posh maternity shop has shiny polyester jackets that aren't meant to be shiny for £120 and various other rich-lady outfits. I look like the *Titanic* in all of them.

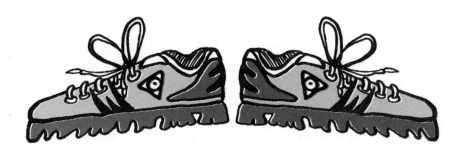

exercise exercise exercise

Moderate exercise during pregnancy is good for you and your off-spring. When we say moderate exercise, we do not mean flinging yourself about like a non-pregnant person with a gym obsession and a desire to run a marathon before lunch. Sensible exercise is good for circulation, relaxation and energy levels, and helps to stop constipation, cramps and backache.

If you're not fit before pregnancy, this is not the time to adopt a strenuous exercise regime. Try things like walking, gentle yoga and stretching, swimming, dancing, antenatal exercise classes, or aquarobics. Look for gyms, swimming and recreation centres or physiotherapy clinics that run yoga or exercise classes designed for pregnancy and have instructors with a special qualification in pregnancy exercise. At the very least make sure your instructor knows you're pregnant. And if in any kind of doubt, check with your midwife or antenatal clinic that the exercise you're doing or about to do is safe for you.

Many instructors are not aware of the special risks of pregnancy. The extra release of the hormone relaxin, which makes your ligaments and joints more stretchy, can make you more prone to injury. Sit-ups are generally a bad idea during pregnancy because they can cause a separation of muscles in your stomach, creating a hernia-like effect.

Yoga

Yoga can help you become aware of how comfortably you are standing, sitting or lying down. Its breathing and meditation practices can relax you during pregnancy and labour. Special antenatal yoga classes can help with many of the discomforts of pregnancy, as well as improving the body's suppleness and strength for labour. The mind-body-spirit approach of yoga can be a good match for the mind-body-spirit-altering experience of being pregnant.

Even if you've been super-fit before pregnancy, you'll need to apply some limitations to your regime. Consult your gym or fitness professional as soon as you know you're pregnant to get some expert advice on exercise modifications, and choose a slower pace, lighter-impact class and hand weights not exceeding half a kilo (1lb 1oz).

If you have played sport regularly before pregnancy, you can usually continue until the third trimester, unless it's a sport that can cause impact injuries, such as football (contesting for the ball), trick rollerblading (falls), baseball (sliding collisions), water polo (being kicked, accidentally or otherwise) and tennis (rabid opponents prone to attacking you with a racket).

Other activities not recommended during pregnancy include horse riding, any kind of skiing, backpacking, and lifting heavy weights and other heavy manual work. Jogging, running and other athletics can be too stressful on joints, breasts and baby, so check your exercise program with your GP or midwife.

You shouldn't exercise while pregnant if you have a history of medical conditions such as recurrent miscarriages, placenta praevia, 'incompetent cervix', pre-eclampsia or heart disease. Other conditions, including diabetes and anaemia, may sometimes mean exercise is not recommended.

when exercising

◎ Wear supportive footwear and a sports bra.

◎ Drink plenty of water before, during and after, and make sure you have some healthy snacks handy.

◎ Remember your centre of gravity is changing, which will affect your balance and co-ordination, so take it easy.

◎ Listen to and trust your body – stop if any activity makes you feel uncomfortable, overtired, hot, dizzy, faint or crampy.

◎ Don't worry if your resting heart rate is higher during pregnancy even when you're not exercising. It doesn't mean you are losing fitness; it simply reflects your increased rate of circulation.

◎ Don't get overheated for prolonged periods – this can be damaging to the foetus, particularly during the first trimester.

◎ Use the talk test to decide if you should slow down or stop. You should be able to carry on a chat while exercising. If you can't talk continuously, or can't talk at all, because of huffing and puffing, then slow down or stop until you can.

◎ You can exercise moderately on all or most days of the week for 30 minutes every day. You can vary your exercise regime perhaps with puffing work outs on one day and some yoga on another with a little aqua at the weekend. (That means exercising in water, not the colour of your leg-warmers.)

⑥ Go gently with abdominal exercises, and support your tummy with your interlinked hands while doing them; about 30 per cent of women have a separation of the abdominal muscles. If this happens, you need to stop any exercising that affects the area.

⑥ Strictly limit exercises that involve lying flat on your back to a maximum of 2–3 minutes, especially from the beginning of the second trimester, and omit them altogether after you reach twenty weeks. The weight of the uterus can compress the inferior cava vena, the vein that carries blood back to your heart from your lower parts, ultimately resulting in a reduced blood flow to your head and to the baby. So if you feel dizzy or faint while on your back, turn onto your left side and rest.

⑥ Don't forget to exercise your pelvic-floor muscles (Kegel exercises, as they are called in the US) – these muscles are like a hammock or sling that sits underneath all your inside organs and has holes in it corresponding to the various openings to the outside. Tighten your pelvic-floor muscles, as though you are trying to stop a wee, three or four times a day. Do as many of these as you can before getting tired. Every antenatal exercise class will tell you how important these are. Doing the exercises will mean faster pelvic-floor recovery after delivery, and will help prevent accidental weeing (also known as stress incontinence) when you sneeze, cough or laugh after childbirth.

⑥ You probably need to do some light abdominal exercises or the spine will be pulled forward by the weight of the baby and throw your posture out. Check with a specialised instructor.

more info on exercise and yoga

 For contacts, see under Exercise in 'Help' (p.404).

BOOKS

Yoga for Pregnancy, Birth and Beyond by Francoise Barbira Freedman, Dorling Kindersley, UK, 2004.

Preparing for Birth with Yoga: Empowering and Effective Exercise for Pregnancy and Childbirth by Janet Balaskas, HarperCollins, UK, 2003.

DVD

Pilates in Pregnancy by Lindsay Jackson, Quantum Leap, UK, 2004.

There is always a danger when learning from a book or a DVD that bad habits or wrong postures can be adopted. If you're at all unsure, or completely inexperienced, consider a couple of lessons in the basics from a qualified instructor experienced with pregnant clients.

your record

✳ What exercise did you do before pregnancy?

✳ What exercise are you doing now?

what's going on

It is possible you might feel the movements of the foetus as 'butterflies' in your stomach from now on, especially if you know what to pay attention to, but you also mightn't feel it for weeks.

You now have about 180 millilitres (6¼ fl oz) of amniotic fluid. Your uterus is kind of like a balloon full of yellowish water. All the joints of the foetus are working and the fingers and toes are all there and waving about. Toenails are just starting to form. The head still looks kind of oversized but the rest of the body is catching up. The downy foetal hair called lanugo has started to grow on the body. (Lanugo means fine wool in some ancient language.) There are various opinions about what the lanugo might be for: it might help keep the foetus warm, or it might be an underfelt for the gooey stuff that eventually covers the baby. Or maybe the foetus is just trying to develop a fashion instinct. Weight: about 110 grams (3¾oz).

M
WIN.
VATS o

WEEK 16

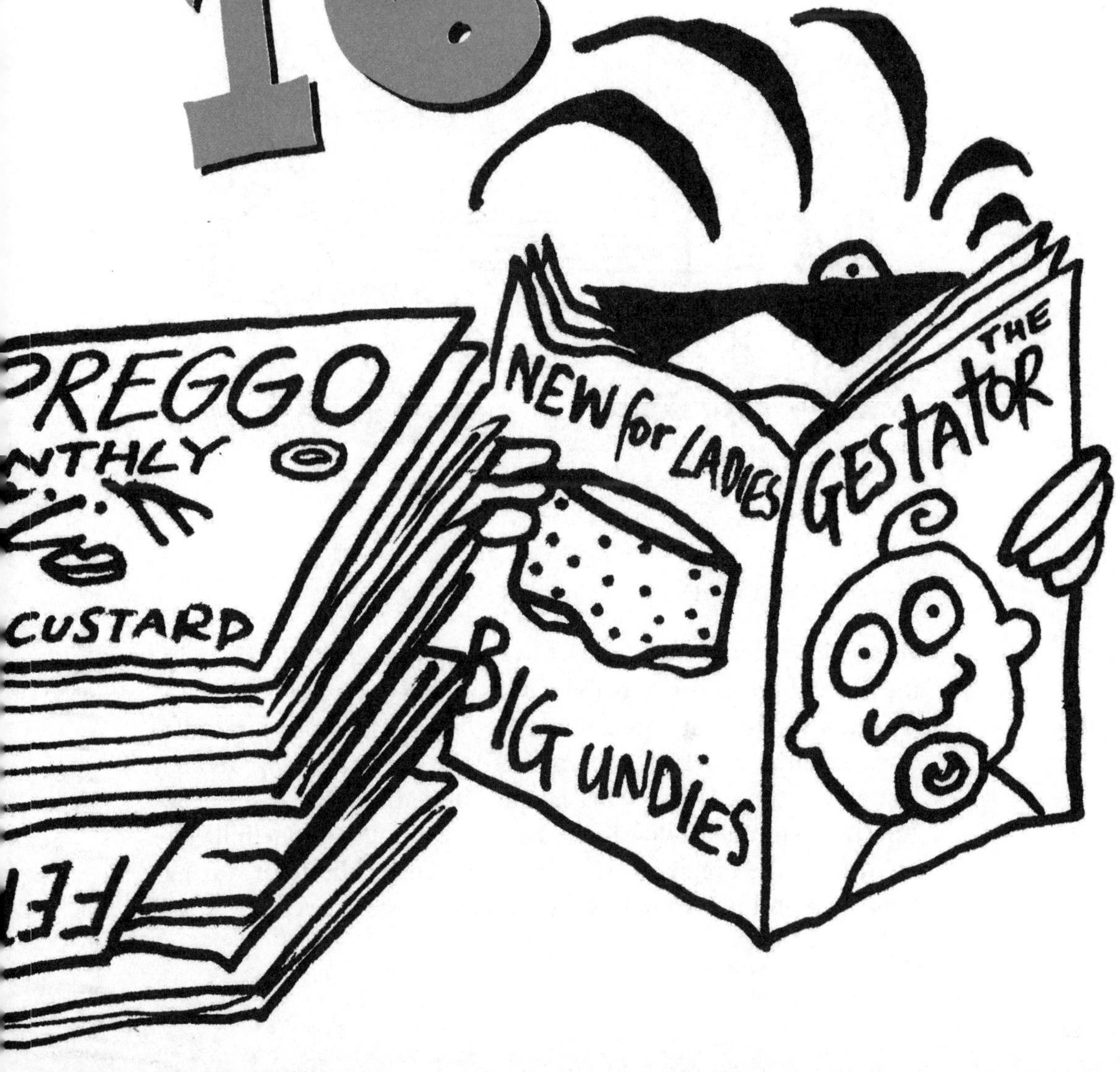

DiARY

No idea what happened this week.
Blinked and missed it.
Oprah's hair's looking tremendous though,
I must say.

Reading foR Dads·to·Be

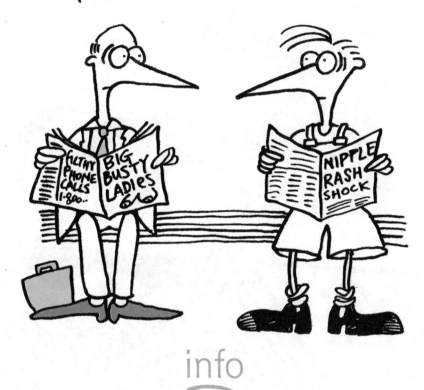

info

'fess up to being pregnant

You're slower, you're more tired, you're more scatty, especially in the first three months, and apparently we've got it to look forward to again in the last three months. (That leaves these middle three months in which everyone tells us we're looking divine, just glowin' up a storm.) Tell people you're tired. Let them help. And let them make allowances. Forgot to pay the phone bill? It's because you're pregnant. Have to sit down on the floor during a meeting and put your feet on a chair and show everyone your undies? Because you're pregnant. Had to buy a new pair of red shoes? Pregnant. See? It's easy.

the pursed-lip brigade

Not married? Married but wearing tight clothes? Planning to go back to work before the baby turns seventeen? Somewhere, somehow, someone will disapprove of you. Get used to it. If you stay home with the baby, some idiots will start asking, 'What do you DO all day?', as if you're just sitting at home watching daytime soaps and eating Mars Bars (ahem). If you're at work, people will ask, 'You haven't put your baby in child care/hired a nanny, have you?', as if it were the same as asking, 'You haven't tied it up and popped it in a tree for the day, have you?'. Apply the same logic as you do for unsolicited advice: it's not about you, it's about them.

stuff you didn't know before

ⓖ Breast milk comes out of the nipple like water comes out of a sprinkler – there are heaps of little holes, not just one. And one breast may produce heaps more milk than the other.

ⓖ What the inside of your navel looks like.

ⓖ You can want to throw up and eat at the same time.

ⓖ You can go and wee all the time and still retain fluid.

ⓖ Sleep deprivation starts well before the birth.

stuff that people don't know

ⓖ It makes people behave nicer to you when they know:

ⓖ You are carrying a quarter again the amount of blood you usually do.

ⓖ In the second half of the pregnancy the baby whacks you in the internal organs all the time, and it's not always a cute little whack – sometimes it's really uncomfortable, sometimes it actually hurts.

⑥ Your feet swell to twice their usual size (well, that's what it feels like).

⑥ You can't get the required amount of deep sleep because you have to wee all night – it's the equivalent of someone waking you up every couple of hours.

stuff for blokes

More than ever, fathers-to-be are keen to attend the birth of their babies – and to act as 'birth partner' (see p.101). Assuming your partner is on for this – and assuming for the purposes of this section that your partner is a bloke – then he's probably reading this book and maybe one of the pregnancy manuals for some serious biology revision. He's maybe even getting a tad jealous at not being the one who's pregnant (roll your eyes until he stops).

During the labour and delivery, the more your partner is prepared for, the better. Especially towards the end of labour, when you may be off with the gas-and-air fairies, he needs to be aware of the birth plan and all the available options to ensure that your wishes are adhered to. If you are planning on NCT (National Childbirth Trust) or other antenatal classes, make sure that you both go along. Blokes can learn a lot at such gatherings and may also find themselves a part of the invaluable support networks that come about through classes. In other words, they can make friends with other new dads and mums in the neighbourhood. This could be handy, especially if all his current group of mates meet down the pub. Life is about to change, big time.

If, on the other hand, your partner won't read or learn anything about childbirth, at least tell him:

a) There's going to be a lot of blood.

b) There's nothing much he can do about the pain, and that's not his job.

c) If he thinks he is going to faint, he should put his head between his knees or stand on tippytoes, or go outside and have a rest. (I say let's see 'im try all three at once.)

MORE FOR BLOKES

www.fathersdirect.com
This UK website is stacked with news and information for dads and expectant dads, including chat subjects (okay – networking, if that sounds more manly). There are articles on the men's aspect of juggling work and family, staying home with the kids and other issues ranging from the sadness of miscarriage to ideas for amusing the kids. A good place to meet other dads, or get specialist help.

BOOKS

Most of the birth and baby books aimed at men aren't much cop as 'how to' manuals for dads who are at home being the 'primary caregiver', but blokes can read the usual books and stuff that's aimed at mums (see Baby-care Books in 'Week 43'). After all, it's the same problems and the same advice. Equally for blokes looking to be a helpful birth partner rather than a quivering wreck, a browse of one of the general pregnancy books (see 'Week 2') is useful. But these two are worthwhile blokey additions.

Fatherhood edited by Peter Howarth, Orion, UK, 1998.

A modern but not too new-manly collection of essays with contributions from the likes of Tony Parsons and Neil Spencer, offering poignant, witty and even philosophical insights into becoming a father. Mirroring the pregnancy tomes, the essays kick off with pre-conception broodiness, then run through the nine months of pregnancy and on to Year One of fatherhood.

The Bloke's Guide to Pregnancy by Jon Smith, Hay House, UK, 2004.

A first-hand account by a bloke who interviewed other blokes about the blokey feelings and experiences they had when their partners were pregnant.

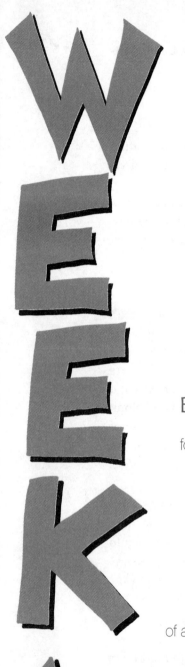

what's going on

You may be sweating, spitting and running like a tap at the nose as well as having those pesky vaginal secretions. Basically you're a leaking bag of various fluids. I'm sorry, but there it is. Find room in your handbag among the lipsticks, spanners and panty-liners for tissues, spare deodorant, spare undies, a couple of wet-wipes, maybe a beach towel. (It's really not that bad.) By now the baby's sex organs are completely formed. The foetal kidneys produce lots of urine: the foetus wees about every 40–45 minutes (at least you don't have to change nappies yet). Icky though it may sound, the foetus takes in some of this wee when it swallows mouthfuls of amniotic fluid. But most of the foetal waste products go through the placental membrane and into your circulation, where it's dealt with by your body's usual functions. Weight: about 150 grams (5^1/$_4$ oz).

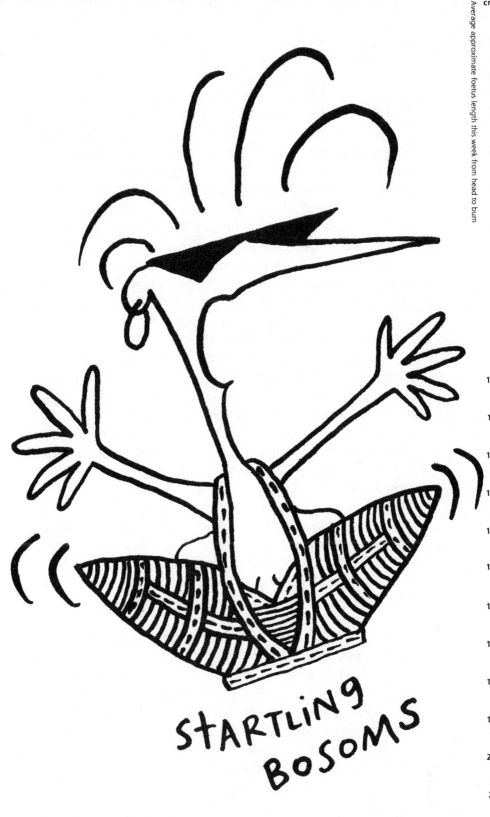

STARTLING BOSOMS

DiARY

My bosoms are getting bigger, and none of my bras are comfy, even the bigger ones I bought. My bosoms used to stick out straight from my body, practically in opposite directions from each other. They were known as East and West. Now they're kind of bigger and lower slung, meaning there's a bit underneath where it gets sweaty. And all these little skin tags have grown there as well. Thank God I found a book that said this was perfectly normal.

Sports crop-tops seemed the best, but now they feel like elastic-bandage boob-tubes three sizes too small. If I'm sitting around at home I don't wear a bra at all. No doubt this means I'll end up having bosoms shaped like tube socks that I can tie in a knot behind my neck when they get in the way. Don't care. Those areas around my nipples I can never pronounce have started to go brown and are getting bumps on them.

Farewell, my strawberries-and-cream nipples, my horizontal, pointy bosoms! Will you now both be called South forever? Why don't I have a photo of you?! Was my youth so misspent that I never even posed for nude photographs? What was I thinking!

I'm feeling very annoyed with myself for not being a supple, lithe, yoga-frenzied woman. The bath in the new house is of such a ludicrous design by some kind of deranged handyman that before I can get in it I have to crawl over about half a metre of tiles or take a huge, dangerous step on one leg. (Well, obviously, otherwise it would be a jump, not a step. I'm losing my mind.) And given that there isn't enough room in the bathroom to swing a cat – actually there isn't even enough room to *shout* at a cat – it won't do. The whole thing is a disaster waiting to happen for a woman whose centre of gravity is changing every day.

I call Pete the plumber to come and fix it. Pete, of course, finds that the bathroom floor is practically rotted through as well and that there's some other piping-style disaster, which means the job turns out to be five times bigger.

One of the reasons I feel like I'm going mad is sleep deprivation. It never occurred to me this would happen BEFORE the little mite arrived. One of the books says this is because I'm sleeping like a baby – not much deep sleep but plenty of REM sleep. That stands for Rapidly Enraged Mother-to-be.

Call me dense, but it's only just hit me I'm not one person who's pregnant – I mean, I am – but I'm also two people. No. I'm not two people but there are two people – a big one and a little one – sharing the same body. Well. That's a bit spooky.

Apparently many people at this stage of pregnancy find that they can have a few sips of wine or beer occasionally without a violent reaction. Geoff poured me an enormous thimbleful of what he described as 'a very smooth cabernet sauvignon' but it tasted like meths to me.

info

breasts

Probably one of the first pregnancy changes you noticed were your breasts getting larger and more tender. They'll keep growing, but extreme sensitivity usually settles down after the first trimester. From here on, the hormones oestrogen, progesterone and prolactin stimulate more growth and the production of some pre-milk stuff called colostrum.

Each breast contains about twenty segments or lobes; each of these is made up of grapelike bunches of glands called alveoli; and each of these is lined with milk-producing cells. During pregnancy your bosoms get bigger because not only do your dormant milk-producing cells and ducts enlarge, your body also grows new ones to help out. (Your original breast size bears no relation to milk production.)

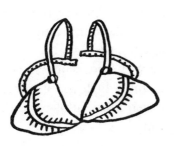
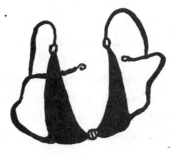

the changes

Breast changes are usually more extreme in a first pregnancy. Your breasts may feel tender, tingling, warm, full, heavy, painfully sensitive or lumpy. You may even have some stabbing pain. You'll be able to see more veins, often blue, close to the skin's surface, carrying the extra blood supply to the area. They're especially noticeable if you have fair skin.

The nipples and areolae (the areas around each nipple) become larger and darker, particularly if your natural skin tone is dark. Most nipples and areolae go a shade of brown, even if they have been pink before. This can happen gradually to the entire area, or in patches. Each areola is dotted with sebaceous (oil-producing) glands called Montgomery's tubercles (those little bumps), which secrete a fluid that keeps the nipples supple. The glands become more prominent during pregnancy, so you get a bumpier effect.

You may have a small amount of colostrum – a thin, yellowish liquid – leaking from your nipples towards the end of pregnancy, and even earlier on, but not everyone does. This can cause wet patches, but can be soaked up and hidden by breast pads, otherwise known as nursing pads; you can buy these in the baby section of the chemist or supermarket. Actual milk production won't start until after the baby arrives.

bras

Wearing a well-fitted supporting bra during pregnancy is recommended. You'll probably need to increase your bra measurement and cup size by at least one size. The increase might even be more, depending on the overall weight gain and whatever your breasts feel like doing. (For example, you might go from 34B to 36C.) You can buy bras to fit your changing size, even though it might mean buying a new size a couple of times during the pregnancy. You don't need a maternity bra or new size while your present bra fits well, is comfortable and gives you enough support.

Good features of a maternity bra include wide straps, a wide band of fabric under the breast and a high cotton content. Anything that digs into the skin is even more intolerable than usual, so make sure you get a comfy fit.

Maternity bras often fasten at the front between the cups; or where the straps meet the cups at the front; or they don't fasten at all, but rather stretch so you can just pop a bosom out the bottom to breastfeed. Whatever suits you best. If you started with big bosoms, you'll probably need more support than the stretchy crop-top style. It is advisable to wait until the last few weeks of pregnancy before getting fitted for a nursing bra, as there may still be changes in your rib measurement. Most bra-fitting services suggest that you wait until the baby engages deep in the pelvis before trying to find a bra that will fit after the birth.

afterwards

Don't be sucked in by cosmetic surgery hype that breasts are 'deformed' by breastfeeding and need to be 'enlarged' with sacs of plastic and saline. Sharky cosmetic surgeons don't really care about your bosoms, they just want your money. And there are many possible hideous side effects, including rupture, pain, scarring, lost nipple sensation and inability to breastfeed again.

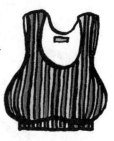

Likewise beware the faffy marketing techniques of the cosmetics companies trying to sell you 'bust firming' and 'breast cream' and 'body treatment' moisturisers. (Often the names are in French or pseudo-French.) They will not prevent your breasts from changing shape or sagging. These creams don't affect the tissues inside the breast, and many are a shockingly expensive waste of time. A cheap moisturiser that smells nice is just as good at keeping the surface of your skin moist, and just as likely to keep your breasts firm – that is, not at all.

Often these creams and oils have ingredients that feel tingly or make the skin seem tighter – the same tightening feeling can be achieved by putting eggwhite on your breasts and waiting for it to dry. Don't be fooled – neither eggs nor creams are a match for Ms Gravity once she's decided to make her presence felt.

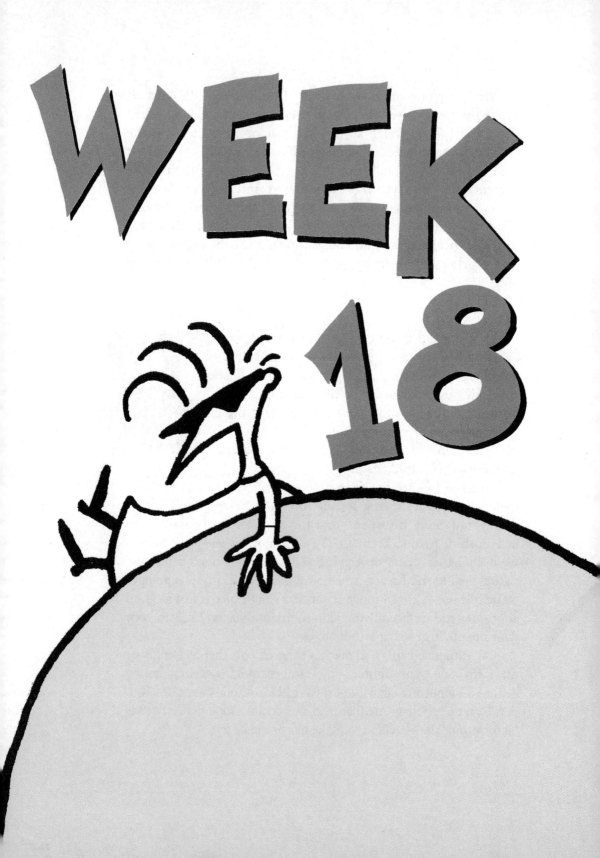

what's going on

You'll find many pregnancy books tell you that this is the week you'll start to feel a first baby move around. Don't hold your breath: you might not feel it move for weeks yet, and that doesn't mean there's anything wrong. Babies mostly move when you're resting at night: basically after 8pm and before 8am. When you move around during the day, you rock the baby to sleep. Use pillows to support your growing tummy while you sleep.

According to some pregnancy experts, this week the foetus can make facial expressions. Oh yeah? Like what? Astonishment? 'Euwww yuk, that amniotic fluid tastes bad'? Anyway, the foetus is definitely able to move around a lot, swing on the umbilical cord (well, that's what it looks like) and can bite its own fingers or do the hokey-cokey if it feels like it. There is lanugo hair all over the body, and blood cells start to form in the bone marrow. Tastebuds are forming.

Weight: about 200 grams (7oz).

Average approximate foetus length this week from head to bum

cm
1
2
3
4
5
6
7
8
9
10
11
12
13
14
15
16
17
18
19
20
21
22

DiARY I 'pop along' to a group physio lesson at the maternity hospital. It is mostly couples, except me, and exactly the sort of thing I hate – name tags and a white board and splitting into two groups to workshop questions such as 'What does fitness mean to you?' and 'Will exercise help?'. (Duh, I think. 'Course it will.)

I am very annoyed to discover that mad exercising in the last few weeks of pregnancy will not actually guarantee a short labour. This seems to be another major design fault of this whole caper, along with painful childbirth.

A woman called Anthea, wearing a black velvet Alice band on her long blonde hair and shoes that cost more than all the rest of the clothes in the room added together, tells the class smugly that she is still going to gym every day and doing a special program of exercises and weights. She looks bloody shocking – has a grey pallor and is scarily thin for someone who is up the duff. Lorraine the physio asks gently if her gym instructor is RSC qualified for pregnancy fitness. No, Anthea says, rather patronisingly, explaining that it's a very superior sort of gym and they do know she's pregnant and IT'S FRIGHTFULLY EXPENSIVE.

Later in the class when Lorraine explains an abdominal muscle injury that causes bits of your organs to poke through like a hernia under the skin of your tummy, Anthea squeals in recognition, 'Oh my GOD, I've got that!', and goes a bit quiet for the rest of the class. One imagines the very superior gym is about to receive a call from her frightfully expensive lawyer.

We practise (a) sitting on giant inflatable balls to strengthen our squatting muscles and straighten our backs, (b) sprawling on beanbags, and (c) a relaxation technique that I fail at miserably. Not for me relaxing in a hospital room full of strangers lying on nylon carpet with the fluorescent lights temporarily off, thank you. We are informed about the importance of pelvic-floor exercises and I just know I'm not going to be able to apply myself enough to do them. I've tried. I did six in a row one Saturday and got bored. We all pass around a plastic pelvis and stare at it as if it might suddenly have something to tell us.

Here's what I learn in group physio at this point:

✳ The average female pelvis is ludicrously small for what's expected of it.

✳ Pelvic-floor exercises exercise the pelvic floor (hello). (The pelvic floor is the trampoliney bit that is stretched under all the pelvic organs.) The main jobs of the pelvic floor are to stop all your organs from falling out of your fanny (well, they wouldn't really, but it would all get a bit saggy in there); contracting around the holes to prevent unscheduled leaking, especially during coughing or sneezing (that is, it's a continence accessory); and allowing your vagina to contract rhythmically if you are in any way interested in sex, which is hard to imagine.

✳ How to exercise the pelvic-floor muscles without anybody noticing. My favourite instruction was 'Your buttocks should not be moving'. I often think that.

✳ They now say to work your pelvic-floor muscles to fatigue three to four times a day, rather than five times thirty times a day or thirty times five times a day, which was the old-fashioned advice.

✳ It is difficult to have a mid-class snack while the physio is explaining to a young woman how to sit when you shit. (Tragically I walked away, so I'll never know.)

✳ Nap when you can, even for 15 minutes.

✳ Bend and rotate your arms backwards like you're doing a chicken dance, when you can. Also put your feet up when you can and, if you can't, flex them back and forth. Both of these will keep your muscles flexible and help your circulation.

✳ Don't hunch over your stomach. Sit backwards on a chair, with a pillow between you and the back and your legs to each side, or sit on a giant inflatable ball, which you can buy from physio supplies shops.

✳ If you have to pick something up, use the lunge position (bend at the knee, one leg in front, keeping your back straight).

If you vacuum, hold the cord behind your back with one hand, which automatically keeps your back straight. When you're at the sink, stand on one leg and put the other foot on the shelf under the sink, as long as the shelf is low enough for you to feel comfortable. Anthea says what are we thinking of, we should all hire a housekeeper. (I suggest we could dress her in a long, black frock and call her Mrs Danvers.)

✳ A diagram of a uterus looks like a bagpipe with a tent rope on it.

✳ Being fit may not ensure an easy labour, but it will mean a better labour and recovery than you would have had if you were unfit.

✳ Don't go into spas and saunas. Their temperature can be raised to levels harmful for the foetus without you realising.

✳ Don't get really hot and then jump in a cold pool, or otherwise shock your system with sudden temperature changes.

✳ Because the relaxin hormone goes into overdrive during pregnancy and slackens all the ligaments, joints and muscles, don't overstretch or bounce on stretches.

I think this is more to do with the stage I've reached of pregnancy than my heroic efforts on the gym mats, but I suddenly seem to be sleeping a lot better and floating through the days. If I didn't know better I'd say I was on drugs.

Another thing I have started noticing: people who warn you against unsolicited advice already have their own. 'Don't listen to any busybodies,' they say. 'What you'll need to do is . . . '

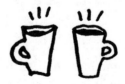

info

repelling unwanted advice and comments

When people give you that firm advice – 'You must have a nanny', 'You must always look after the baby yourself', 'Men can't look after babies', 'You must use cloth nappies' – remember it's about them, not you. They're usually just telling you what THEY did and insisting that you do the same, maybe partly because that's all they know and partly because if you do it the same way it will make them feel better. Your experience will be different from everybody else's. Listen, but don't automatically follow their advice.

The advice thing starts as soon as you tell people you're pregnant, and continues throughout parenting life. Having babies is such a universal experience that everyone has opinions to share, whether you want to hear them or not.

You'll hear things about whether you can tell if you're having a girl or boy based on how sick you are, how much your baby moves or what shape your tummy is; why you should insist on seeing an obstetrician or listen only to midwives; why you should/ shouldn't use pain-relief drugs during childbirth; how to avoid an episiotomy/caesarean/cracked nipples; why you must/mustn't breastfeed; why you should always use/never bother with cloth nappies; how you make your baby sleep through the night (pick it up/ignore it/give it a stiff gin); how to avoid nappy rash; why you must go straight back/never go back to work; what sort of child care is best; what sort of schooling is best; what to do when your child is arrested in its mid-30s. The list seems infinite.

Some advice will be useful and compatible with your own ideas, and some won't. Read books where you feel in tune with the basic philosophy, and choose a couple of friends to listen to. In the end you'll find that having to deal with your own, real baby will provide the best information.

Another mind-boggling thing is that people want to touch your tummy, and sometimes they don't even ask if it's okay. This

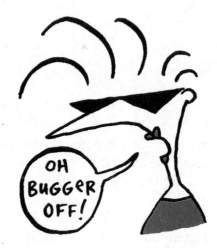

is easier to cope with than the advice. You can say, 'I'd rather you didn't', or grab hands that are heading towards your belly.

at work or parties

Sometimes people, even in a meeting at work, will bang on about anything to do with pregnancy, including cervical mucus, in front of anyone at all. (Make sure this isn't you.) You can learn to get out of these mortifying situations by saying pleasantly and firmly, 'Let's stick to the agenda, shall we?' Even if it's a lie, you can always try, 'Oh, I've got a rule – no pregnancy talk at work/parties/whatever', then gently disengage and move away. You can go to the loo and come back if you think someone will have changed the subject in the meantime.

strangers

Advice can be worse in your first pregnancy because people assume you want their opinion, and you have no ammunition to defend yourself against it. You can give strangers a distant smile and no verbal response. A lot of pregnancy/baby chitchat when you're out and about is from people who are just looking to pass the time of day or strike up a conversation. These ones are easily dealt with: 'Gosh, is that the time? Must fly.'

friends

Advice from friends is usually offered with good intentions, and they can give you some invaluable insights and shortcuts. Store away anything that seems useful and ignore anything you don't like the sound of. Alternatively, you can always tell friends you'll come to them if you have any questions, or that you're sick of everybody giving you advice and could they please shut right up before you slap them.

the older generation

Take with a grain of salt any of the pregnancy and baby-care advice from parents or parents-in-law, which is likely to have a long-expired use-by date. It's worth having a tactful chat early on about how you see their role in relation to the baby. Without putting too fine a point on it, they need to understand that as far as the baby goes, you're the boss.

Unfortunately, some members of the older generation, including grandparents, may have fixed ideas about how things should be done (the way they did them). Here are some of the outdated notions you may have to firmly explain are not acceptable.

BEFORE THE BABY ARRIVES

'Eat lots of lamb's liver.' (No. Too much vitamin A can damage the foetus.)

'Morning sickness is a myth.' (It isn't.)

'You should try to hide your bump.' (Oh for God's sake!)

AFTER THE BABY ARRIVES

'Breastfeeding/bottle-feeding is bad for your baby.' (It's your choice.)

'There's no need to use a baby seat in the car for every trip, particularly short ones.' (This is potentially lethal and is just not on.)

'Put the baby to sleep on its tummy.' (This is a dangerous – and a possible cause of sudden infant death syndrome, SIDS. See p.371.)

'Throwing the baby into the air is perfectly okay.' (No, this can be as damaging to the brain and eyes as shaking a baby.)

'Put honey on a dummy.' (It rots teeth and can create a 'sweet' dependency.)

'Hitting, smacking and threats of violence teaches kids a bit of respect.' (They are more likely to teach the child to hit other children and creatures smaller than they are.)

'That child is being "bad".' (This targets the child, not the behaviour.)

'Of course dropping around without ringing to check if it's convenient is all right.' (Aaaargghhhh!)

'Give small children lollies and sugared soft drinks as a treat or a reward. And milk or juice in their night-time bottles is fine.' (All these are a major cause of children having to have all their first teeth removed under anaesthetic.)

'Always leave a baby to cry/never leave a baby to cry even for 30 seconds.' (Both of these are extreme.)

'Insist on a sleep routine/refuse to follow a sleep routine.' (Whatever works for you and your baby is fine. But you might want to check some of the books recommended in 'Week 43'.)

Grandparents might say, 'But we did this with you and you turned out fine.' Rather than replying, 'Well, that was bloody lucky then, wasn't it?', try saying, in the case of safety issues, 'You did the right thing then, but they've done all this new research and the right thing to do now is . . .' When all else fails, just say, 'I really need it to be done this way.' On the subject of safety, if a friend or relative is likely to ignore your wishes, it's best for you to be there whenever they have access to the baby or your children.

solicited advice

Advice from experts and pregnancy books is often conflicting, which can be confusing. And you only need to experience the different midwife shifts at a hospital when you're learning how to breastfeed to find out just how varied even professional opinion can be. It can be tricky to filter it, and – as always – you need to assess the individual you're dealing with, whether it be a physiotherapist conducting an antenatal class or a breastfeeding consultant or a paediatrician after the baby's born.

Find women who you relate to who are pregnant, or who have had children, especially recently. Ask them anything you need to know, and they'll tell you their experiences. But bear in mind you're just researching – your experiences will not be exactly the same, though you may get pointed in a few directions. New mums will have a few hints about settling babies or the best nappies, that kind of useful stuff. Mums whose kids are older have usually forgotten the details.

your record

✳ Write down all the unsolicited and solicited advice, useful and useless you get.

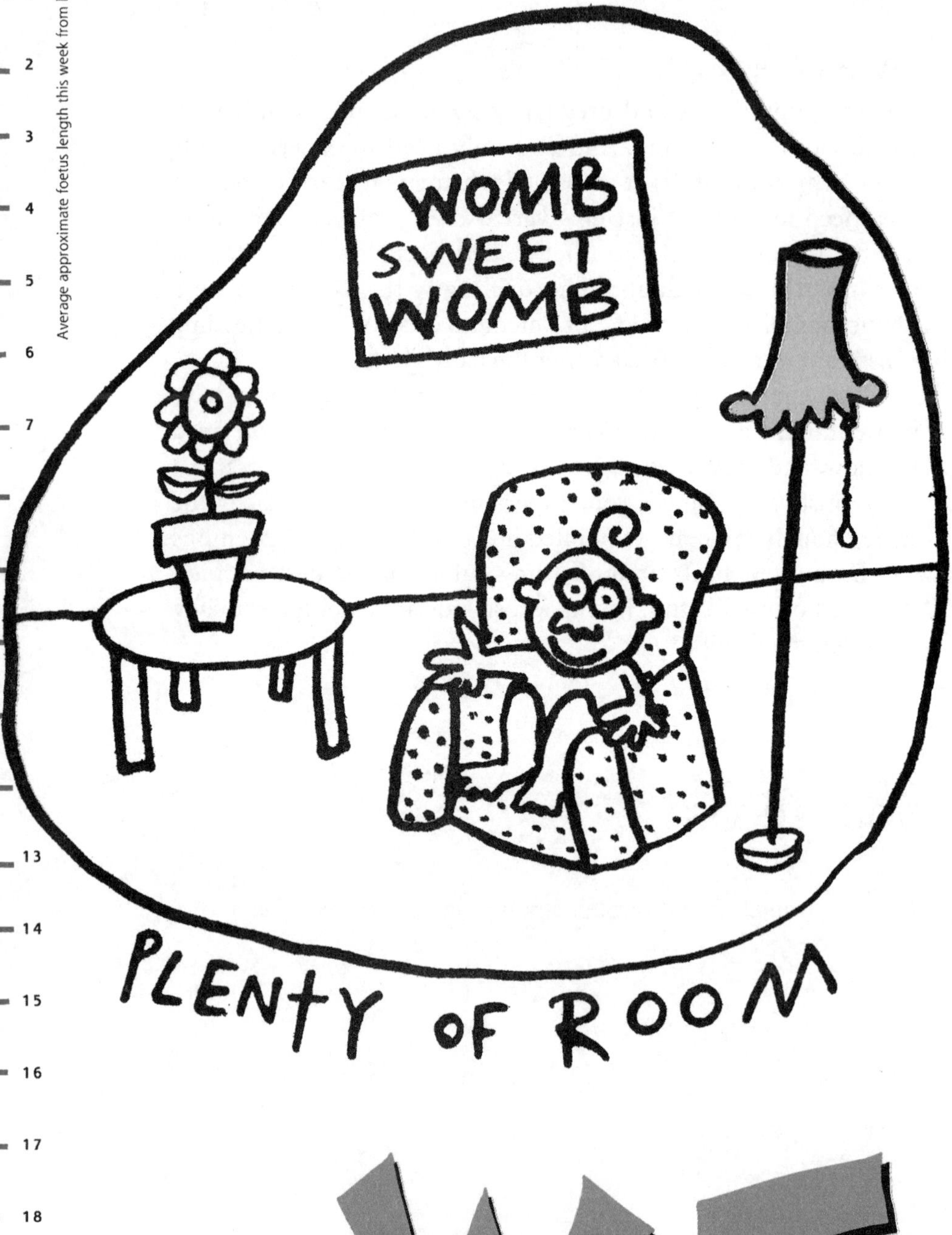

what's going on

Your waistline is missing, presumed obliterated. You may have backache, skin pigment changes, and a tendency to vague . . . somethingorother. The foetus still has plenty of room to move around in the amniotic sac, but it's a tighter fit than, say, a pear in a bucket of water – that's why, if you haven't already, you will feel movements any time from now on. Its muscles have developed enough for the foetus to be doing loop-the-loops, swinging around with its umbilical cord. The foetus is putting on brown-coloured fat deposits, which produce heat to keep it warm.

Weight: about 260 grams (9oz).

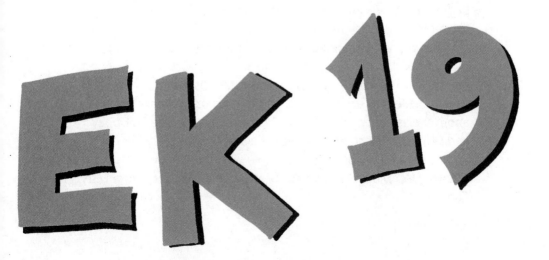

EK 19

DiARY

I have been reading Sheila Kitzinger. She abandons comparing the foetus to fruit for a moment to solemnly declare, 'You may notice that you are putting on weight on your buttocks'. Actually I've been noticing that for the last nineteen weeks, sunshine. If they're going to get any bigger, people will start to think I'm shoplifting a futon.

The finance experts in magazines and on the radio all suggest that when you stop using contraception you should start saving for all the stuff you're going to need, especially because one person is probably going to drop an income for a while. Accordingly, we are spending money like it's the last day on earth.

I have £82 left in the bank. We've got security screens, we've got built-in wardrobes coming, we've got trees going into the garden. We've got new maternity clothes. For some reason I'm in a demented frenzy and keep wanting to buy towels even though we've got enough. Must be some innate memory of all those films where the baby comes early and some gnarled old trusty shouts, 'Boil some towels and splice the mainsail!' Or perhaps I'm thinking of pirate movies.

Back, legs and neck all painful. Get hysterical. Ring the chiropractor at home. Make an appointment for the next afternoon, so of course by the next morning after a reasonable sleep (only four or five wees during the night!) most of the symptoms are gone.

Rush from the chiropractor to the midwife for my regular check-up. I can't wait to listen to the heartbeat again. I am beginning to get quite worried because I can't feel the baby move like all the books say I should by now. Maybe Cellsie's gone out.

Thankfully there are no infuriating mothers in the waiting room. I hand in my wee sample and sit on my own, remembering my weekend of feeling weepy, hideous, fat, disgusting, spotty and vilely repellent in every degree, and getting really freaked out about the sea of cellulite. So far I've been Sneezy, Sleepy, Dopey and Grumpy. I'm hoping for the full complement of the Seven Dwarfs before the confinement. There wasn't a Weepy, sadly. Or a Crappy. Or a Dippy. Spotty never got a look in. Or, indeed, a Fatty. Can't think why.

Try this out on the midwife (it's Niki this week), who says I could be Happy. Then she tells me somebody has already made the Seven Dwarfs joke in a book she can't remember the name of. Great. So now I'm Plagiary as well.

I tell Niki about my anxiety at not feeling Cellsie move, even though I've nearly reached 20 weeks: 'All the books say you should have felt the baby move by now.' Niki's opinion on the matter, basically, is bugger the books (except that Niki probably never says bugger), I'll feel it soon enough.

I realise that I don't know whether you keep feeling the baby once you've felt it for the first time or if you have to wait another week. Niki says once you feel it you feel it every day. She puts the little instrument on my stomach and it amplifies the baby's heartbeat. It makes me grin.

'It sounds groovy,' I say. 'Kind of swishy.'

'I always think it sounds like Rolf Harris,' she says. 'That wobble board thing. Anything else worrying you?'

'Yes. I am 78 kilos.'

'That's okay.'

'Am I putting on too much weight?'

'No, and you can't diet.'

'Yes, I know. I was just wondering whether I should hire a wheelbarrow to get around in.'

Quite often in the street I suddenly find myself rubbing my stomach in the unselfconscious way men scratch their scrotum or stick their hand up between their buttocks to arrest some jockettes making a bold upward bid for freedom. And I don't care who sees me. My stomach sticks way out in front and people ask, 'When are you due?', and I say, 'August', and they look at me as if I've got a rhino up my frock. Their next question is usually 'Is it twins?'

If it wasn't for the phone, I'd never talk to anyone. All my childless friends are flat out at work (so am I) and the ones with kids are worse. I never go out at night any more, and when I do I leave parties at about 10pm, stone-cold sober, wishing people wouldn't smoke. Francine the beauty therapist was right. My life really is over . . .

info

maternity clothes hints

⑥ Always remember: this is a TEMPORARY wardrobe. Don't spend a fortune unless you're a diamond heiress. Design and maternity clothes just don't seem to be words that go together. Can you recall any shop you ever bought clothes in before you were pregnant with a maternity wear section? Thought not. You really have to make the most of an indifferent lot.

⑥ Borrow everything you can from a previously pregnant friend, but only things you know you'll wear. Don't clutter up your drawers with stuff that doesn't fit or you would never wear. Write down who has lent you what – with the label and description recorded – so you can give it all back. (Some friends will just say you can pass it on down the line.)

⑥ Don't borrow anything really flash if the person you're borrowing from wants it back. You never know what's going to happen to it, and you probably won't be able to replace it.

⑥ Check out the racks in the following sections: sports, dance wear, men's, and full-figured women's clothes. Bear in mind that in the last month or two of pregnancy just 'big' may not do it. You'll probably need at least a couple of items that have the properly designed stomach bits you only get in maternity clothes.

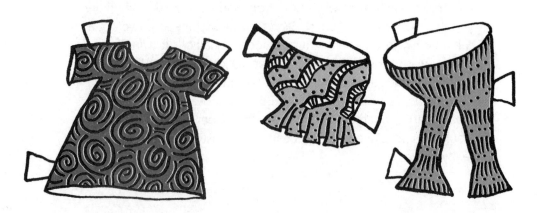

⑥ Don't worry if your maternity wardrobe is all black, or all navy, or all incredibly boring in some way or other. At least everything will match. You'll be so sick of the sight of everything by the time you give birth, anyway, that it doesn't matter.

⑥ The maternity fashion police will tell you not to wear overalls or stirrup pants because they are unflattering. May I just say that from about the thirty-second week of the pregnancy, you might as well be wearing an armoured tank: nothing is flattering.

⑥ To cut down on searching every morning, look through your wardrobe ONCE, now. Put all the possible maternity clothes up one end of the wardrobe and clear a drawer for the non-hanging possible clothes and maternity undies and bras. As each item of normal clothing outlives its usefulness, put it in the normal-person part of the wardrobe or chest of drawers.

⑥ Work out what the weather will be like in the last four months or so of the pregnancy and plan accordingly.

winter

See if any of your friends have a suitable, A-line shaped overcoat that you can borrow to get you through. If you're going to need to wear huge socks, you're probably going to have to buy a pair of gigantic shoes for the duration. A basic winter maternity wardrobe could include:

1 frock for best
1 skirt
2 pairs black trousers
4 pairs opaque black tights
gigantic jumper
maternity jeans
2 maternity-sized bras – maybe one pale and one black
gigantic cotton underpants

summer

Forget that polyester was ever invented. Go for cotton, or microfibre or a rayon if it's the cool, floaty kind. Corner a big bloke and confiscate all his T-shirts and shirts. A basic summer maternity wardrobe could include:

1 frock for best
1–2 everyday gigantic frocks
large T-shirts
large 'men's' shirts
2 maternity-sized bras – maybe one pale and one black
loose maternity trousers
gigantic cotton underpants
shawl, wrap or giant jumper for cold evenings:
use a horse blanket if necessary

undies

◎ The most important word on undies is cotton.

◎ Undies can either be worn under the belly, if you like a bikini style; or if you find up-to-the-waist styles more comfortable, you can probably just buy bigger sizes of your favourite brand – if or when these become tragically inadequate, you may need to invest in maternity knickers.

◎ Women who have bad backs, are overweight, or are carrying twins, may be advised to wear a maternity girdle to give some extra support late in the pregnancy. These can be supplied by the local obstetric physiotherapist (at your local hospital) and you can be referred by your GP or midwife. Maternity girdles should not be designed to make your stomach look smaller.

◎ Real tights usually just don't fit at all as you progress in size. But why doesn't anyone make matt-black opaque maternity tights that don't fall down so you don't get that sagging gusset thing happening? Until they do, you could take a tip from Superman and wear your underpants OVER your tights to keep them up.

shoes

Yes, your feet are getting bigger – firstly, they're probably puffed up with extra fluid (and if you go on a plane they puff up like balloons), and secondly, they're probably broader because of all that extra weight you're carrying. The ligaments in your feet are softer and stretchier than usual, so your feet will 'spread' and well-fitting, comfortable shoes are essential.

⑥ Your feet may end up flatter and one size bigger permanently. You may want to wait and see before buying lots of hideously expensive new shoes.

⑥ If you wear socks, buy thin ones or stocking socks.

⑥ Buy a new, larger, all-purpose, flat-heeled pair of shoes to 'live in' for the duration – many very pregnant women wear sports shoes. Or pop a couple of canoes on your feet.

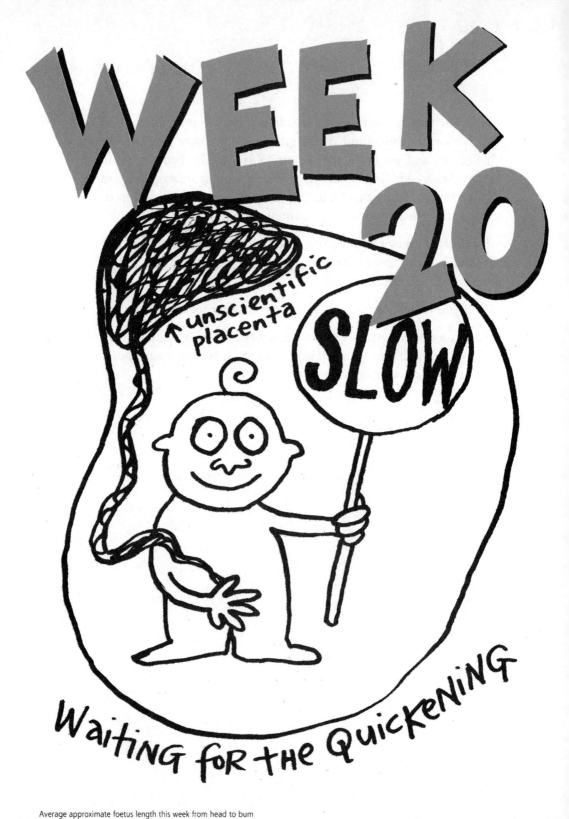

Average approximate foetus length this week from head to bum

cm 1 2 3 4 5 6 7 8 9 10 11 12 13 14

what's going on Probably by now you will have felt the baby move, but maybe not. It's usual to laugh or cry. Doing both at once is perfectly fine. It might still be too early for anyone else to be able to feel the movements from the outside. For a while, it's your little secret bond.

The foetus puts on more muscle and tests it out by moving around. One book says your baby is as heavy as 'a medium-sized Spanish onion' (do let me know if you find a Spanish onion weighing 320 grams). The skin's sebaceous glands (needed, of course, to make pimples later) become active and make the oily stuff called vernix caseosa that covers the skin. It's the foetus's do-it-yourself wetsuit made, disgustingly enough, of fatty material and dead skin cells. (If that doesn't make you feel sick, how's this: doctors say the coating looks like cheese.) Vernix caseosa waterproofs the skin against the amniotic fluid, and protects the foetus from scrapes when it bangs into the wall of the uterus.

Weight: about 320 grams (11^{1}/$_{4}$ oz).

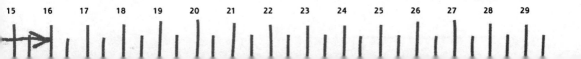

15   16   17   18   19   20   21   22   23   24   25   26   27   28   29

DiARY I'm not depressed any more but I still haven't bloody well felt the baby move and it makes me really anxious. I feel very cheated about it not kicking and really cross with the books for making me feel like a freak because I haven't felt 'the quickening'.

Beck says, 'You have felt the baby move, but you just don't know you have. You probably thought you were going to fart or something.' How romantic.

We go out to dinner and I have two glasses of very nice champagne (I seem to have lost the all-alcohol-tastes-like-meths sensation) and am so sloshed I sleep for 11 hours and only go to the toilet four or five times. Remarkable.

Feeling suddenly bigger and paradoxically less fat. Probably because it all seems like it's out the front there, now. I really feel like I'm carrying weight, though – when I try to run, this galumphing, hilarious big tummy precedes me like a cartoon beer belly. Geoff says soothing, private things like, 'You are *not* a fat old baggage. You are the Tummy Princess.'

Suddenly feel connected to other mothers a bit – certainly more than I ever have before. Not all mothers. Well, obviously. Not Pamela Anderson Lee or the Queen or anything.

I saw Peter X in the street today. Nothing like the wildly startled look of an old boyfriend who's about to say, 'Hi, you look well', and then has to restrain himself from fainting as he realises you're pregnant and he doesn't know what to say. His eyes rolled around in his head like the old master in Kung-Fu – lots of white. Poor thing. I suspect that just for a split second he thought it might have had something to do with him – until he came to his senses and realised that six years' gestation is probably pushing it.

Yesterday I paid for all my literal slackness in not doing my pelvic-floor exercises. I sneezed and wet myself. Not a huge gush, but enough to make a tiny splash on the floor. Luckily I was standing on the wooden floor at home.

When I sneezed Geoff said, 'You look absolutely mortified.'

'Well, I just wee-ed,' I explained helpfully.

Geoff's old friend Luke and his wife, Sita, call to offer a pram. Excellent. Uncle Mike insists that he will buy us an eco-friendly cot, which is nice (secondhand cots can be both grotty and kitsch) but a mixed blessing. He will no doubt complain forever about how much it cost and express the view that the baby should be sleeping in a hammock in the open air.

My friend Susanne's getting on in her pregnancy now. She just rang to say she was in the shoe shop and a woman told her she had good posture. Susanne, completely vague and stuffed full of pregnancy info, meant to tell the shop assistant that's because when she walks she 'leads with her sternum', the breastbone. Unfortunately what she actually said was she 'leads with her perineum', which is the area between the vagina and the anus. No wonder the shop assistant looked startled.

Susanne's not putting on enough weight and I've got plenty extra. We're considering a transference.

info

weight gain

Weight gain is an important part of a healthy pregnancy. You'll find pregnancy 'experts' are all over the shop when it comes to saying how much weight you should gain. The right weight gain for you is different from the right one for somebody else (you know, depending on your height, weight and body frame when you became pregnant, and whether you give a stuff about it). The ranges nominated for a one-baby pregnancy vary from 12 kilograms to 16 kilogrammes (26–35lb). Many slender women put on 20–30 kilos (44-66lb) during pregnancy and then lose it again afterwards.

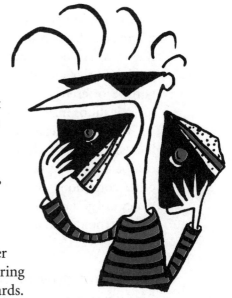

About a third of the weight gain is baby, placenta and amniotic fluid; the rest is new bits of you – increased blood volume, breast growth, fluid and fat. The body needs to build up stores of fat during pregnancy, which is then used in breastfeeding. The weight you gain will probably go something like this:

baby, placenta, amniotic fluid: 4.5 kilograms (10lb)
increased size of uterus: 1 kilo (2lb 3oz)
increased breast size: 0.5–1 kilo (1lb $1^1/2$ oz–2lb 3oz)
increased blood: 1 kilo (2lb 3oz)
retained fluid: 1 kilo (2lb 3oz)
increased fat and protein stores: 3 kilos (6lb 9oz).

Most of the weight gain is in the fourth to the seventh month of the pregnancy. At the birth you can lose up to 12 kilos ($26^1/2$lb) at once, and in the days following, the excess fluid will also be lost through sweat and urine.

You may be weighed every time you visit the midwife or obstetrician, and they may give you advice on diet if they think you are gaining too much. But these days you'll more likely encounter a tape measure. There is evidence to suggest that measuring the growth of the uterus rather than your weight gain is a more accurate estimate of foetal growth. The measure is stretched from your pubic bone to the top of the uterus. Either way if you're not gaining enough weight or if the uterus is not getting bigger and they are concerned about foetal growth, you will be offered an ultrasound scan to check this and further investigations may be made.

Your obstetrician or midwife will be on the alert for any rapid increase in weight during the last ten weeks of pregnancy, which can be a sign of pre-eclampsia (see the info in 'Week 31'). Some other conditions associated with too much weight gain in pregnancy are gestational diabetes, high blood pressure, varicose veins, haemorrhoids and uncontrollable Magnum addictions.

more info on weight gain
See Eating and Supplements in 'Week 2' and Exercise in 'Week 15'.

your record

✳ You might like to create a time capsule for your child with a few snippets of your life before they arrived. It's a bit of a boy thing, but how about knocking out a few lists for posterity: best ever books and movies, the clothes you were into when you could get into them, a record of the mates you see most of (closest mates can change alarmingly after a child). Maybe even throw in a few world events. Like Palace's first away win of the season, says Geoff.

WEEK 21

what's going on

You could start to get heartburn and indigestion. Get used to people judging your size – 'You don't seem very big' or 'Oh my God!' – sometimes on the same day. However, you will probably have a second (for some women, third) routine ultrasound scan at around this time, which should be both reassuring and amazing.

The foetal eyelids are still fused closed (until week 27), but the foetus can hear sounds from within and outside your body. The brain has been developing very quickly, but its surface is still very smooth, not like the textbook pictures of adult brains we're used to.

Weight: about 390 grams (13^1/$_2$ oz).

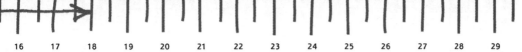

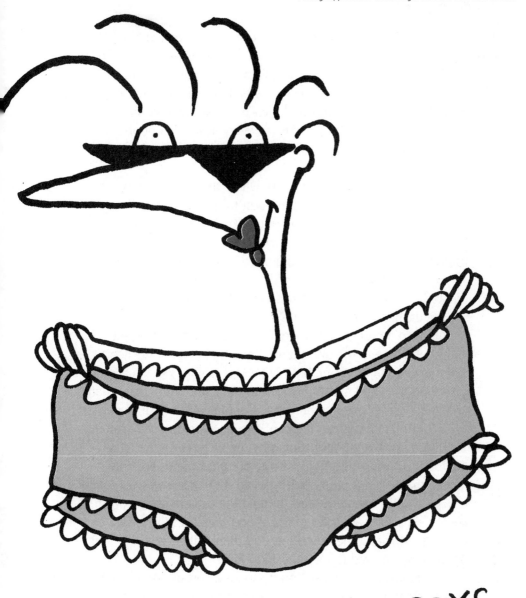

You CouLd catCH StiNGRaYS iN MY UNDeRPaNTS

DiARY

I have new moles and skin tags everywhere. It's like my skin is hyperactive and throwing out extra bits wherever it can. Basically, I'm getting extra tags and moles in every area I already have them, plus a whole new bunch of tags under each breast. My hair also appears to be attempting an Afro at every available opportunity. It seems to be growing faster and getting thicker, but perhaps this is an optical illusion.

My tummy's sticking out about where the rest of the world used to be, so when I squeeze through to get out of the lift at work and automatically calculate I've got a 10-centimetre clearance I actually rub myself against someone, who starts to look very frightened at the idea of being groped by a pregnant woman.

But work is not a big item on my agenda this week, for I'm due to have my '20 weeks' ultrasound. I'm actually closer to 21 weeks but, hey, who's counting?

Jill, who'll probably be a godmother without the God bit, and Geoff come to the ultrasound. I'm a bit nervy. In my heart I feel that everything is fine but my head is saying, well, things do go wrong. Maybe I have more of Aunt Julie about me than I had imagined, some little microprocessor implanted to flash signals at me: 'TERRIBLE things can happen'. Maybe everyone gets scared.

It all turns out all right. Going by the pictures on the screen the foetus is twenty weeks four days, but ultrasounds are only 'guesstimates'. Jill is pretty gobsmacked. I think she was expecting it to be a fairly static side view. Instead the camera goes in from all angles – top of head, soles of feet – and measures the length of the thighbone and the arm bone, and thankfully everything's all right and connected to the other right bits.

The foetus face still looks pretty spooky, sort of like a skeleton face, while the shot of the spine makes our little darling look like the remains of a mackerel on a dinner plate. It's hard not to think it's really waving or having a chat or playing peekaboo when really all it's doing is instinctively having a rowdy time, practising grabbing, sucking and Morris dancing. The ultrasound operator takes quite some time and is very thorough, checking the four valves of the heart, measuring a whole lot of circumferences and lengths and widths. He speaks very quietly to his assistant, who types it all into a computer. But he says reassuring things to us, too, at intervals, pointing out the features like a tour-leader on a trip around Rome.

The scan left me feeling happier and more relaxed than I can remember, though more quiet-reflective than punching the air. Nonetheless, it left me confident enough to agree on a shopping trip for baby clothes with Aunt Julie, and even she seemed affected when I showed her the little polaroid snap they gave us. No horror stories were brought up, although she did tell me encouragingly and at some length that ALL first babies cry CONSTANTLY and wriggle all the time and drive their parents mad.

On our round of the department stores, I queue behind a woman with a small child and say 'Hello' in exactly the same tone Aunt Julie uses. Reel back in horror and hope I won't automatically start trying to feed small children grey mince on rice and boiled chops four nights a week. A few minutes later say 'boo' to another strange child just as if I am channelling Aunt Julie, who is at that moment looking at a pink floral suit and saying, 'This is lovely, dear, unless it's a boy.' (She is very worried about cross-dressing babies.) The child seems to take it rather well and in the jaunty manner it was intended.

Shopping for baby clothes is actually just like being size 16 in a shop for grown-up women where all the sizes are 8 and 10. Everything's teeny tiny. Except there are slightly more snap fasteners at crotch level than usual. When shopping for myself I can still go into a shop and say, 'Yes, I'll have one of those in size ginormous, thank you.' If they have them. At this stage you could catch carp in my knickers.

Anyway, back to baby gear. Some kids' clothes are £30 a throw, even £60 a throw, for something that they must grow out of in a nanosecond. I'm thinking I might just coat my child in Vaseline to keep it warm. There are T-shirts and romper suit things you can buy with 'Baby' written on the front – you know, in case you think you've given birth to a ferret, or you get confused and start dressing your bedside lamp. 'No, that's right, tea-cosy on the teapot, T-shirt on the BABY.'

And there are these hair bands with flowers on that go around a baby's head, and basically they're used on a baldy baby to indicate that it's a girl. Oh, say it loud and say it proud: 'The kid's bald.'

People keep asking me if it's going to be a boy or a girl and I say, 'Yes, I believe so. So I've been led to understand. But we're not fussy. We're just hoping for a life form of some description.' They say, 'Well, you should find out so you know what kind of clothes to buy for the baby.' I'm like: is it going to matter? Is somebody going to accuse a 4-month-old child of cross-dressing? 'You perverted infant, you're dressing like Julian Clary – get a hold of yourself!!'

And sometimes people ask, 'What are you hoping for?' to which I confess I have said, on two occasions, 'A giraffe. They're up running around the paddock an hour or so after birth and starting to feed themselves.' I'm yet to get a laugh on that one.

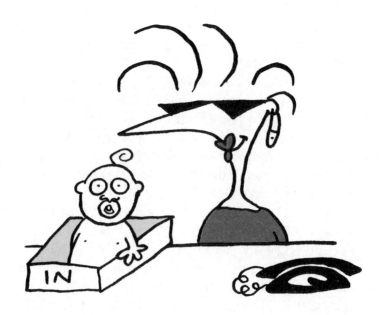

info

at work

In a healthy pregnancy and a healthy workplace there is no reason why you shouldn't keep working for as long as you want to and your doctor and midwife agree, especially as the money will come in handy pretty soon. How close to your due date you work will depend on how you feel.

Most women value some time alone before they begin the horror! the horror!... oops.... the extremely rewarding and divinely bondworthy, magnificent experience of childbirth and caring for a newborn baby. It's common to take maternity leave for at least the last four to six weeks of the pregnancy, and longer if you can afford it. You'll probably feel really tired and uncomfortable in the last few weeks. Resting well, exercising gently, eating right and thinking serene thoughts during the last weeks of the pregnancy certainly won't hurt.

On the other hand, if your body doesn't really function unless you're having six meetings a day and dealing with 42 emails, then keep going in. The only real rule is that you do have to stop work when your labour begins. Well, maybe not the really early stages.

It depends enormously, of course, on your job. If you have to do a lot of standing up, working in the last few weeks can get really difficult. Even a desk job can become hard. You might just want to lie on the couch and read magazines or watch videos. From week 32 your heart, lungs and other vital organs are work- ing really hard and getting more and more squished up by the growing uterus. The strain on your back, joints and muscles is increasingly intense, and you might be vaguing out a lot. Not to mention that by week 36 that baby head bouncing on your cervix can make you jump around and swear – not always good during a meeting.

Some doctors recommend that if your job has you on your feet more than four hours a day, you should stop work by week 24, and that if you need to stand half an hour of each working hour you ought to stop work by week 32.

Other work conditions that should be discussed with your doctor are possible exposure to teratogens – substances or environmental factors that could harm your baby (see the info in Looking after your embryo in 'Week 4') – work that involves lots of lifting, carrying or bending, or shift work, which can upset sleep and eating patterns.

Being pregnant at work should probably be dealt with like any other personal issue: don't blab everything to everybody, especially gossipy people and ones who couldn't care less and drop off for a nap at the first sign of the word 'trimester'. This will also allow you to feel more professional for the time you are there and when you come back.

Regardless of what the law requires of them, managers can vary dramatically in how they view the whole deal of pregnancy and maternity leave. Bosses in some large companies have done cost-benefit research and realised it's cheaper and smarter to give valued employees leave, then welcome them back with flexible working hours, than drive them out and start training new people (who may also get pregnant). Other bosses try to sack you as soon as they find out: this is illegal.

If you want to have flexible working hours when you return to work you should be able to sit down with your employer and put your case forward. They have to seriously consider your request and it would be considered unjustified by the Employment Tribunal to refuse.

While you're at work, busy trying to be your same old reliable, efficient self, you might really be feeling very different, hiding how you feel and worrying that you might overlook something important.

Here are some suggestions that might help.

ⓖ Keep a stash of healthy snacks at work, which are useful for keeping your blood sugar up and nausea at bay during the first trimester, and for general nutrition the rest of the time.

⑥ Make yourself comfortable. Put your feet up when you can. Sit rather than stand. Practise squatting for labour during private moments. Have regular walks and stretches if you're bent over a desk for much of the day. Drink plenty of water. If you feel really tired, use your lunch hour to sleep in a spare office, organising to have someone wake you up at the end of the break. If you do this, don't forget to make time to eat.

⑥ Take it as easy as you can. Ask for some time working at home if you can.

⑥ If work is stressful, try yoga or meditation classes and learn some good relaxation techniques.

⑥ Keep the best work diary you could imagine and religiously consult it every morning. Make lists. Invest in Post-it notes for reminders. Get colour-coded folders. Get other staff pals or an assistant to remind you of things, including 'Go and have lunch'.

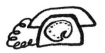 If you think you're being discriminated against, check your rights with your union, or see a lawyer or government department dealing with employment. Many of your rights are protected by the Sex Discrimination Act but you must act quickly to take your case to the Employment Tribunal as disputes usually have a time frame within which they will consider a request.

your record

✳ Is being pregnant affecting your work? If so, how?
✳ Describe your job or what you do all day.
(Your child will be interested to know eventually.)

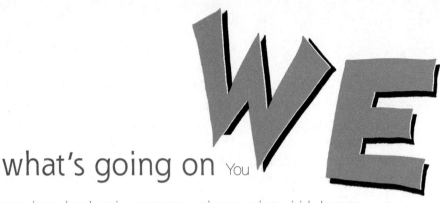

what's going on

You may have back pain, cramps, varicose veins, vivid dreams, and feel strangely calm. You also put on the most weight in the second trimester. But of all the weight you put on, a relatively small proportion is the weight of the actual baby. The rest is stuff you need such as blood, amniotic fluid, larger bosoms, necessary fat stores and, um, cheesecake.

Downstairs there may well be some exhibition somersaulting going on. The inner ear has reached adult size. There are now eyebrows and head hair (unless you've got a baldy baby). The lungs are starting to produce stuff called surfactant, a detergentlike substance that will help them to function properly by keeping them expanded after a breath. Weight: about 460 grams (1lb).

Average approximate foetus length this week from head to bum

| cm | 1 | 2 | 3 | 4 | 5 | 6 | 7 | 8 | 9 | 10 | 11 | 12 | 13 | 14 |

fig (a) doing pelvic-
floor exercises

fig (b) not doing pelvic-
floor exercises

DiARY My horoscope this week says: 'Dating is invested with potential. Those who are pair-bonded ought to beware sudden attractions to deeply inappropriate types.' In my case, I presume, this would mean . . . anybody else in the entire universe.

Geoff talks to all the men at work about weird things their wives do when pregnant. I don't have enough people to talk to about this stuff. Most of my friends who aren't childless have forgotten what it's like to be pregnant. Even my lesbian friends who want to have kids haven't got around to working out how yet. We are about to leave the baby-free zone.

I've been organising a nappy-wash service for Susanne for when she gets out of hospital with the new baby. I've been sending out a form letter to all our friends.

Dear Friends

As you may have noticed, Susanne Anderson is about to have a baby any minute now. Possibly at this very moment. What you may not know is that newborn babies need their nappies changed up to sixty times a week.

Yes.

Horrible, isn't it?

To help deal with this rather confronting fact, we have organised Susanne a gift account at Eco-Nappy – which will deliver clean nappies (and take away the other kind), as soon as she gets home from hospital. (She has expressed a firm wish to receive a gift of nappies rather than flowers, which will only make her sneeze.)

You might like to contribute a week's worth of nappies (£16.50) yourself or as part of a cartel. Please fill in the enclosed coupon, add a cheque and send it straight to Eco-Nappy. Susanne's account number is 62240. Don't forget to add your name to the coupon so Susanne will receive a card with your name on it.

Love, Kaz.

I am prostrate with exhaustion and self-admiration after such efficiency. Then I realise I forgot to put stamps on the letters.

This not-feeling-the-baby-move business is getting embarrassing. Beck, with absolutely no tact in sight, tells me I'm a 'bit remedial'. She assures me again that I have felt the baby move but haven't realised it, and tells the story of a large woman who came into casualty when Beck was a nurse.

The woman was complaining of terrible, sudden, intermittent abdominal pains. (You know what's coming, don't you? Well, she didn't.) The ambulancemen told the nursing staff the pains were coming at regular intervals and were probably labour contractions, although the woman kept saying she wasn't pregnant. Beck said to her, 'But haven't you felt the baby move?' 'It's just wind,' the woman said, shortly before being joined by her offspring, whom she regarded with some astonishment.

I've popped into Beck's clinic, after another visit to the chiropractor, to see if I'm in early labour or just constipated. What a glamorous job she has.

'I'm not giving you a laxative without feeling what's going on,' she says. 'Otherwise you might be having a baby instead of a poo.'

Charming.

Speaking of wind, am nearly crippled by it on a jaunt along Oxford Street, shopping for baby gear this afternoon, and have to walk around bent in half and rubbing my stomach. People look rather concerned but I can hardly announce: 'It's all right, move along, I think I just need to do an enormous FART.'

Once again some of the baby clothes have Paris couturier prices, and although I am careful I end up spending £85 on small hats, vests, cotton jumpsuity things and oh, all right, a couple of expensive cute things like a red denim jacket and matching leggings. Bought a few light blue items. Not because I think I'm having a boy but because that pale pink makes me feel queasy.

I think it's better if I stay out of babies' and children's wear departments. It will be cheaper, and I don't want to end up with a child resembling anything remotely like those demented-looking blond children with bowl haircuts you see in glossy kids' wear brochures, dressed in velvet frou-frou knickerbockers with matching bow ties, looking like their parents would have seizures if they got a speck of mud around the knees. I'm thinking of dressing Cellsie in a plastic mac from dawn till dusk and just hosing him or her down before bedtime.

info

skin

A whole lot of stuff happens to your skin when you're pregnant. Everything is working overtime, generally resulting in more oil, sweat and pigment (colouring) being produced. More blood is flowing closer to your skin, making it warmer; and increased oil gland secretions, giving skin a shinier appearance, add to the pregnancy 'glow'. Retained fluid can give the skin a fuller, smoother appearance than usual. Necessary fat stores mean more cellulite on buttocks and thighs for the duration.

MoLe fRENZy

glow

glow

glow

grow, grow, grow

It depends on the individual: although many women find their skin looks better than ever during pregnancy, some may be prone to pimples or acne, while others may find themselves with dry, scaly skin. Oestrogen slows down oil production, but progesterone promotes it – and they are both very active during pregnancy. Most skin changes, including some skin tags, are temporary, but some are permanent: you may end up with darker nipples forever; a few more moles and stretch marks will stay, but fade to be hardly noticeable unless you run around naked under fluorescent lights.

pigmentation changes

Pigmentation changes, also known as melanin or colour changes, are caused by increased production of melanocyte-stimulating hormone (MSH), which acts on the cells that affect the colour of your skin. These changes are usually more obvious on dark skin. The theory is that darker nipples make it easier for breastfeeding babies to find them. If you have fair skin and red hair the changes will probably be slight.

linea nigra

The dark line called the linea nigra, which divides your tummy into halves along the site of the stretching rectus muscle (from your navel down to your pubic hair), often appears by week 14, though sometimes not until weeks later. (The line is actually there before pregnancy – imaginatively and inaccurately called the linea alba, Latin for 'white line' – though it's not particularly noticeable on any skin colour.)

The area around and inside your navel can also become darker. So can existing freckles and moles; and the skin under the eyes and arms, between the thighs and of the genitals may also be noticeably darker during pregnancy. Some pregnancy experts say the vagina turns purple. But who's game to look? It doesn't matter what colour it is. (Tell a lie. Lime green would be a worry.) Oh, let's just take their word for it.

irregular patches

Irregular patches of slightly different-coloured skin might turn up on your face; these are called chloasma, or by doctors who used to watch 'Zorro', the 'mask of pregnancy'. The patches are dark in women with light skin and light in women with dark skin.

Folic acid deficiency is linked to too much colour change in the skin. Exposure to the sun will intensify changes such as the face patches. A hat and a 15+ sunscreen cream will protect you.

stretch marks

Stretch marks that look like thin pink, red or purplish lines on pale skin, and paler brown lines on dark skin, are the result of collagen fibres in the skin tearing and breaking. They can happen on breasts, tummy, thighs and bottom. (The same hormone that makes ligaments relax during pregnancy, relaxin, also decreases the amount of collagen in the skin fibres, making them more fragile.) After pregnancy, stretch marks gradually fade to silvery lines in the skin, usually barely noticeable.

You can't stop or heal stretch marks. They are caused by the skin being forced to stretch a lot and quite quickly, and they are generally worse in cases of rapid, excessive weight gain. How many you get and how quickly they fade will largely be determined by the skin and body type you inherited. Some skins have more elastin and collagen than others.

Gradual weight gain may help to minimise stretch marks, and a good diet that includes plenty of protein and vitamin C will help keep skin in a generally healthy condition. Many people swear by vitamin E cream, but there's no scientific research that proves it helps, and many women who use vitamin E cream still get stretch marks.

skin tags

Skin tags are little extra bits of skin that often develop in places where there is some friction, such as the bra line under your breasts, or under your arms. They are caused by small areas of skin getting overactive. Some women lose them a few months after birth, others get to keep them forever (dermatologists can remove them if you're bothered). Guess you'll just have to wait and see what happens to yours.

visible veins

Some people develop spider veins: threadlike, wiggly red lines, usually on the cheeks. They are small broken blood vessels caused by rapid dilation and constriction of the blood vessels when circulation increases during pregnancy. Blue lines under the skin, on the breasts and on the tummy just show some of the extra blood you're carrying. They will go away after the baby arrives. Bulging varicose veins in the legs can be painful. Your doctor or midwife can tell you how to avoid them (the regular advice being to put your feet up when you can and wear special 'support' tights). The veins may eventually disappear but in severe cases you may need to have them surgically removed.

rashes and spots

Heat rashes can be caused by the combination of increased circulation, body temperature, sweating and skin friction in pregnancy. Rashes might cause itchiness. It may help to dress in cotton clothes that allow good ventilation and to wash using a non-soap alternative or special oil (ask your pharmacist).

Red spots sometimes appear on the face, arms, torso, palms and soles of the feet. These too are caused by increased blood flow through dilated vessels, and go away after pregnancy.

Some medications for acne and psoriasis can be very dangerous to the developing foetus, so you should discuss alternative treatments with your doctor. On the bright side, conditions such as eczema and psoriasis often improve during pregnancy.

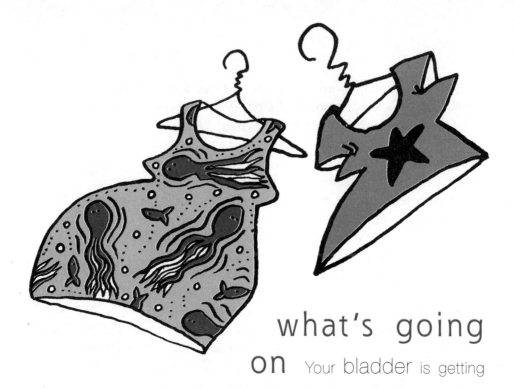

what's going

on Your bladder is getting squished up even more, so you may need to wee more often. You might feel practice labour contractions from now on, called Braxton Hicks (or they may not start for weeks, or you might not ever experience them).

WEEK

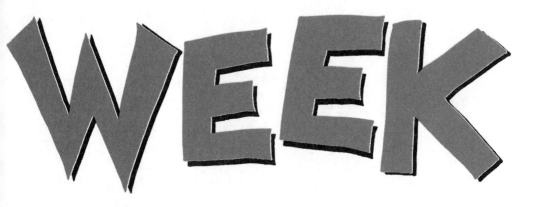

Average approximate foetus length this week from head to bum

| cm | 1 | 2 | 3 | 4 | 5 | 6 | 7 | 8 | 9 | 10 | 11 | 12 | 13 | 14 |

The foetus is growing like gangbusters, and the brain is maturing. Some researchers believe the foetus has started to think. Others, to be safer, say we can't really tell when this happens, and it may be much later. (And anyway, it's probably just stuff like 'I think I like to suck milky things' and 'La, la, la, whatever'.) The skin is growing very quickly, but there's not much fat yet developed for plumping up underneath it, so the bambino looks a bit pruney. Weight: about 540 grams (1lb 3oz).

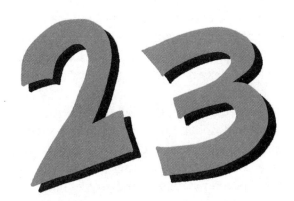

23

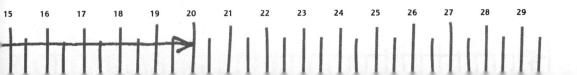

15 16 17 18 19 20 21 22 23 24 25 26 27 28 29

DiARY

Just ate entire giant bar of chocolate. Feel sick. This won't stop me from having lunch, mind you. By this stage I find I am in need of some even more simply enormous underpants – the kind of thing you could wave if you were surrendering. I find it somehow soothing not to think about the size of my bum. The only time I can get a sense of weightlessness is in the bath. I'd rather be swimming, even though it would resemble the opening sequence of *Free Willy*. But the public pools don't seem very appealing and I've let my healthclub membership lapse. Hey ho.

Susanne's baby has arrived. She's a very beautiful girl with gigantic feet and no name, but never mind that: Susanne did the whole labour as Warrior Woman without pain-killers! She went into hospital after several hours' denial that she was in labour, and had the baby within the hour. All went swimmingly, directed by an Asian trainee midwife under the strict supervision of her mentor. Susanne said it felt like she was being observed and marked out of ten. As it turned out, she must have had at least straight 8s. At the end, when the pushing didn't seem to be going anywhere, the midwives were joined by an obstetrician who marched in, put a suction cup on the baby's head and pulled it straight out.

Susanne said she was in shock afterwards and that she hadn't been prepared for the pain, or for such a quick labour. She felt overwhelmed and shaky and thought she'd rather die than ever do that again, but a few days later she'd kind of forgotten. She had the 'baby blues' on Day 4 when the real breast milk came into her breasts, but she reckons that wasn't too bad – she just let herself cry all day without feeling weird about it. She looks terribly glamorous and serene in her silky nightie, and the baby seems to be an old hand at the breast.

Susanne's maternity ensemble reminds me I don't have anything suitable to wear in hospital. I head off to Oxford Street again to get myself a nightie and dressing-gown because a T-shirt, hiking socks and an old overcoat obviously will not do. I also try to buy a back-supporting maternity-girdle-type thing. But when I mention the girdle, the saleslady asks sternly through cat's-bum lips, 'Has your doctor told you to get one? They're not recommended these days. Have you told your doctor?'

'I don't want one to hide away my stomach, I want it to support my back.'

'I see,' she snaps. 'We haven't got any.'

Have I got this Nesting Thing bad. All afternoon I daydream about moving the furniture. Why can't I live in a minimalist house like the ones in *Elle Decoration*? I've been following the magazine advice to 'de-clutter', but all this seems to mean is I've put most of the things I unpacked after the move back into boxes. Mercifully, I am removed for a while from the house by the necessity to travel up and down the country to promote the new fashion range. Most of this is talking to buyers but I get to do a bit of radio along the way, including a humilating slot at Classic FM, where, while I'm waiting, an assistant catches me eating a muffin out of a paper bag and returns with a plate so I won't 'have to be a savage'.

Living in a big city like London is really no fun in this condition. I flew up to Manchester and back at Heathrow, the queue for a taxi stretched into the far distance, full of business people who looked at me as if I was an alien.

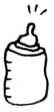

The evening paper had a feature about breastfeeding in public being 'just exhibitionism' that sent me into a fury. I mean, really. You'd think that mothers spend their days pushing their prams around the streets in string bikinis, and removing their nipple tassels to flaunt themselves the way it was written. Does breastfeeding really remind people of Carry On films and Barbara Windsor? I think not. Then again, I'm not sure I didn't find the letter the following day from the chairwoman of the Breast Police even worse: she said she found mothers who *bottle-feed* their baby in public offensive because they were depriving their babs of breastmilk's vital ambrosia. A nice thing to read for those mums who would love to breastfeed but can't. It's odd how engaged I suddenly find myself in this debate. I don't think I'd have given the article a second glance a year ago.

But I've become almost obsessed with the baby thing. I've even been browsing the preggo mags, while waiting for trains. The piece I liked best was a tip for how to tell your partner that you were pregnant by having a special dinner with a table decorated with white flowers called baby's breath. Geoff, at least, being a professional, could tell baby's breath from a head of cauliflower, but even he'd be unlikely to make the connection.

What I liked less about the mags were the aerobicised chicks adorning most of the pages and reminding you of the crucial need to maintain a fitness program. I haven't done any side-lying crunches, don't know what an isometric abdominal is, and haven't done any pelvic-floor exercises. Which means by Christmas I'll be incontinent, broke and 487 kilos. What I want to see is a few of these pregnancy magazines with women who were more than size 10 to start with and who've just had two nights of insomnia and half a black forest cake; and instead of male models, I want to see proper blokes looking unshaven, and shell-shocked after seeing their first ballistic baby poo.

I think it's time for a bit of a holiday.

info

travelling

The best time for holiday travel is the middle trimester – you're probably not queasy, there's not much chance of labour starting, your energy levels are up, you're not too huge to get comfortable and you're less likely to be mistaken for a large wildebeest in the dark. Plus, you are still travelling on your own. After the baby comes, it seems to be increasingly hard to leave the house, even to go to your mum's for the weekend, without two suitcases of wipes, nappies, toys, plastic bags, spare clothes and a portable kitchen.

Most women travel without any problems at this time, but there are things you should consider in advance, especially if you're looking to go beyond Europe, or travelling long-haul. Most urgently, you should check with your GP that you don't have any conditions that preclude some travelling – such as high blood pressure – and that you can safely have any vaccinations you need for your intended destination.

That done, think twice about going somewhere unusually hot or humid, or host to a frenzied-mosquito festival. Pregnancy has already raised your body temperature. In addition, high altitude destinations (over 2,000 metres or 6,500 feet) are not recommended because of the lack of oxygen for you and your baby. Machu Pichu will just have to wait.

In fact, popping over to the other side of the world on any long flight, especially in economy, is not a great idea. A long-haul flight will multiply the discomfort and side effects of anything you may already be experiencing, such as fluid retention and puffing up (and crawling over people to get to the loo). And importantly, long periods of cramped inactivity on planes can raise the chances of a dangerous blood clot. If you do go on a long-haul flight, remember to move around as much as possible to keep your circulation going, and follow any relevant safety advice offered by the airline.

If you are lucky enough to live in a developed country, this is probably not the time to visit a developing one if you can avoid it. You might not be able to have the vaccinations you'll need (most vaccinations are off limits until after Week 12), and you'll be exposing yourself and the baby to disease and the sort of medical care they make scary films about. Malaria, in particular, carries an increased threat to you and your baby, and you should get expert advice from your GP and MASTA (see p.211) before travelling. If you are heading for regions where gastro bugs are common, pack diarrhoea medication recommended by your GP for use during pregnancy, don't let yourself dehydrate, and drink lots of reliably bottled water. Better, though, is to plan a holiday that allows for good diet, rest and relaxation. You probably need it.

⑥ If you travel anywhere overseas, get top-grade travel insurance that includes full medical costs – especially important if you are going to the US – and allows you to cancel if neccessary for a pregnancy-related reason. If you have an annual policy you may find it has become invalid: be sure to check. If you are less than eight weeks pregnant, many companies won't provide cover; the Post Office is one of the few that does.

⑥ If you are booking with a travel company, ask them how to find a doctor at your destination who speaks your language. Carry a brief medical history, including your blood group and allergies. Many people carry their own maternity notes. If you do need any medical help while overseas, it's vital the doctor knows that you're pregnant before treating you or prescribing anything.

⑥ If you are travelling in the first trimester, read the sections on miscarrriage (p.68) and ectopic pregnancy (p.58), so you are informed if you're away from home. Travel doesn't create any additional risk of miscarriage but it is important to ask yourself what would happen if you have a miscarriage while travelling and need high-tech emergency hospital care.

⑥ If you plan to travel late in pregnancy, check if any country you're travelling to requires proof of the due date of the baby. Without this in writing from your doctor, they may refuse entry.

by car

You can drive all through pregnancy as long as you don't rule yourself out for severe vagueness. (Driving yourself to the hospital in labour, however, is not on).

⑥ Take snacks, drinks and a back support cushion if driving for long distances (and likewise on train trips). The only snacks you can buy in most places have the nutritional content of a battered Mars Bar and three times the calories.

⑥ Stop, stretch and have rest breaks, and don't hold back if you need to wee: make sure you stop regularly and go to the toilet.

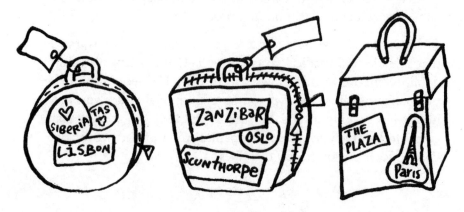

⑥ Put the seatbelt's lap strap underneath your belly and the sash between belly and breast.

⑥ You can sit on a folded towel for the last couple of weeks of pregnancy in case your waters break when you're driving, so the amniotic fluid doesn't ruin the upholstery.

by plane

Most airlines refuse bookings from pregnant passengers during the last four to five weeks of the pregnancy in case you give birth prematurely on the flight. Restrictions and medical certificate requirements vary from airline to airline. Ask the airline in advance what they require: your GP or midwife can give you a certificate of pregnancy or a letter stating that in their opinion you are fit to travel. Don't think you can fox an airline by just turning up – they may make an arbitrary decision not to let you fly if you can't 'prove' your due date.

If your blood pressure is high, or you are severely anaemic, or you have experienced vaginal bleeding, you should not fly at all during your pregnancy. If you are expecting twins (or more), have had a previous premature delivery, or have increased uterine activity (contractions), flying is not advised beyond Week 24.

It's not safe to fly in an unpressurised aircraft when pregnant because of the lack of oxygen. Large planes all have pressurised cabins but smaller planes (used for short hops around the Greek islands, for instance) may not, and you need to find out about this from your travel agent. Oxygen levels can fluctuate even in pressurised aeroplane cabins, so if you are feeling lightheaded ask the flight attendant for some oxygen.

Assuming you're on for a flight, here are some tips:

⑥ If taking a short holiday or trip, try to limit yourself to hand luggage to save having to wait on arrival.

⑥ When booking flights, say you are pregnant and ask for an aisle seat (for access to the toilets and leg stretching) near the front of the plane (you can get on last, get off first and have better air quality).

⊚ Check with your doctor to assess your risk of deep vein thrombosis (DVT) developing during air travel.

⊚ Ask an attendant to put your hand luggage up in the rack for you. Take plenty of walk and stretch breaks. Elevate, flex and rotate your feet while you are sitting, to help your circulation.

⊚ Avoid dehydration by drinking plenty of fluid – water, diluted fruit juice or milk – but not alcohol, tea or coffee. Bring your own healthy snacks and a drink, in case of delays.

⊚ Wear comfortable shoes and thin socks because your feet will swell even more than usual on a long flight, and put on support pantyhose if you have varicose veins. Puffiness may last for a day or so afterwards (see the info on swelling and fluid retention in 'Week 28').

staying away

⊚ Take your own pillow in a bright-coloured pillowcase (so it's harder to forget and leave behind) – this will leave other pillows for propping under your tummy or between your legs.

⊚ In your handbag carry a few essentials such as tissues (you never know when your nose will run or stuff up or you'll need toilet paper), ear plugs and an eye mask.

⊚ Don't even think about high heels.

⊚ Lighten your load as much as possible. Some marketing geniuses make small cosmetic travelling kits for this very purpose. Cute but expensive – you can make up your own. Put all cosmetics, shampoos and so on in tiny plastic bottles (you can buy them at chemists) or get sample-sized sachets, and take just enough for what you'll need while you're away.

⊚ Pack light, versatile clothes: a perfectly fine three- or four-day business trip can be accomplished with one black microfibre frock (microfibre doesn't need ironing and black won't get grubby so quickly), two pairs of tights, one pair of microfibre or cotton black pants, two T-shirts or shirts with short or long sleeves, two pairs of socks, four pairs of undies, two bras and … um … a jacket. Unless somebody else will be available to carry your luggage at all times, plan to be able to have everything in a carry-on-the-plane-sized bag. Or have a small bag on wheels and ask someone to get it off the carousel for you.

If you're travelling past the first trimester you're probably very pregnant-looking by now – so if you'd like to avoid people asking you lots of questions on your train, bus or plane trip, read some erotic fiction with lurid book covers. You'd be surprised how much people leave you alone.

more info on travel

The Rough Guide to Travel Health by Dr Nick Jones, Rough Guides, 2004.
Okay, we're biased but this is a genuinely useful pocket guide with lots of advice on travel during pregnancy (including the low-down on vaccinations and malarial prophylactics), plus country-by-country tips for trips. It has handy sections, too for travel with – BABIES!

MASTA (Medical Advisory Service for Travellers Abroad). www.masta.org
This advisory service is run by the London School of Hygiene and Tropical Medicines. It offers a Traveller's Healthline (0906/822 4100) which you can phone up and leave details of your trip (including state of pregnancy). You will then be sent a list of recommended vaccinations (payment is through your phonebill).

CDC (American Center for Disease Control and Prevention). www.cdc. gov
This excellent US government website is packed with advice and links, and includes up-to-date outbreak and immunisation advice, as well as specific sections on pregnancy, babies and children.

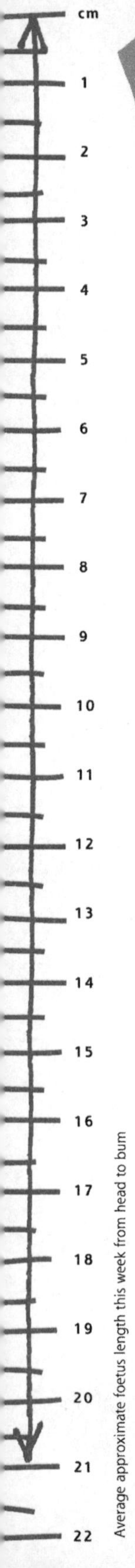

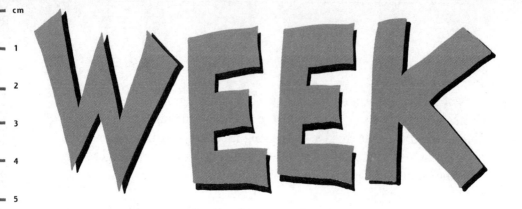

WEEK

On the left margin (vertical):
cm scale from 1 to 22

Average approximate foetus length this week from head to bum

what's going on You may be feeling constipated. Changes in blood flow can mean your blood pressure drops and you may feel faint. This can happen when you lie flat on your back because the weight of the uterus can compress the big fat vein (the inferior vena cava) that carries blood from your lower parts back to your heart. If you do feel weird, stop lying on your back and you'll feel better again.

Many babies born at this stage have survived with the help of hospital intensive care, but this is by no means guaranteed. The biggest problem is that the lungs aren't really finished, so if the foetus came out early it would need help to breathe. The foetus still looks thin compared to the roly-poly Anne Geddes postcard-style baby, but is starting to get plumper. Weight: about 630 grams (1lb 6oz).

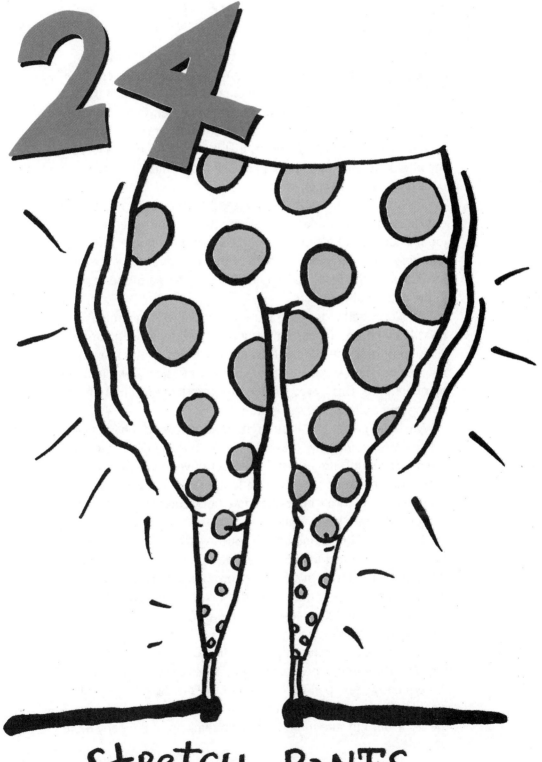

STRETCH PANTS

DiARY

I'm thinking more about the baby. The great festival of nesting continues. Beck says every time she rings me up there is another workman in the house. This time it's the carpenter, Crazy Axel (he doesn't call himself Crazy Axel, but he should). Crazy Axel makes built-in wardrobes in large pieces that he unloads off a trailer onto the pavement and then realises none of them will fit through our door unless he saws them in half.

Installation brings a whole new sense of horror, with great big bits gouged out of the wall, and Crazy Axel's habit of leaving the job for hours at a time and walking back into the house without knocking. After three or four days of this, he drives away, leaving the job unfinished and his mobile phone in the wardrobe. It rings in the middle of the night.

Why do I bother to make those few social calls to remind myself I still have friends? I distinguish myself by leaving parties when most other people are arriving. It's impossible to keep up my previous, non-pregnant pace – but hard to slow down to a real pregnant pace. This leaves just the uncomfortable feeling of being boring and guilty at the same time.

My brain is suet and I can't remember anything. I have stuck Post-it notes around my computer screen so many times it looks like a clown's ruff. I'm also still really sensitive to smells. I try to go to the supermarket again, but one foot into the deli section and I nearly faint and throw up at the same time. Luckily I don't try fish – my head might have rotated.

Back home, I'm sitting on the couch watching the Teletubbies (practice) when I feel a sort of a feeling that could be some lunch rearranging itself, only it's too low down, and might be a fart but isn't, and come to think of it, I've felt it before. Eh-oh! It's Cellsie! I feel intensely pleased with the world, and can't help patting my tummy in reply.

People are still trying to get us to find out if it's a girl or boy. An article in the local paper asks, 'Does discovering your unborn baby's sex spoil the surprise or does it allow for sensible planning?'. It says three-quarters of British women want to know the sex – but I'm sure it has to do with thinking of the baby more as a person, so you'll take any info you can get. If the doctor could tell whether or not the kid was going to have a natural talent for footie, you'd probably want to know that too – partly because there are so many unknowns and undercurrent worries that any hard and fast information can seem comforting. Apparently, people are more likely to find out the sex of babies when they have already had a child or children. I suppose that's the one thing they are not pre-warned about.

I squeeze into some old stretch pants and wear them down the street. And I do mean stretch pants. They are so thin that the tight grey lycra shows my bum crack (a fact helpfully imparted by Geoff when we arrive at the tube station) and threatens to simply twang off my body at any moment. A rather narrow squeak for me, if I can use the words 'me' and 'narrow' in the same sentence.

info

childbirth education classes

where?

Ask your midwife or GP for their recommendation regarding childbirth education classes. Book an antenatal class as early as possible in your pregnancy to make sure you get a timeslot that suits you. Classes available vary greatly from place to place across the UK. They may be run by your hospital, by your local midwife or health visitors, by your own GP or health centre. The National Childbirth Trust (NCT) also runs classes, usually in the evening and at the home of whoever is running the course. For more on NCT classes, see p.60.

man watching birth video

why?

The aim of antenatal classes is to prepare you and your birth support partner, psychologically and practically, for labour and delivery. Well, as prepared as you can be if you've never done it before. And these classes are full of first-time parents. (Already-parents are probably at home having a lie-down.) The classes often have a couple of weeks dedicated to stuff that happens after the child is born – breastfeeding, baby care and safety for L-plate parents. In some areas there are classes especially for women whose first language is not English, classes for single mothers, twins groups, and classes for teenagers.

what?

Also known as parentcraft or prenatal classes (or to several men of my acquaintance as the horror video club), antenatal classes usually comprise five or six weekly sessions in the third trimester of pregnancy. Ask about the style of the class before you book in. Some are run as a series of lectures; others may have an open structure, allowing for discussion. Some offer hands-on sessions for practising breathing and massage techniques; others may encourage the sharing of feelings about pregnancy and childbirth, or involve lying around on lumpy, brown corduroy beanbags discussing your innermost feelings with total strangers.

Other antenatal classes focus specifically on fitness or yoga during pregnancy and after delivery. These classes can be found through hospital antenatal clinics, local sports or recreation centres. The Active Birth Centre (see p.402) also has a list of registered yoga teachers for pregnancy.

Ideally the person running the class will impartially present the pros and cons on issues such as hospital and home birth, and available pain relief, without saying things like, 'Anyone who has an epidural is a big wuss' (or the reverse). If the class seems to be going in a direction you don't like, try another one – or give up. You're not back at school. Good classes should ensure you develop realistic expectations about what labour will be like, providing a balance between childbirth as a joyful, amazing event and the things that might go wrong or go against your picture of the ideal birth. Ask lots of questions: classes are there to give you the information you want.

Typical classes will provide information on how to recognise the onset of labour: when to come in to the hospital or birth centre, or call in the homebirth troops; pain relief; and body positions that might help during labour. They almost always show videos of childbirth; provide a tour of a birth centre or labour ward; and include advice on antenatal and postnatal exercise, caesarean section, induced labour, the partner's or labour support person's role, breastfeeding, unsettled babies, how to reduce the risk of sudden infant death syndrome, and how to recognise postnatal depression.

who?

You'll find that pregnancy and childbirth books often talk about the various schools of childbirth theory, such as Sheila Kitzinger's psychosexual approach (birth as an earthy, sexual, visceral woman-baby thing), or Janet Balaskas's active-birth model. In practice, antenatal classes tend to provide a combination of the most helpful elements from various schools of thought as they relate to the experience and philosophy of the hospital maternity department or group. The classes run by the NHS are usually provided free of charge except for refreshments. The NCT classes cost around £150 for you and a birth partner.

Perhaps the best aspect of attending a class is that you form friendships with other new parents in your area. Classes are also handy for preparing your birth partner and make it less likely that s/he'll be asking questions during the real thing such as 'What happens now?' and 'Can I have some of those drugs?'

your record

✳ Spend a day with a parent and small baby.

✳ When you've had a good lie down, record your overwhelming impressions.

WEEK 25

what's going on

The foetus is about due to start putting pressure on your ribs and also on your digestive system. You could get pains down the sides of your tummy from now on as the uterus stretches. The foetus looks pretty much like a baby at birth. It will definitely have developed its own sleeping patterns: usually awake when you're asleep and vice versa as your movements soothe it to sleep. (This is why babies can be rocked to sleep once they come out.) The foetus may be startled by loud music and start kicking you when it hears a certain tune. Or maybe it's dancing. This is a good time to play it music, talk to it and see if you get a reaction.

Weight: about 720 grams (1lb 9oz).

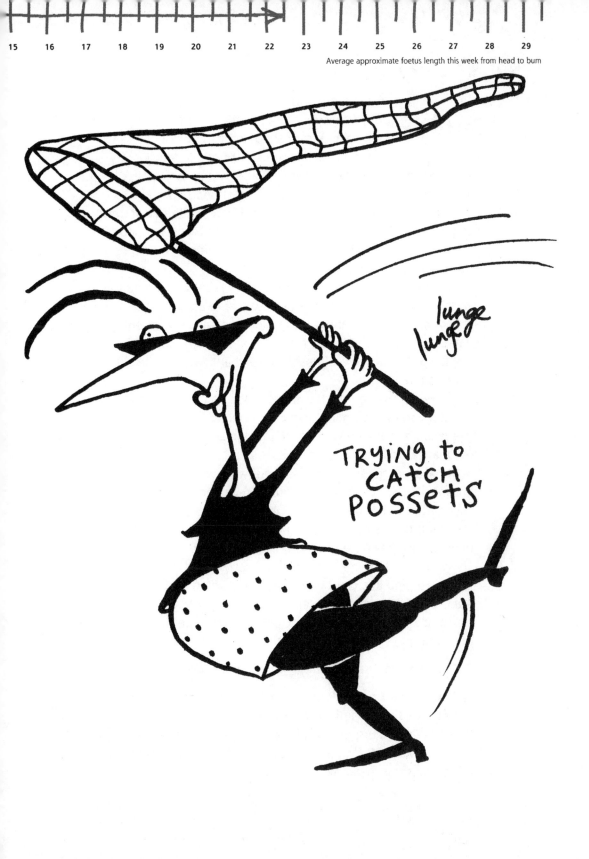

lunge
lunge

TRYING to
CATCH
POSSETS

DiARY I keep forgetting where I am in the middle of sentences: it reminds me of all those times recovering from endometriosis operations, when the general anaesthetic seemed to temporarily wipe out most of my vocabulary. I have covered the house with a confetti of Post-it notes, and I keep paper and pencil AND a tape recorder next to the bed at night. I have written down really helpful stuff like 'Remember the thing', and I mumbled odd unintelligible words into the tape recorder before standing on it on the way to the loo for the nine-hundredth time.

Geoff inquires whether, now that I'm pregnant, I intend to eat his head. Turns out he has been watching a wonders-of-nature program on the telly about black widow spiders. I point out loftily that the praying mantis eats the head – the black widow eats the whole lot. He looked a bit taken aback that I have this detailed information.

A weirdy man on the bus tries to look up my skirt. I feel like saying, 'Careful. You might meet someone coming the other way!' I've heard about men who are affected in an unseemly way by pregnancy, and here is the proof.

It takes some effort to think about what will happen after the baby arrives as I can't seem to stretch my mind past the concept of childbirth, but it must be done. Oh my God. It's not just that I'm pregnant; there's actually going to be another person along any minute, and they haven't even got their own room.

Actually I don't really mind if the baby spends the first few weeks sleeping in a cardboard box, but it would probably upset Aunt Julie. We have completely run out of money, but these are some of the things the books seem to think we should be purchasing:

✳ A gigantic industrial-strength washing machine.

✳ A fridge with a freezer big enough to store frozen casseroles for the weeks after the birth. The fridge-freezer we have is a legacy of the old shared-house days and is a lot more used to ever-emptying bottles of vodka and tubs of ice-cream with a spoon frozen into them. Does this mean we're not ready for a baby?

⁕ A Moses basket (aka crib). This is the one thing Susanne says I will need, too: a nice basket with sheet lining, and a stand and handles so you can cart it around from room to room. I quite like the idea of having a baby in a basket and it seems you can use it instead of a cot for the first few months.

⁕ 'Muslin squares for catching possets'. This one mystified me for a while but it turns out the squares are a technical terms for 'bits of cloth to put over your shoulder that the baby can vomit onto'. That's something to look forward to.

⁕ 56,000 nappies

⁕ A changing mat. Susanne says this is the other must have. It's a plasticy padded thing, available in a range of baby-cute designs, which you lay your baby on to change its nappy. Apparently it limits the spread of poo around your house.

⁕ A 'bonnet'. I presume they mean hat. Or is it compulsory to get something with bobbles on it?

⁕ A 'nursery', a word which previously had connotations only of seedlings. Will need to strip Geoff of personal space and manhood by taking over his 'office' to achieve this.

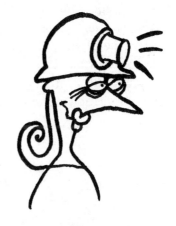

⁕ A dimmer switch, 'installed for night feeds'. Have a dimmer switch installed?! Seems extreme but it's apparently pretty useful. On the other hand, I might just make do with an old lamp, or park the cot near a window that lets in street light. Or perhaps I could gaffer tape a bicycle lamp to my head.

⁕ A small sink with running water – some pregnancy books actually suggest you install one in the corner of the room. Oh and while the builders are in, perhaps a turret or two might be nice.

info

baby clothes

The exact quantity of clothing you'll need will depend on things such as whether you have a very vomity baby, how often you will be washing, and whether you use cloth or disposable nappies (cloth nappies tend to create more clothes washing because their 'containment' is not as efficient as that of disposables).

It's not a bad idea to get your baby's clothes and nappies in before you get too big to go charging around shops and bargain outlets. Here's what you'll need.

nappies

A newborn baby needs about sixty nappy changes a week on average. Later you use fewer nappies, but more goes into them. (That was delicately put, wasn't it?)

Cloth Depending on your washing plans and which type of cloth nappy you are planning to use, you will need 15-20 nappies, at each stage of your baby's growth. The shaped Velcro nappies are ideal for tiny babies as the fasteners make for easier changing and no grappling with nappy pins or snappy fasteners. Get ones with extra protection at the side against leaking.

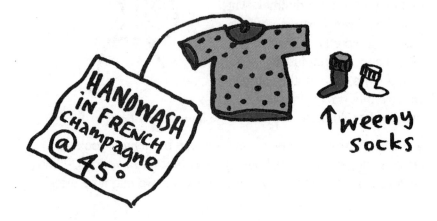

HANDWASH iN FRENCH CHampagne @ 45°

↑weeny socks

Cotton cloth nappies should be used for tiny babies, and then you can move on to towelling ones (more absorbent) after a few weeks or months. When the baby first arrives, you protect each nappy with a liner. These can be either disposable or cloth, which you can wash and use again. You will also need plastic pants. For tiny babies the tie-on type are best being just a shaped plastic sheet with ties – easy to use. Later you can try plastic pants with elasticated legs and waist. You can get these from chemists or baby shops. You can just throw the dirty ones in the nappy bucket or washing machine, rinse, and shake off the water afterwards.

There may be a nappy laundering or delivery service near where you live. The service will deliver clean nappies and take away dirty ones – however many you need. Order the delivery to arrive the day before you are due home from hospital, to ensure there is no chance of being caught without nappies if the company doesn't visit your area on the day you get home, or your area is scheduled for afternoon delivery.

Disposables If you opt (like most people) for disposable nappies, you might sleep a bit easier if you buy 'eco' brands, which have less chemicals and are more biodegradable. As with cotton nappies, disposables come in a range of sizes: you'll need to start with 'newborn'. In addition to a pack or two of nappies, your baby starter kit needs to include a couple of small towels, muslin squares or cloth nappies to cover the changing mat, which is otherwise a bit too plasticky and cold to put a baby on.

basic newborn-baby wardrobe

ⓖ 6 vests with wide or envelope necks.

ⓖ 2 cotton sleep suits .

ⓖ 6 front-opening babygros (stretch suits), with or without feet depending on the time of year.

ⓖ 2–3 pairs of cotton socks, or stretchy, pull-on, machine-washable bootees – forget ribbons, forget handknits. You won't need socks at all if the weather is very hot, or you plan to use babygros with feet all the time, though in colder weather they can be worn inside the stretch suits to keep the feet snug.

⑥ 8 muslin squares, which are easily washed and dried and become indispensable – used as over-the-shoulder protection after feeds, general mopping up cloths, placed on the changing mat for the comfort of the baby and put in the Moses basket to collect dribbles from the mouth (so cutting down the need for endless laundering on the crib sheets).

⑥ Bibs – you don't need these straight away, and the number will depend on whether your baby vomits a lot, possets (does small vomits) or dribbles a lot. To be honest, all babies dribble a lot. Get big towelling bibs, not the plastic-backed ones which are stiff and no good for wiping faces. Velcro-fastened bibs are much better than ribbon-tied ones or ones you have to pull over a baby's head. You'll need about eight bibs once the baby starts eating solid foods but that's a way off. For breastfeeding, people usually just have a cloth nappy or a muslin square handy to mop up possets.

⑥ 2 shawls or blankets.

summer baby

The baby may need grow-suits with short sleeves and legs, or may be more comfy with short-sleeved cotton nighties during the day, or even a vest and nappy as long as the insects are kept away.

A summer baby won't need much in the way of blankets but a couple won't go astray for cool nights. For hot nights, substitute a few soft, absorbent muslin squares.

winter baby

The baby will need three to four outer items: cardigans or jackets are easiest to change, though an all-in-one warm, padded suit can be valuable. If you use jumpers or windcheaters, make sure they have two buttons at the neck or are very stretchy. Fabrics such as velour, thick cotton jersey, or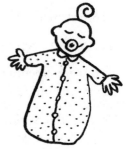

thermal materials are more practical than woollen knits, which are harder to wash and dry and can be itchy. You'll also want one or two hats.

hints from mothers

⊚ Buy natural fabrics.

⊚ All clothes you get should be able to be soaked, machine washed and tumble dried, if you use a dryer.

⊚ Get long vests, even if they seem too long – the shorter ones end up looking like crop-tops. Good vests have really generous neck and arm holes so that you can get them on your baby quickly and easily.

⊚ Babygros (also called all-in-ones, stretch-suits or jumpsuits) are much easier to change if they have press-studs that run from the neck to the crotch and right down the inside of both legs of the suit. DO NOT BUY A SINGLE THING THAT BUTTONS DOWN THE BACK OR LACKS CROTCH FASTENERS. Remember, you need to go up a size in babygros as soon as they fit snugly, or they will start to hurt your baby's feet and stop legs stretching out properly.

⊚ If you buy those headbands with a bow on them for a girl baby your child will look like a demented Easter egg in a nappy.

⊚ A small baby doesn't need shoes except for show. Warm, snug socks are fine – it's not going hiking any time soon.

⊚ A surprising number of bonnets have long cords on them. Don't buy them – they're too dangerous. In fact, don't buy anything with cords or flappy tassels or long strips of loose material – they are all strangulation risks.

⊚ A tiny baby hates being dressed and undressed. Choose soft, stretchy cotton or cotton-blend clothes. Many people use envelope-neck nighties for newborn babies in preference to stretch suits, to help make changes quicker and less traumatic:

they are easy to get over the head, and provide handy access to the nappy at the other end.

⑥ Go to bargain places, but consider why any clothes on sale might be bargains, or seconds. Small marks that will wash out are fine, but clothes likely to spontaneously combust are not.

⑥ Borrow as much as you can. If it has to be returned, keep a list! Don't ask people to lend you baby clothes – they will offer if they want to. Sometimes they are keeping their baby clothes in case they decide to have another one, and it's all too psychologically confronting to give away their supplies.

⑥ Buy or borrow the minimum number of tiny-sized clothes: they don't get worn for very long and big babies can skip the newborn size and go straight into 0–3 month size.

⑥ Babies grow out of things so quickly, you could well match up with someone with a slightly bigger baby and someone with a slightly smaller baby to become part of a clothes chain.

⑥ If you don't have friends with spare baby clothes available to borrow, and you're on a budget, go to charity shops or NCT secondhand sales. Launder everything well, particularly if it has been stored in mothballs (napthaline) or camphor, both of which are poisonous, or in dry-cleaning bags, which retain fumes.

⑥ Cheaper chain stores can have very good babies' and children's wear departments: sometimes the best clothes are the cheapest because they're not fiddly and made for show. At this early stage they won't need to last unless you're passing them down the line to other children. Don't overbuy, even though the clothes are so cute; your baby will grow quickly.

your record

✳ What clothes have you bought your baby?

✳ What music have you played the baby, and which songs prompted a kicking reaction?

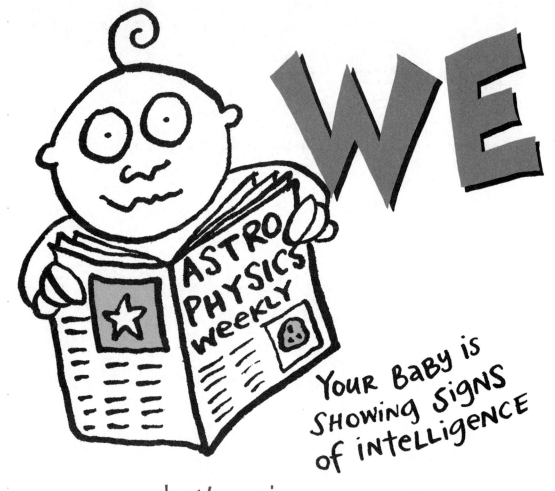

WE

YOUR BABY IS
SHOWING SIGNS
OF INTELLIGENCE

what's going on Get lots of rest and exercise. (You should also get gifts consisting of large gems, but this is unlikely.) If you haven't worked it out already, stop wearing shoes with heels, and don't do any climbing or hurling yourself about: remember your centre of gravity has changed and you need to protect your tummy. You will be steadily gaining weight.

Average approximate foetus length this week from head to bum

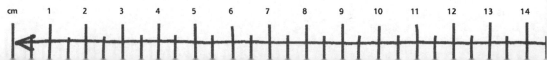

cm   1   2   3   4   5   6   7   8   9   10   11   12   13   14

EK 26

This coming month the foetus will really spend time putting on more fat and muscle. Each week its chances of survival outside the uterus increase as it makes more surfactant for the lungs. According to one pregnancy expert, this week in the uterus your baby 'is showing signs of sensitivity, awareness and intelligence'. So if you put a little calculator in there your foetus could probably estimate the cost in Euros of 5600 nappies. It can detect light even through its still-closed eyelids, smell (sadly for the foetus the only thing on offer is the amniotic fluid, which smells like a swamp), as well as hear, and possibly play the slide guitar. The baby will recognise other voices from now on: friends, Daddy, aunties and Dusty Springfield singing 'Son of a Preacher Man'.

Weight: about 820 grams (1lb 14oz).

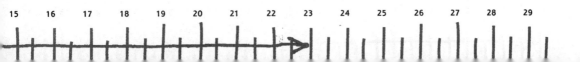

15 16 17 18 19 20 21 22 23 24 25 26 27 28 29

DiARY Are the leg cramps causing insomnia, or can I feel the leg cramps because I'm awake in the middle of the night? What a fascinating philosophical question. Beck says there are two things that might be causing sore calves: blood pooling in the veins, or lack of calcium or magnesium – in my case probably magnesium as I am taking enough calcium to turn into a tusk. For the itchy, runny nose and sneezing, she suggests a special garlic-and-horseradish dose.

'What about this gigantic tummy?'

'That will settle down in a few weeks.'

My tummy is now not just a big ball out the front, but a bulge all around the sides. And did I mention shocking heartburn and indigestion? Pregnancy is an absurd strain on the body, and we just don't expect that any more. We expect there to be a pill or an exercise or a mantra or a caring discussion that will alleviate 'discomfort' – and 'pain'. Nope. It's just a pure and simple pain. I'm sorry, but I'm not finding this a sublimely spiritual experience. It's a deeply PHYSICAL experience.

The feeling of a baby moving must be different for everybody. Some books say it feels like wind, or feathers, or gentle patting. Sometimes I think it feels like someone's twanging a ligament as they might test out a harp string; sometimes it's like a bit of inside bongo work – all these feelings still all very low down in my tummy. Although the bump seems to start under the bosom, the top of the uterus is actually just at navel level. All the stuff above is displaced bits making way for the uterus.

This morning's paper reports that a computer-driven baby doll is being used to help teenagers realise how much work a baby is. The baby doll is taken home from school over a weekend, and is programmed to cry constantly or several times, day and night. A special sound indicates how often the nappy must be changed, and the student must decide how often the baby needs to be fed. One girl who had the baby doll for the weekend said, 'It really put me off having kids.' You should try pregnancy, love.

What an incredibly raunchy life it is: so far this week I've had half a glass of red wine, nine Frosty Fruits and a Magnum, some calcium tablets, and I'm about to get my daffodils in. AND

WHAT'S MORE I am becoming a stately pregnant lady and am now so considerably fattened up that that THING has happened. That THING where your thighs rub together up the top. If I wore corduroy trousers while I was walking, I'd sound like a sword fight.

info

baby equipment

You're about to enter the world of safety warnings – try to keep in mind that most babies are robust little critters, but they still need to be protected. All the baby-wrangling gear listed below needs to be safe and should conform to the various British and European Standards (BS/ES). Always check for the label.

If you're going to do a lot of this shopping on foot, do it now while you still feel energetic. The major items can be bought at department stores and specialist baby shops (some of which will hire gear). Smaller stuff can be bought at supermarkets or chemists. You can get secondhand baby equipment through trading papers, secondhand shops, NCT sales, friends, and notices on baby health centre pin-boards. If you get stuff secondhand, replace any worn straps and all of the Velcro.

car seats

Baby restraints (car seats) are compulsory for transporting a baby in the front seat of a car. It is illegal to carry your baby in your arms in the front seat of the car. The best way for a young baby to travel is in a rear-facing infant car seat either on the front passenger or back seat. This is held in place by the adult safety belt. Make sure it's correctly fitted and make sure you know how to use it before you make the first trip home from hospital. Some of them are surprisingly tricky to work out, with impenetrable diagrams and instructions in German. Don't buy a secondhand car seat unless it's in excellent condition and you know its history.

When you come to use a rear-facing baby seat, do not place it in the front passenger seat if your car is fitted with an air bag: this is a danger. And if you carry your baby into a house asleep in the seat (as you will), don't leave the baby where you can't see it, and make sure the baby's head doesn't slump forward.

baby's bed

Whether you choose a carrycot, Moses basket or cot for your baby's first weeks, it should conform to the British Safety (BS 7551) standard. This is no time to skimp or save money: peace of mind means a safe baby and a better sleep for you. Whatever device you choose will need a firm, well-fitting mattress, two mattress protectors made of waterproof-backed fabric, and at least three sheets. You can buy fitted baby sheets of towelling or flannelette (it's not necessary to buy the sheets made of fine linen with ittle duckies embroidered on them); or you can cut up adult bed sheets. Pillowcases can be used for crib sheets. Two or three cotton cellular blankets that can be firmly tucked in are safe and easy to wash. Duvets are a hazard for young babies as they can cut off the air supply and smother a baby. Pillows and cot bumpers are also dangerous and not recommended for newborn babies.

Carrycots and Moses baskets are only for young babies – your baby will need to move into a cot (or, gulp, stay in your bed) by the time it is four months old. But baskets are useful in that you can carry them around, and take them on weekends away. When choosing a basket, make sure it has a tight-fitting mattress and a firm, secure base. Also, be careful when carrying it in the early weeks, when you're less than 100 per cent fit – there is a risk to your back lifting it from the floor. Bend those knees.

Rocking cribs – pricey but cute – are good baby sleep pads, particularly for a baby that fusses and frets. The soothing movement helps to settle the baby. But don't feel you're missing out overmuch if you can't afford (or borrow) one. That same motion can be replicated by gently patting your baby in a cot, or rolling the baby in a pram back and forth over an arm's length.

A well-swaddled newborn baby can be comfortable in a cot. And a slightly older baby can be 'dressed' for cot sleep in a quilted-cotton sleeping-bag with arms (these are sold at most babyware outlets), which is handy if they have a tendency to kick off the sheets and blankets in their sleep. Your baby should be placed at the foot of the cot, so there is no danger of it wriggling under the blankets.

A cot mattress should be firm and fit snugly: make sure there's no more than a 2.5cm (1in) gap between the mattress and the sides of the cot so that the baby can't get stuck. You should really buy a new cot mattress, unless you're getting a good one from a friend, and you should be wary of dodgy old foam ones (where the foam can easily squash away from the edge of the cot). If you can afford it, you might prefer to buy a cotton cot mattress.

Other important factors for cots include the spacing of bars, the security of a drop side, the efficiency of wheel brakes, what the cot is painted with (old lead-painted 1950s models are dangerous), and the position of the mattress relative to the height of the sides. Most cots have a base with an adjustable height. This reduces awkward stretching in the first few months and can be lowered once the baby can sit up.

Oh – and did I mention that cots can be a bugger to set up (they tend to arrive flat packed with ropey instructions). Don't leave it till you're in labour and if you have a DIY accomplished friend, eat your pride NOW.

pram or pramette

Technically a pram means one of those huge, old-fashioned vehicles, with gigantic wheels, that a Mary-Poppins-style nanny would push around with the sixty-seventh Earl of Whatever inside. Pramettes are the newer, lighter designs that can often be converted into a stroller (buggy). But no one except shop assistants ever calls them a pramette – they're all prams to us. As with cots, when you buy or borrow one, you need to consider safety, as well as cost, durability and adaptability.

The most popular pram, these days, is a convertible pushchair or buggy that folds flat – making it suitable for the newborn baby (who cannot yet sit up, or indeed hold its head up). These kind of buggies are relatively light and compact and therefore easy to transport and store. To accommodate a young baby, they should have a fully reclining seat and be able to face either forwards or backwards (the position you generally start with for newborns). They usually come with the added extras of rain cover and sunshade (as if). Some models are designed as a combination of car seat, carry cot and pushchair.

Three-wheeler buggies with all-terrain wheels have been sweeping the market over the last few years. Do you need one? Probably not, unless you just have to keep jogging, or your local streets are rutted with holes (some friends living in Sarajevo rated their all-terrain buggy very highly). But all-terrain buggies work well and if you have a dodgy back you might find one easier and more comfortable than a regular buggy. Have a try in the shop.

Ease of use should be your number one consideration. Is the pram light and easy to fold if you are going to put it in the car or on a bus? Fold it up and down yourself a few times in the shop and see how you get on: if you can't do it empty, it won't be easier with a babe installed. Is the pram comfortable for you and your partner to push? Is the handle height right, or adjustable? Make sure your pram comes equipped with a five-point harness for the baby, good brakes and a shelf or basket underneath large enough to hold your baby bag or shopping.

You should also decide, before going shopping, if you want the buggy to convert to a stroller later on. Don't be too hung up on this. Buggies for older babies and toddlers are lighter and more portable than convertible prams and if you can afford one, or have one lined up from a friend, you'll want to change over.

⊚ Note that prams are designed for tooling around the streets, or standing next to you when you're hanging out the washing or writing a Booker Prize winning novel. they're not good for leaving in another room unattended (ditto carricots, baby car seats and sofas) just in case the baby wriggles into trouble.

light for night-time feeding

It's worth considering either a dimmer setting for the main light in the baby's room – this isn't difficult or costly to install – or a small, low-wattage lamp, which provides just enough light for you to change and feed by. There's a theory that nipples and areolae darken after a pregnancy because small babies see contrasts rather than colours, and can more easily spot the feeding station in low light. A dim light helps to say to a baby, 'It's still night-time. Have a quiet feed, no chatting, do the business and back to sleep.'

Recent US research indicates there may be an association between shortsightedness and a light left on in a baby's room all night in the first two years of life. If you need a night light, keep it very dim and indirect.

changing mats and tables

You will be changing gerzillions of nappies, so it makes sense to do it as comfortably as possible. The minimum requirement is one or (if you live on more than one floor) two plastic-covered, hard foam changing mats. These have built-up sides to help contain the baby and you can put them on a bed or a table or dresser (waist-height is easiest for changing). These mats can be scrubbed down and disinfected and thrown in the car to protect your friends' homes from baby poo. There are also disposable mats on the market but they're not very environmentally friendly.

If you can afford it – or borrow one – a changing table is a handy thing, though go for a solid timber one with lockable wheels; the wire ones are too flimsy. Timber ones usually have a few shelves underneath, which are useful for nappies, a change of baby clothes and the baby wipes.

As you'll soon realise, everything you need to change a nappy must be placed within reach of the changing table beforehand because you can't take your hand off a baby on a changing table.

bath venue

Early on it is as easy to wash a baby in a clean kitchen sink or bathroom basin (being careful of taps which remain hot), as in a special baby bath. However, plastic baths are cheap and you can place them in the bath when you use them.

More importantly, you'll need two or three soft bath towels, for wrapping a baby in after a bath. You can buy towels with a hood to keep baby's head warm, though these are better in theory than in practice. For drying sensitive newborn-baby creases and crannies you may prefer to use a muslin square.

For toiletries, buy a baby bath liquid or soap alternative, or an unscented bath oil; blunt-ended nail scissors; a nappy change lotion; cotton balls, nappy wipes or wash cloths. Ask around to find out what products people recommend, then buy small sizes to test on your baby.

feeding gear

You'll need nursing bras and nursing bra pads if you breastfeed. The pads soak up any leaking milk before it hits your clothes and can be bought as paper-based disposables or fabric washables.

Some women find breast pumps useful for expressing milk in order to have a night off; or when their breasts are painfully full; or they need to go to work. Electric ones are better than hand pumps for expressing often; say, for going to work. You can buy or hire from chemists. If you're planning to leave the occasional expressed breast-milk feed, you'll also need one or two bottles and teats, a sterilising unit (or you can just boil things) and bottle- and teat-cleaning brushes. You can freeze portions of breast milk in special plastic bags available in chemists.

For bottle-feeding, you'll need six to eight bottles and teats, bottle- and teat-cleaning brushes, a sterilising unit and an insulated bottle-carrier. Bottles are supposed to be always kept very cold and then warmed just before use.

nappy buckets

Two nappy buckets with a lid are essential if you're washing nappies yourself. But everyone needs one because any clothes and bedding that come into contact with baby poo should go in a bucket of water and sterilising soaking powder before machine washing. Sterilising agents have a use-by date, so check this if you are using leftover product.

even more stuff

You might find some of the following items useful:

⑥ A baby-changing bag – any big bag that has a shoulder-strap handle will do, but some are specially designed to fold out like a portable changing table. (For details of what goes in it, check out the info in 'Week 43').

⑥ A baby-monitor – like a one-way walkie-talkie set, this is helpful if the baby is sleeping (or not!) out of earshot.

⑥ A sheep's fleece or two – these are conforting for babies and non-sweaty. Some people like to have them under the cot sheet, or thrown on the floor or placed in the pram for the baby to lie on. They need to be washed regularly, otherwise they can harbour gerzillions of dust mites, but they can be machine washed and tumble dried.

⑥ One or two quilted or flannelette baby sleeping-bags – these washable, zip-up bags are very cosy in a big cot or a pram in cold weather, but make sure you remove any dangly lace, ribbon or drawstrings.

⑥ A pouch or sling – great for comforting a fretty or crying baby while getting on with whatever else you need to do. Wearing a pouch or sling is a good way to have walks or go shopping when the baby is little, though it can be hard on the back when the baby starts to stack on weight. A baby should only spend 1 or 2 hours in it at a time. Try it on before you buy it: look for well-padded shoulder straps, sturdy fabric, a head support and secure and easy-to-use clasps. Babies outgrow slings by 5 or 6 months.

⑥ A few months further down the track you will need a high-chair, and you may also want to buy a mobile, a travel cot (which doubles as a playpen), a fold-up pusher, a baby jumper, a backpack, and a large aircraft hangar to put them all in.

what's going on

Hurrah, you're in the third trimester. Hire a brass band: bah de bah, bah de bah. If people don't stand up for you on public transport, say 'Excuse me, I'm pregnant. Could I sit down?'. About twelve people will rise from their seats as if given 140 volts up the fundament. Your moles may be getting bigger and you may have small skin tags, especially under the arms and breasts. You need a lot more fluids from now until the birth. You can forget about moving gracefully. People will not be saying, 'Aren't you Audrey Hepburn?' You need to put your feet up when you can: at work, if possible on another chair – better still, make the boss massage your feet.

The foetus has grown so much it is running out of room, and it takes a little longer to manoeuvre about and turn upside down and sideways. Babies born now have a very good chance of surviving (they're called 'viable' in doctorspeak). The foetus has been practising breathing here and there, but from now on its breathing will become more rhythmic and constant. Folds and grooves appear on the surface of the brain, which is developing very quickly. (Of course if the foetus

is born early, all this developing will continue outside the uterus,

usually in an incubator with ventilators and other monitors

attached.) Weight: about 920 grams (2lb).

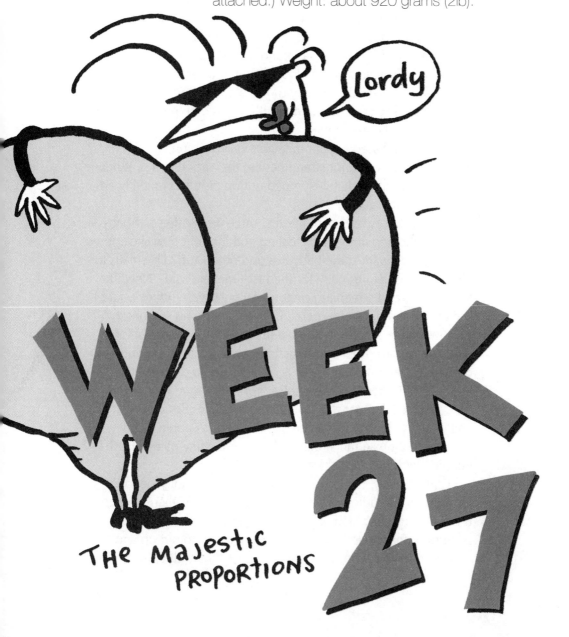

Lordy

WEEK
27

THe MaJestic
PROPORTIONS

DiARY It's true, you can spend an entire week in a dressing-gown, although I accessorise it differently at work. I find when teamed with battery-operated earrings and a beehive people tend not to notice the dressing-gown. I have developed approximately sixteen billion skin tags and my moles are all getting bigger. I am looking like a currant bun, so instead of calling Cellsie Cellsie we have started to call it Chelsea (a relative of the currant bun – how very droll).

Maybe I'm practising not getting much sleep because I wake up for an hour or so every night and lie there with vaguely aching legs, listening to the blood swishing in my ears, or to my heartbeat. It is very disconcerting. My blood sounds like languid wobble-board music and I don't really want to be reminded of Rolf Harris in the wee hours.

I have purchased a giant inflatable ball to sit on, which is supposed to be good for strengthening the back muscles. When it arrived, Geoff immediately jumped on top of it and rolled head-first into a bookcase.

Jo rings to say she spent the first three weeks after her baby was born looking at him and feeling nothing, but now she adores him, and do I want some babygros and other stuff? Liz emails to say she looked at her baby for the first time and said, 'Now I have to put this weird screaming creature on my breast? What would I want to do that for?' I'm grateful people are being so honest.

I'm getting scared about how much has to be done before the baby is born. After two hours' sleepless panic in the middle of the night about coping with it all, I decide to drop another day at work: if I'm not fooling myself, I'm not going to fool anybody else. (Maybe I can get that on a letterhead.) Besides which, at the end of every day my feet smell like the world is ending – they have swelled up so much that all I can wear is my pair of Hush Puppies, with the elasticky bit cut.

Outrageously, my favourite midwife, Anne, had gone to Paris in some sort of ludicrous attempt at a private life when I visited the clinic. I spent bloody ages in the waiting room looking at pictures of thin people in magazines, then had to put up with another midwife, who while clearly competent and replete with all her marbles doesn't have Anne's bedside manner, and indeed doesn't even help me to sit up after examining me. She tells me that I have put on 14 kilos since the start of my pregnancy, adding that 'Most people have put on 8 to 10 by this stage.' Why she didn't just call me Mrs Blimpy I don't know.

I have a blood test which checks for glucose levels, anaemia and antibodies.

Afterwards I go to visit Beck to say, 'Help me, I'm Mrs Blimpy.'

She says, 'Bollocks!' (I do love a medical adviser who says 'bollocks'.) 'Some people put on 20 kilos when they're pregnant.'

However, we agree that if I can nourish the baby and not get fatter myself, this will be a lot easier to carry around. So I must take the special pregnancy multi-vitamin-calcium supplements. I must stop eating Magnums, and stop toasted muesli for breakfast. I must have porridge with some apple or half a banana in it.

'Can I have sultanas in it?' I whine piteously.

'You can have four,' she says.

I strike her.

Then I go out to dinner and have lemon tart with ice-cream. Oh well, sod it.

info

safety

The only way to childproof a house is to never let a kid in it. But you can try to make it safer.

The older the baby gets, the more dangerous the house gets. Baby books will tell you what tricks your baby is likely to be up to next. Remember that there's a wide age range for milestones: your baby could be an early roller; your toddler could be an early climber.

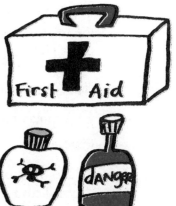

As said in last week's info, every baby-relevant item needs to be safe: cots, prams, car seats, baby chairs, toys, changing tables, clothes, dummies –

the lot. Remember when you are preparing the house for small persons that the most common causes of death and injury in little kids include car and pedestrian accidents – often in their own driveway – drowning, suffocation, falling, burns, poisoning and electrical accidents.

You will need to organise:

⊚ A tamper-proof cabinet for any garden poisons and chemicals, and a first-aid kit placed higher than a child on a chair or the bench could reach.

⊚ Cupboards in which the following have been moved to a higher position: household poisons such as cleaning agents and detergents; medicines; alcohol; batteries; pesticides; mothballs and camphor; soaps and shampoos; cigarettes; matches and lighters; cosmetics and perfumes; essential oils; foods that could cause choking, such as peanuts and marshmallows; plastic bags (and go through wardrobes to get rid of drycleaning bags); glasses and other breakables; objects with sharp bits – babies and toddlers can be gymnastic and inquisitive. You can also get baby-proof catches to 'lock' cupboards.

⊚ Smoke alarms (get them now).

⊚ Electrical circuit breakers and power-point covers.

⊚ No keys left in house cupboards or doors.

⊚ A bathroom heater fitted high up on a wall.

⊚ Hairdryers kept away from water.

⊚ Fire guards for heaters and open fires.

⊚ A cooker hotplates guard.

⊚ Kettles and irons should be out of reach.

⊚ Electrical cords that are placed off the floor and out of reach – curled cords on kettles and irons are good.

⊚ TVs, screens and computers should be topple-proof.

⊚ A fire blanket for the kitchen.

⊚ Stair and doorway barriers.

⊚ A high shelf in the child's bedroom or playroom and a toy box with a lid.

⊚ If you have a pool or a pond in your garden you need to fence it in or cover it over. Your baby might walk before 12 months and crawl way before that. Always empty toddlers' paddling pools and baths after use, and keep a lid on nappy buckets at all times. Babies can drown in a tiny amount of water.

other people

Never hesitate to ask people to: smoke outside the house; stop drinking hot tea or coffee while nursing your baby; support the baby's head properly when holding; and not bounce the baby up and down after a feed. They'll probably be glad of the instruction: many non-baby-savvy friends want some guidance.

Grandparents or older friends and relations may need a firmer hand. Practices from their own parenting days, such as ignoring a baby safety restraint in a car, are unsafe. Their homes will also need to be checked.

prevention

⊚ Read the info on baby clothes in 'Week 25' and on baby equipment in 'Week 26' for safety hints.

⊚ If you have a toddler in the house, a nursery door lockable from the outside with a bolt (not a key, which could get lost) can prevent the sibling helpfully throwing toys or food in with the baby when its asleep, or tossing the baby out of a cot like a toy.

⊚ Never leave a small baby unattended with another small child or a dog. Never put a child, a dog and food together.

⊚ Always remove bibs before putting a baby to bed.

⊚ Sterilise anything that goes into your baby's mouth until at least 6 months old – okay, you don't have to boil your nipples.

⑥ Put cots, prams and baby chairs out of reach of any dangly curtain ties or blind cords and stoves, heaters, fires and electrical plug points.

⑥ Turn all saucepan handles towards the back of the stove.

⑥ When you are travelling or at someone else's place, you might need to bring safety stuff with you, and be vigilant particularly where there are other young children and dogs.

⑥ Don't leave a baby to feed unsupervised from a propped-up bottle.

⑥ Don't attach a dummy to a baby's clothes with a ribbon or string.

⑥ Don't leave a baby, even for a second, unsupervised on a changing table.

⑥ Never leave a baby or young child in a bath, no matter how briefly.

emergencies

Keep a contact list near the phone or add emergency numbers to your direct-dial system. The numbers should cover your local doctor and NHS Direct. Babysitters should be told about it. You can do an infant and child first-aid and resuscitation course with the Red Cross, the St John Ambulance Service, at your local hospital or get an instructor to come to your playgroup.

Add a thermometer and baby paracetamol to the family medicine cupboard and/or the baby bag. Ask your GP when you can use the paracetamol.

more info on safety

 Advice on safety issues and accident prevention is dispensed by the Child Accident Prevention Trust, 4th Floor, Clerks Court, 18-20 Farringdon Rd, London EC1R 3HA; Tel 020 7608 3228; safe@capt.demon.co.uk

your record

✳ What baby equipment have you bought?

✳ What have you borrowed, and from whom?

✳ Are you passing down any heirlooms or toys?

what's going on For you, just more of the same, really.

Your baby may be hiccuping. It will usually decide to party while you are resting or asleep. Its eyes are partially opened – quite sensibly as who would want to open their eyes wide in a fetid old swamp of amniotic fluid? The baby is now covered all over with vernix, so it looks a bit like one of those long-distance swimmers smothered in gunk. Except babies have got more brains than to try to swim from Dover to Calais. They just hang out in the uterus growing their bodies so their heads don't look too big. Weight: about 1 kilo (2lb 3oz).

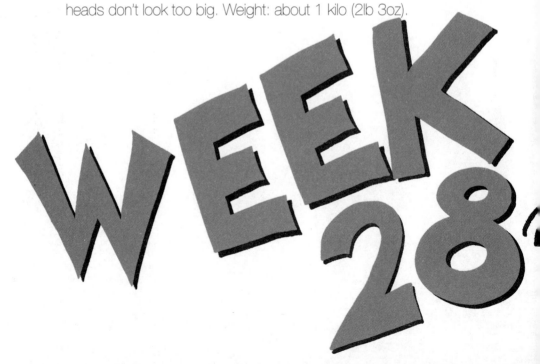

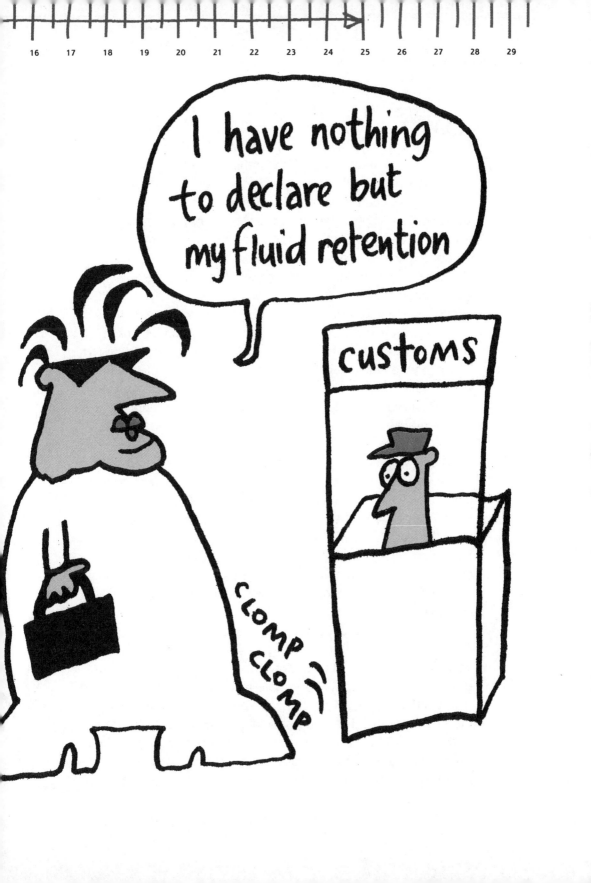

DiARY

My feet hurt to walk, and my tummy's really starting to pull forward, so of course it's time to go travelling again. I'm at Fashion Week in Milan. The usual lot get all the publicity, and if anyone mentions Romeo Gigli to me again I shall have to have them killed. There's nothing wrong with a lacy wisp of froth and a scrinch of lace webbing between your headlights, but it's not like you can actually DO anything in it other than accept your best-supporting-actress award. As one does.

Planes always make my feet swell up, but now it seems to work on the whole body. My fluid retention after I get off the plane at midday is clearly visible to the naked eye. Have gone quite bullfroggy around the face, and the indent marks on the ankles where the socks finish are like trenches. Luckily Beck had suggested I pack some dandelion-leaf tea, which I make at my hotel in a coffee plunger I buy in the lobby shop. The tea tastes as well as looks like lawn clippings. I get so desperate, I make it up and plunge mid-afternoon instead of waiting until morning, and am weeing all night. It works, though.

People now have their routine off pat: 'When are you due?', followed by 'Do you know if it's a boy or a girl?', followed by 'Is it your first?'. I go to a very Fashion Weeky cocktail party (vodka ice lollies instead of devils-on-horseback – but not for me) and meet the lead singer of a band whose name I forgot the moment he told me, who asks 'Is it exciting?' I think this a much better question and earbash him until his eyes glaze over and he staggers to the refreshment tent for more lollies, supported by an elfin keyboard player.

It's becoming harder and harder to manoeuvre the body around, and I am sad to say that grunting while changing position is by no means unknown. I do it on the plane home and gross out the chemical-weapons salesman sitting next to me. I find it very difficult to believe that Geoff would want to have sex with me, and he admits that he doesn't want to ask because (a) I seem so tired, and (b) my body seems rather preoccupied, but he does want to have sex with me because he loves me. This is the sort of answer people should win a three-piece suite for on quiz shows.

We try having sex but it is really quite an absurd proposition. It is impossible to avoid the conclusion that there are three of us involved. Well, there are. I wish I could unstrap the Chelsea bun for a couple of hours. I can now see cellulite on my thighs without having to pinch the skin together. Geoff says 'It's for a reason', and 'It's temporary', and 'It doesn't matter' (give the man another sofa, please), but if THIS is what size I am at six-months pregnant, I am terrified to think of me at nine months. Especially the little matter of getting it OUT.

Sometimes the Chelsea bun kicks really hard and I get a shock. 'Sit down in front!' yells Geoff. And quite often I am forced to move because the baby is clearly going to make the position untenable by stretching against me somewhere uncomfortable. It's odd that so many women say they love to feel their baby move, but they never tell you that sometimes it's really horribly uncomfortable and sometimes it even hurts. Last night in the bath things got really freaky when my rounded tummy momentarily went up into a tentlike shape with a point. At any moment I thought Sigourney Weaver might appear in a singlet.

To add to the glamour of my relationship, apparently I am snoring like a tractor with a coke habit every night.

I have a marvellously glamorous moment in a restaurant debriefing the boss about Fashion Week. As I squeeze between tables on the way to the toilet, I attempt to keep my bump off a nearby table and instead sweep my arse along the table behind me in a majestic arc, taking the two menus and a good bit of the tablecloth with me. Talk about dignity.

info

third-trimester hassles

These three complaints can start earlier, but usually bug pregnant women the most in the last three months.

heartburn

What is it? Heartburn is that burning sensation you feel behind the breastbone, sometimes accompanied by the taste of small amounts of regurgitated food and stomach acid. It doesn't affect the baby.

Why does it happen? Because of the high levels of progesterone during pregnancy, which relaxes muscles, the muscular valve between the stomach and the oesophagus (the tube connecting stomach and mouth) relaxes, and so stomach acid flows up into the oesophagus and sometimes the mouth. It doesn't help that later in the pregnancy your uterus is encroaching on your tummy and squeezing it upwards.

What can you do?

⑥ Eat several small meals slowly, rather than wolfing three main ones.

⑥ Avoid spicy, highly seasoned, fried or fatty foods, chocolate, coffee, alcohol, carbonated drinks, spearmint and peppermint, and anything with lots of chemical additives.

⑥ Wear loose clothing around your tummy.

⑥ Don't fold yourself up on the couch because that squashes your tummy, and bend from the knees, not the waist, to pick things up.

⑥ If the heartburn is worse when you lie flat, try elevating your head by at least 15 centimetres (6 in) with pillows, which will help to stop the yukky stuff flowing up into your mouth.

⑥ Try not to put on too much extra weight.

⑥ Don't smoke.

⑥ Try foods such as milk or yoghurt or acidophilus drinks (sold in all supermarkets) which help to neutralise the stomach acid.

⑥ If none of this helps, ask your doctor to recommend an antacid that is suitable for use during pregnancy. (Avoid preparations containing sodium or sodium bicarbonate.)

backache

Why does it happen?   Progesterone and relaxin relax the ligaments and joints of the spine and around the pelvis. This jollies everything along for childbirth, but makes it hard to have good posture, especially when the weight of the baby puts pressure on your lower back and weakened tummy muscles, and pulls the spine forward.

Lower back and leg pain can be caused by the pressure of the enlarging uterus on the sciatic nerve. The pain may pass as the baby's position changes. If it is very severe, you may have to go to bed for an extended period (not as much fun as it sounds).

What can you do?

⑥ Avoid standing and sitting for long periods of time. When you are standing, tilt your pelvis forward so that your bum tucks under, and keep your shoulders back; when sitting, get yourself well back into the seat, and put your legs up on another chair if possible.

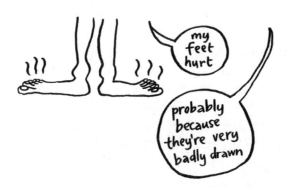

⑥ Do some gentle stretching exercises recommended by your hospital obstetric physiotherapist or by a yoga teacher experienced in pregnancy.

⑥ The flatter your shoes, with good support, the better. This is no time for sparkly, aqua-go-green, platform thigh boots. Sadly.

⑥ Avoid twisting movements such as using a vacuum cleaner, or sports such as tennis, badmington and squash.

⑥ Bend from the knees when lifting things.

Avoid gaining too much weight – hate that one.

For backache itself

⑥ Have a massage.

⑥ Relax in a warm bath or aim the shower spray at the painful area.

⑥ Apply a warm (not hot) hot-water bottle or heat pack.

⑥ If the pain is severe, ask your doctor to prescribe an analgesic safe for use during pregnancy.

⑥ If the pain is really bad, ask your midwife or GP to refer you to the obstetric physiotherapist, or to recommend an osteopath or chiropractor specialising in backache during pregnancy.

swelling and fluid retention

What is it? Swelling (also called oedema), most noticeably of the fingers, legs, ankles and feet, occurs because the body retains more fluid during pregnancy. (Your face can also swell, due to the effects of natural oestrogen and cortisol, a steroid hormone, changing the distribution of fat in the body.)

Some fluid retention and swelling is perfectly normal and should cause no more than mild discomfort. However, if you feel that you are excessively puffy or if the oedema persists for more than 24 hours at a time, you should see your GP. There may be nothing wrong but it can be an early sign of pre-eclampsia (pregnancy-induced high blood pressure; for more on this, see info in 'Week 31').

Why does it happen? Hormonal changes can prompt the kidneys to hang onto salt, leading to fluid retention. There is much more fluid in your body to maintain the level of amniotic fluid, and increase the water level in your blood to help the kidneys to get rid of waste.

Hot weather, standing or sitting for long periods of time and high blood pressure are the most common causes of mild oedema. It also occurs more commonly later in the day, as fluid pools in the ankles and feet – that's gravity for you. In the mornings you might see more puffiness in your eyelids and jawline. It is more likely if you're carrying a multiple pregnancy or excess weight.

What can you do?

⊚ Sit down and elevate your legs higher than 90 degrees; or better still, lie down – on your left side, or on your back supported by a cushion so that your back is tilted 10 degrees or more.

⊚ Wear comfortable shoes.

⊚ Avoid socks or stockings with elasticised tops.

⊚ If the oedema really bothers you, try wearing support tights (these are available in pregnancy fittings with extra tummy room) – and remember to put these on in the morning, when the swelling is less.

⊚ Don't add salt to any food and check the salt content of preprepared foods.

⊚ Drink plenty of water to flush the body free of waste products. Drinking extra water won't increase fluid retention – it may even reduce it.

⊚ If your fingers swell, remember to take off any rings before they become uncomfortably tight.

more possible tests

gestational diabetes

This is a temporary form of diabetes that can arise if the body does not produce enough insulin to keep pace with the increased blood sugar caused by pregnancy. (Some pregnancy hormones act against insulin.) It's routinely screened for by testing the urine at each antenatal check-up and by a blood test, usually at 28 weeks of pregnancy.

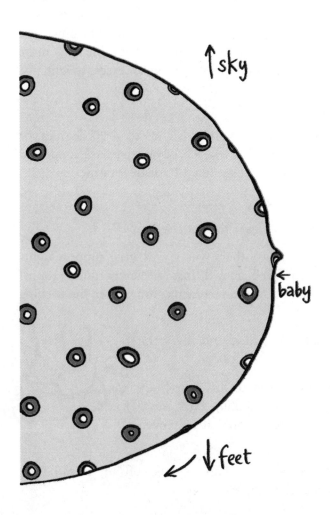

group B streptococcus (GBS)

This bacteria can be found in the vagina and although it will cause no problems for the mother, babies can become really sick if they travel to the outside world down a vagina with GBS present. A vaginal swab is usually routine if it is thought that the baby is in any risk of coming into contact with the bacteria. For instance if you go into labour early, or if the baby's waters break prematurely or before labour starts, or if you have had a previous GBS infection. If the bacteria is found you'll be prescribed antibiotics to clear it up. These are given to you during your labour so that the baby benefits too.

anaemia

Your blood sample will also be checked for haemoglobin levels (indicating anaemia – insufficient iron). See 'Week 2' for more information on iron supplements.

your record

✳ Have you had heartburn? Backache? Fluid retention?

✳ What have you done to treat it?

WEEK

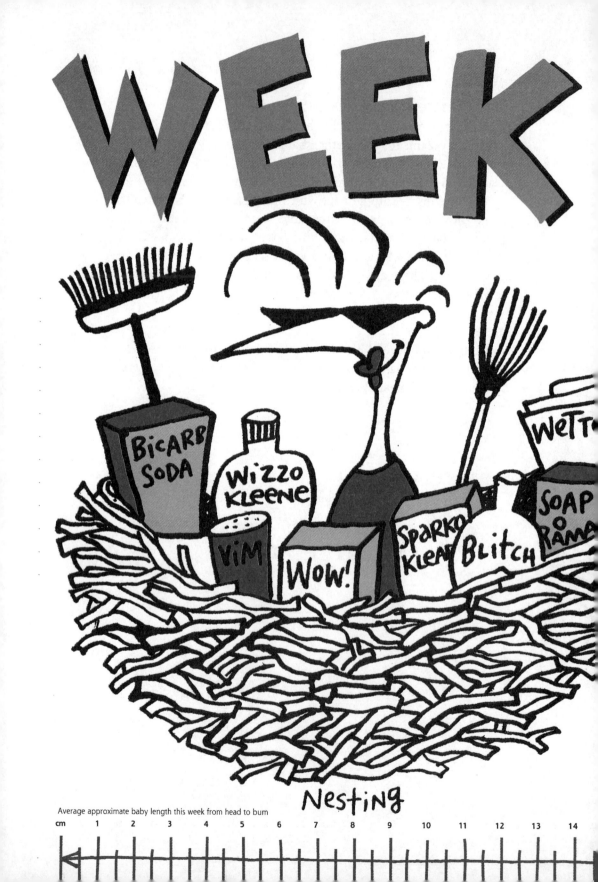

Nesting

Average approximate baby length this week from head to bum

cm 1 2 3 4 5 6 7 8 9 10 11 12 13 14

29

what's going on You may be hard-pressed to find a **comfy sleeping position.** If you feel uncomfortable lying on your back, especially into late pregnancy, that's because the baby is pressing down on the main vein that pumps blood back to your heart. If it doesn't make you uncomfortable, sleeping on your back is fine. Most women who feel discomfort or faintness, even when they're asleep, will automatically move position. (Incidentally, you shouldn't be examined by a **dentist,** or **massaged,** while flat on your back: make sure there's a cushion under your right hip so you're slightly tilted to the left. Nothing makes a dentist flappier than a fainting pregnant woman.).

The baby is looking very babyesque at this point – **plumper** and **rounder.** The newborn-baby breathing rhythm is developing steadily; it's more regular, with fewer **stops** and **starts.** Weight: about 1.15 kilos (2lb 8oz).

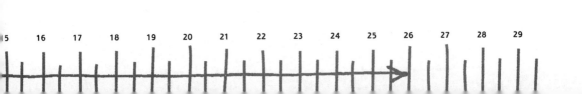

5 16 17 18 19 20 21 22 23 24 25 26 27 28 29

DiARY

I think I've contracted interior design nesting instead of cleaning nesting. (Typical. Even when I'm nesting I don't want to do the dishes, I'd rather arrange some vases in the hallway. Tremendously useful skill around the house.) I am still putting things in boxes and hiring large young men to come to the house while Geoff is at work to move furniture from room to room. Maybe it's not just about making a nest, but about chucking out stuff from the past, stuff you don't need, and working out what you do want.

My thoughts seem to be getting more and more random. I found myself obsessing, while going through my email at work, about the catering arrangments at the hospital. What if I delivered Chelsea bun in the middle of the night? Would there be a kitchen open somewhere that could rustle up some cheese on toast or even an ice-cream scoop of NHS mashed potato? Or do I need to get Geoff to bring along a few provisions and a camping stove? Will have to ask the midwife about that one.

I have discovered that pregnancy makes you sweat more – if you're not retaining it, you're leaking it, or sometimes both at once. Not to mention all that extra blood in there. I tried a strong antiperspirant, but it only blocked my pores and I felt like I was carrying a marble around in my armpit for a couple of days. I had to go without any and then went back to deodorant. I can remember at sixteen weeks when I skipped ahead in the books and thought, 'God, look at twenty-eight weeks.' It seemed so far away. But now I'm here, in a flash. Better take some photos while I'm looking pregnant.

Weeing a zillion times a night, too. Trying to remember to do pelvic-floor exercises. Too boring for words. And my shoes have started smelling awful. I have sprayed them with a perfume called Fracas. Ava Gardner's perfume of choice, Beck told me. I bet Ava never had to spray it in her shoes, though.

Childbirth classes start this week. I don't want to go. For some reason it feels like having to go to Sunday School. I can't stand those things where some earth mother at the front of the classroom asks us all to share our feelings. I've already done the physio classes, dammit. If I wanted to share my feelings with

strangers I'd hire a billboard. I don't want to bond with the group.
They're not going to be there when I have the baby, or when it
grows up. I don't care what they think or what they do, really.
Perhaps I should wear a name tag saying, 'Hi! I'm a Churlish
Bitch'. Geoff, by contrast, seems quite into it all.

Our first childbirth class goes like this: a large, motherly
looking midwife called Melissa in a cuddly blue cashmere cardie
and black leggings gives us all a sticky-label name tag as we walk
in the door. We have to interview another couple (everyone is in
a couple! – what's the world coming to?), and then
introduce them to the class. 'Deborah and Richard are
drug dealers. They conceived accidentally during a
police raid. Deborah intends to take at least a year off.'
Unfortunately not quite that interesting.

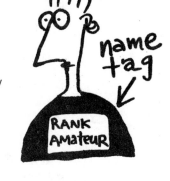

We are divided into men's and women's groups. I
put my middle name on the name tag out of perversity
so Geoff has to keep squinting at my chest and saying
things like, 'Um . . . Georgia is going out to work and
I'm staying home.' I feel it would be more entertaining
if he could just admit he's forgotten the name of the
mother of his child. Anyway, each group is asked to
come up with a list of questions they would like the
class to answer. This almost gets diverting.

WOMEN

Can we eat during labour? (Yes, a bit in the early stages.)

Can we video the birth? (Depends on the midwives and
consultant. Some don't allow videos. Others would wear a
party hat if you asked nicely.)

**What happens if I go for a home birth and then it turns
into an emergency?** (The group will be talking about home
births next week. But apparently the two midwives who attend
a home birth will always call the hospital to let them know
they have a woman in labour, and they'll call an ambulance if
it's needed, and stay with you.)

I want hints to help me in labour. (We'll be covering that.)

When is it really labour? (That too.)

Tell us every single pain-relief option. (Certainly.)

Is there a modem link in the delivery suite so that we can webcam the birth on the Internet? (No.)

Do men ever display the nesting instinct? (Frankly, no.)

MEN

How do we know when it starts? (We'll be covering this.)

What should we expect on the day? (Ditto.)

What support can we give? (All this will be revealed.)

Do WE get any drugs? (Funny how every group asks that.)

What is the man's role during labour? (Do whatever she tells you and be quick about it.)

What if we faint? (Keep up on meals and soft drinks during labour and sit down if you think you might faint.)

How to recognise signs of postnatal depression? (That will be discussed.)

What to have ready at home? (Alcohol. Jewels.)

What if the baby comes early and quickly? (Ring the ambulance and follow their instructions.)

Melissa gives us quick responses to these questions and explains that the first lesson will be on signs that labour isn't far off (maybe hours or days). Signs include the 'show', which is the mucus plug coming out (she says that it might be the size of a 20p piece on your undies, and possibly bloody and mucusy); and the 'waters breaking', which is about a cup of amniotic fluid leaking or gushing out when the membranes break (she says don't get it on the car upholstery because it rots it, so from thirty-five weeks

I'll be sitting on a tarpaulin and four towels in the passenger seat of Geoff's precious van). I ask if it's true the waters smell of pickles. Melissa looks sideways and lets us know it's a sweet smell that's actually, ahem, rather like semen.

Other signs that labour may begin soon are: tummy dropping as the baby's head engages with the pelvis, nesting and cleaning, more Braxton Hicks practice contractions, increased vaginal secretions, pelvic pressure and heaviness in the groin, and a decrease in foetal movements.

Then Melissa points to a chart and explains the following parts of a pregnant woman's anatomy: the vagina ('If you didn't know where that was, you wouldn't be here'), cervix (the bit between the vagina and the uterus), foetus, and fundus (the top of the uterus). She explains that labour contractions begin in the fundus and the pain radiates down to period-cramp territory in the lower abdomen. Our bags should be packed by thirty-five weeks as thirty-eight weeks is considered 'full term'.

Two hours of this and I'm ready for a whisky. Ready, willing, but not able. Next week, apparently, there'll be a video of birth techniques. I can't say I'm overly looking forward to that one.

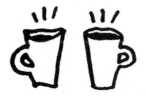

info

what are the signs of early labour?

No matter how much you're feeling like pregnancy has gone on quite long enough, labour is a shock – and premature labour very much more so. However, remember you're living in a developed country with a pretty good neonatal service. If you're living near a major town, your local hospital will be set up for premature babies; if you're in a rural area, you will be transferred to a specialist centre, before the baby is born if time permits, otherwise as soon as possible.

Labour is considered premature if it begins earlier than the thirty-eighth week of pregnancy. Early signs that you may be in labour are:

⑥ Cramps, like period pains, that may be accompanied by nausea, diarrhoea or indigestion.

⑥ Increasing pain or feeling of pressure in the lower back.

⑥ Unusual or persistent achiness or feeling of pressure in the pelvic floor, thighs or groin.

⑥ A watery or pinkish or brownish discharge, possibly preceded by the passage of the thick mucus plug (euuggh!) that has been blocking your cervix.

⑥ Fluid from your vagina (your 'waters breaking'), which means the amniotic sac has ruptured and some amniotic fluid is rushing or trickling out.

late bleeding

Some light bleeding or spotting in the second and third trimesters is usually okay, but you need to have it checked out immediately at the maternity hospital to be absolutely sure. Two uncommon conditions that cause bleeding late in pregnancy are placenta praevia and placental abruption.

placenta praevia or low-lying placenta

The placenta is attached to the lower part of the uterine wall, instead of the upper part, partially or completely blocking the way out. In the late stages of pregnancy, as the uterus stretches and the cervix ripens (becomes thinner and softer, ready to 'dilate' – open wide – enough for the baby to pass through during birth), a placenta attached to the lower uterus can become detached, causing painless bleeding. The risk of having placenta praevia is increased if you have uterine scarring from previous pregnancies or surgery, or there's more than one baby in there; it also seems to be more common among smokers.

If you do have any bleeding, an ultrasound scan will confirm the position of the placenta. If the placenta is low-lying you may need a caesarean at a later stage of your pregnancy and your obstetrician will adopt a 'wait and see' approach. However if the bleeding is severe you may need an emergency caesarean there and then.

placental abruption (abruptio placentae) or placental separation

Placental abruption is when the placenta comes away from the uterine wall too early. The amount of bleeding and also the amount of pain depend on how much of the placenta has come away. The cause is unknown, but it tends to be more common in women who have had two or more children, women with raised blood pressure, and smokers. Sometimes the problem resolves itself and the pregnancy continues as normal. Sometimes the birth must be induced; in serious, sudden cases a caesarean is necessary.

Remember: both these conditions are rare.

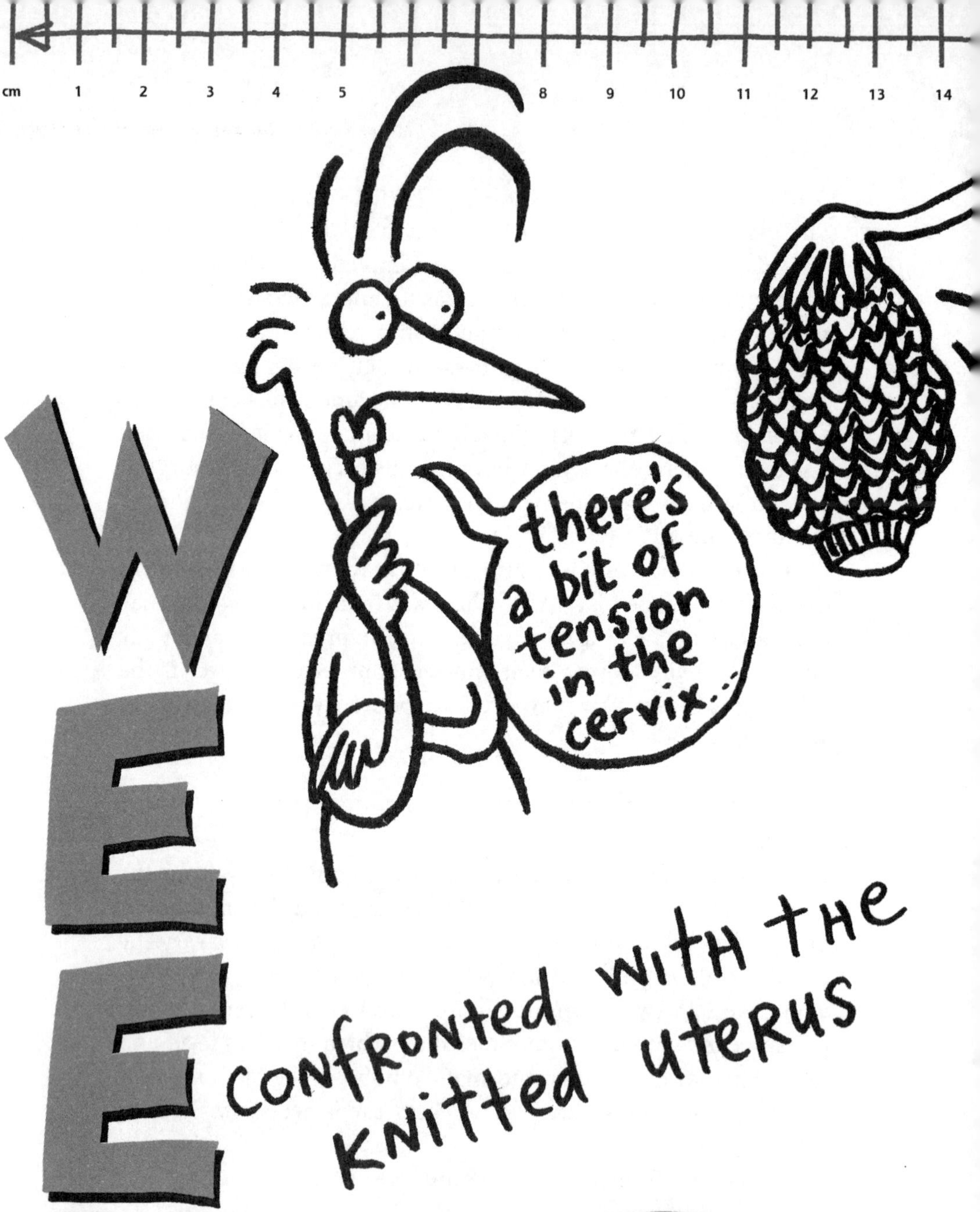

WEEK 30

confronted with the knitted uterus

what's going on
Your breasts are STILL getting bigger. Will they ever stop? Yes. You might be feeling Braxton Hicks practice contractions now, although most people don't feel them until the last weeks. Proper contractions last for one minute each, come at intervals of five minutes or less and go on for at least an hour, and then after a while a baby comes out. So if that happens, you're probably really in labour.

This week and the following three, the baby puts on fat at a greater rate. The skin is still a bit wrinkled, so there's room for the new fat underneath. The lanugo will start to fall out, although a full head of hair may stay. The eyes are fully open, but it can't be very interesting just watching all that hair floating around. Baby hiccuping starts to get more violent: you can feel the jerks. The baby may be jiggled around by the Braxton Hicks contractions. Weight: about 1.3 kilos(1lb 13ozs).

DiARY

Take a day off work and go to spend it with Susanne and her baby (she finally plumped for Teresa). It reminds me that there's a reward at the end of all this. Not that it all seems entirely relaxing. Susanne is full of advice about the changing-table arrangement, the best nappies and nipple creams, etc. I really must start taking notes.

Also go to the clinic and see Anne the midwife. The receptionist takes my name and gives me a big smile, saying 'It must be soon.' 'Soon!' I shriek. 'It's ten weeks away. I can't even begin to tell you what I have to get done before it arrives!'

When Anne examines me, she smiles and says, 'Your baby is big and healthy.' I almost swoon at her feet, and can hardly stop myself from kissing her when she follows up with this advice on my weight: 'Worry about it after the baby is born. The only rule you need to follow is don't eat junk food.'

All the skinny girls at work put on more than 20 kilos during their pregnancy and lose it again afterwards. You can't go on a weight-loss diet during pregnancy. You (well, all right then, I) can stop eating a Magnum a day though, which might help. I tell myself that it's more dangerous for a baby if I don't put on enough weight during pregnancy than if I end up looking like a pivotal protagonist in *Moby Dick: The Mini-series*.

For a fashion designer, I've got bugger-all to wear. Even if I could find anything good to fit, shopping is no fun any more because after walking for 15 minutes my feet feel like someone's been whacking them rhythmically with a baton for an hour. However, on the way back from the clinic, I step inside a posh babycare shop and accidentally spend £120 on things like blankets and vests and tiny baby-socks. The worst of it is I feel weepy looking at the stuff and have to brush away the tears even as I reach for my credit card.

Geoff is being a prince – well, a prince's servant – still doing all the dishes and cooking most nights. (He tends to cut things up into infinitesimally small pieces, but never look a gift dinner in the mixed metaphorical mouth, I say.) Meantime, the delivery vans are queueing around the block. More shelves. A changing table.

Second week of childbirth classes. And tonight our special project is: Normal Labour. Melissa is slightly less perky and it turns out she's been delivering babies for the past 36 hours. Still, a cup of tea and she has rallied, giving us a pep talk about having faith in your body and the pain being part of a natural process. I don't really believe in this. I have always thought childbirth was actually a design fault, though it is strangely comforting to know that millions of women have done it. To accompany her explanation of the mechanics of birthing, Melissa produces a very startling pink knitted uterus with a cream cuff on it, which represents the cervix. I don't know where she got the pattern.

What Melissa says, waving the knitted uterus to emphasise her points, is that the average for a first-time labour is 12 to 16 hours. The time is counted from the start of getting regular contractions. (Statistically, second and subsequent babies slither out after about 6 hours.) I'm still not clear about this 12 to 16 hours. It seems to be roughly made up of 10 to 12 hours waiting for the cervix to dilate to 10 centimetres (first stage), and then say 2 hours pushing and shouting at people (second stage). After that there is a third stage of labour, when the placenta comes out, which nobody seems particularly interested in. If an injection of oxytocin is given this takes between 6 and 10 minutes. If it comes out naturally, it's usually under an hour.

Melissa says that your waters can break at any time before or during the labour, even right at the very end. I think this was news to us all. At first the contractions last for 20 seconds, like a period cramp. They increase from 20 minutes apart to 5 minutes apart. During the last bit of the first stage, the contractions are very intense and 3–5 minutes apart.

The second stage of labour is heralded by the 'transition' – when the cervix is almost completely dilated (about 10 centimetres): wide enough for the baby's head to fit through. Ow. Ow ow OW. The contractions are only 2 or 3 minutes apart and last for up to 90 seconds. This is usually the stage when women scream for an epidural and are often refused.

'If you're abusive we know you're nearly there,' says Melissa.

If it's bad, adds Melissa, this is a stage when you can be shaky and vomit from the shock and stress, and you flake out for those tiny minutes between contractions. At this point most of the men in the class move closer to their partners and take their hands. (You can tell they're thinking, 'Oh you poor dear', and then, 'Glad I don't have to do that bit.') They will not be so free with their fingers during the real thing: support people are advised that only two fingers be gripped by the labouring woman as any more fingers are easier to squish together, and even break.

The final push, apparently, feels very like the urge to poo, and during this birthing stage, Melissa tells us, women often keep changing positions – we are no longer slotted into stirrups. Some women have their baby on all fours or a birth stool, or sitting up on the bed. Squatting is popular elsewhere in the world but it is not something we do a lot of, so unless you're on one of those giant inflatable birth balls they have in some labour rooms it will probably be too much for your leg muscles.

'Once the head is through, that's the hard bit done – unless you've got a really big baby and then the shoulders can be difficult.' Melissa then talks about the third stage of labour, which involves the expulsion of a large stuffed red stocking, with a veil around the edge that makes it look like a giant jellyfish, and a twisty grey dressing-gown cord hanging from it, which is the placenta and umbilical cord. 'Often we ask the dad if he wants to cut the cord,' Melissa says. For some reason every woman in the class packs up laughing.

Then we watch two videos. The first one is narrated by a serious bloke who says things like 'some of the joy and happiness brought about by this happy event' and 'this stained mucus plug' as if he were reading the regional news. This happy event and the stained mucus plug are both brought to us by somebody called Helen, who wears a yellow jumper until the second stage of labour, when she changes into a mauve silk negligee (bad move, really). At the hospital Helen wanders the corridors like Lady Macbeth and then ends up panting, which Melissa has said is not good so early in the labour. Another midwife turns up in a rather fetching lycra top and holds one of Helen's legs while Michael, her husband, holds the other. Being in labour is probably the only time a woman wouldn't even notice this happening. Then midwife one squirts some cold detergent on Julie's private parts, which Melissa says is shocking behaviour as it gives Helen quite a fright. 'We like to give you a quick, warm wash,' she says. And finally it's birth time, with the midwife holding the baby back so it doesn't come out in too much of a rush, and tear Helen. The head comes out a very grey-blue and turns slowly before the rest slips out.

The Helen video is 15 minutes long, which seems perhaps a little misleading. Nonetheless, nearly every man in the room has gone into shock and half of them have tried to crawl into their partner's lap – forgetting that, with a seven-month pregnant woman, lap space is at a premium.

We watch a second video from Brazil, showing a sequence of women giving birth in the squatting position, under the guidance of a man in a white coat. Only the highlights are shown, the babies slipping out and being caught, rather like a kind of football world cup round-up. The women then scoop the babies up as if they do it every day.

This seems a bit of a fantasy, but light relief after Helen's fifteen minutes of glory, and I broach the subject of a move to Brazil on the way home with Geoff. He's in a kind of trance and doesn't seem to hear a word.

Back in bed, poor old Geoff is squished into an area the size of an envelope. I waddle to the toilet about six times a night and have taken to having under-desk naps at work. And the mood swings! Geoff never knows whether he's coming home to Medusa or Mrs Bunnikins. One of the male models looks at me in the lift at work and blurts out, 'What happens to all that stomach . . . afterwards?' 'I'm giving it to the Salvation Army,' I reply.

Still, this was probably the perfect week to consider the realities of childbirth as I am just changing from major denial (well yes, I know I'm pregnant, but I don't think I actually want to go through giving birth) to major denial (look, I know I'm pregnant, but I really don't want to think about how this baby everyone keeps saying is so HUGE is going to get out).

info

premature birth

why does it happen?

Most premature births are deliberate – a planned intervention by the obstetrician due to concern over, most commonly, a mother's high blood pressure (this is referred to as PET) or a baby's slow growth (referred to as IUGR). However, a relatively small percentage of pregnancies results in unplanned premature labour. It is not always clear why this happens, though possible factors may include:

⊚ Over-distended uterus caused by more than one baby, or too much amniotic fluid.

⊚ Incompetent cervix (this means your cervix isn't staying tightly closed enough).

⊚ Early rupture of the membranes of the amniotic sac ('waters breaking').

⊚ The mother has a urine infection.

Premature labour also tends to occur if there is a serious problem with the baby in the uterus, but such problems will usually have already been observed and acted upon.

how early is too early?

Any baby born before thirty-seven completed weeks is considered premature, or preterm. With specialist care, babies as young as twenty-four weeks can survive. By thirty weeks, there is a 90 per cent survival rate, and more than 80 per cent of these babies will be fine after a bit of special care.

If there is enough warning, the aim would be to try to delay the labour or delivery for twenty four hours so that the mother can be given steroids to improve their baby's lung development. Some drugs, known as tocolytic agents, can be effective in stopping the uterus contracting. Delaying tactics would also be used if mother and baby needed to be transferred to a hospital where a specialist neonatal unit could care for the baby at birth.

special care
Premature babies are often delivered by caesarean section, particularly if there are complicating factors such as pre-eclampsia, signs of foetal distress or breech birth (bum-first baby). However, if the problem is a mother's high blood pressure, the baby will be induced in a vaginal birth. Labour tends to be quicker than normal with premature babies.

⑥ A neonatal paediatrician will be part of the medical team at any premature birth: in other words, a specialist in premature babies will be there. Your baby's condition may be assessed using a test of responses at 1 minute and again at 5 minutes after birth, called the APGAR score.

⑥ Your baby will need help with temperature regulation and possibly breathing. Therefore it will be placed in an incubator and taken to the hospital's intensive neonatal care unit where it may be ventilated. The care unit is normally attached to the maternity unit and found in the same building.

⑥ If antenatal steroids were not received by the baby and its lungs are not developed enough yet, surfactant-replacement therapy may be used. This involves using an artifical protein in place of surfactant, a substance that normally completely coats the lungs in the last weeks of pregnancy to prevent them collapsing.

⑥ Some small babies have difficulties in feeding. They have a sucking reflex but cannot feed for long periods and tire easily. They will need to be fed small frequent amounts, usually through a tube. If your baby can take milk, you can express your breast milk so that this can be given. Those babies who get their mothers' milk do better and so you might want to consider breast feeding, if feasible. This is something positive you can do that will really help your baby's progress.

⑥ Premature babies grow and thrive better if exposed to the mother's voice, massage, skin-to-skin contact with parents or carers ('kangaroo care'), soft music, recordings of heartbeats, and water beds or hammocks that simulate movement in the uterus. You and your partner will be encouraged to be with your baby as much as is possible and your relatives, too, can help with the constant care.

common premature characteristics
Premature babies differ from full-term babies in a number of usually temporary ways.

⑥ Obviously, premature babies weigh less than full-termers.

⑥ They are small, red, wrinkly and frail, with relatively large head and hands.

⑥ Their skin is pale, and blood vessels can easily be seen underneath because there is not much fat.

⑥ There is a layer of fine hair (lanugo) on the body.

⑥ Their motor functions, including breathing and feeding, are less efficient and their cry is not as lusty as that of a full-term newborn baby.

⑥ They tend to be irritable in the early days, though this can be combated with soothing care, soft noises and love.

your record

✳ What experiences have you had of childbirth?

✳ Have you been to a birth? What was it like?

✳ What videos and descriptions have impressed you either
positively or negatively?

what's going on

Hello stretch marks here, there and possibly everywhere! What a splendid mauve, perhaps an attractive aubergine colour, or is it hot pink? Mind your posture, as your tummy will be putting you off balance.

The baby can blink or close its eyes when a bright light is shone onto your tummy. There's a lot of brain action going on: receiving and sending lots of signals through the nervous system, maybe testing out the idea of thinking, possibly wondering how long it has to hang out in a hairy swamp. The baby's definite awake and sleeping times are still usually roughly the opposite of yours. Weight: about 1.5 kilos (3lb 4oz).

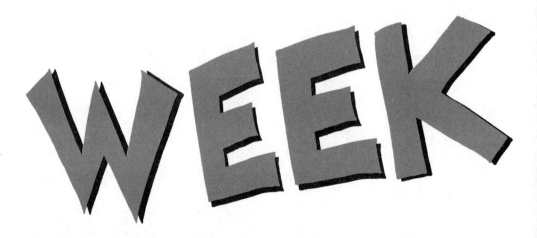

Average approximate baby length this week from head to bum

| cm | 1 | 2 | 3 | 4 | 5 | 6 | 7 | 8 | 9 | 10 | 11 | 12 | 13 | 14 |

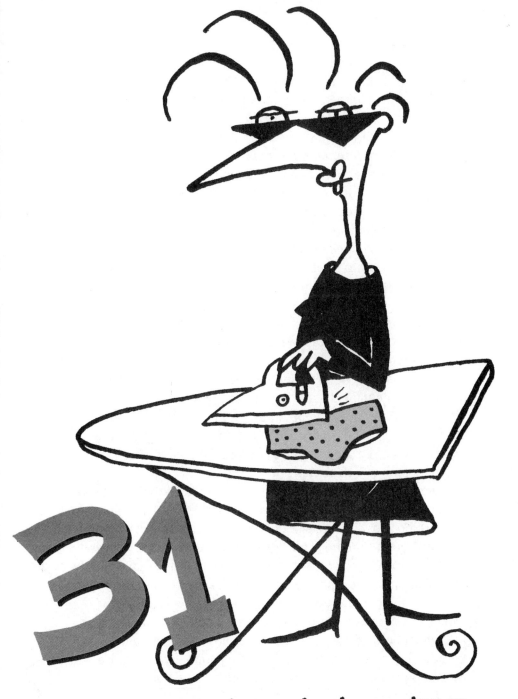

31

Guard against madness —
DON'T IRON YOUR UNDIES!

15 16 17 18 19 20 21 22 23 24 25 26 27 28 29

DiARY

I'm a little breathless because my lungs are all squished up. Unfortunately this does not make me sound like Marilyn Monroe singing 'Happy Birthday, Mr President'; it's more like an over-exerted warthog. Also, I have a constant ache where the ligaments from the baby area extend down to the groin. Leg cramps keep waking me up at 4am, and I can't get back to sleep.

Beck says it's probably not magnesium deficiency but a circulation problem and maybe I should walk shorter distances every day instead of half a mile from the tube, every other day, when I decide not to splash out on a taxi home from work. Maybe I get worse cramps during the nights when I don't walk.

During my walk today a huge truck pulled up near the park with rolls of wire in the back, and a big burly bloke in a reflective vest got down from the cab, walked around to the passenger seat and collected a 2-year-old girl with a Milly Molly Mandy haircut. 'Come on, darling,' he said. And they went to feed the pigeons.

It made me think that having children brings out the best kindness and the worst temper in us. And I hope it will bring out the best in me, not the worst. Or at least when it brings out the worst there will be someone else to take up the slack while I go and bite some telegraph poles.

Geoff and I spend the best part of an afternoon looking at cots. It's amazing – some of them even LOOK dangerous, having gaps that a rhinoceros could practically climb out of. Not much more to buy now, but it would be nice if the washer-dryer fairy paid a visit.

Never speak too soon about household appliances. Just after I write that bit I notice that the enamel is flaking off the toaster onto our toast, so no doubt I've been ingesting bits of plutonium or aluminium or something. Then this creepy guy turns up to service the central heating boiler, which I thought should have a new fan because the old one sounded a bit like a jetfighter landing. He opens up the front and says, 'It's a wonder you're not dead.'

'Excuse me?'

'This thing's been leaking carbon monoxide. You could have nodded off to sleep on the couch and never woken up. I'm surprised you're still alive.'

Well. When I finally managed to rustle the repairman out the front door, I burst into tears and call Geoff, only to get his mobile. Damn, damn, damn, he is probably down the back of the garden centre explaining succulents to some dopey businessman, so I call the midwifery department at the hospital, where FINALLY, just before I think I'll go mad, a midwife assures me that unless I have experienced the symptoms of carbon monoxide poisoning (severe nausea, severe headaches and severe lethargy and faintness) nothing will have crossed the placenta, and even if it has the likely result will have been a lack of oxygen getting to the baby, similar to what would happen if I smoked or walked around in the traffic all day, in which case the baby might be a little small.

'No,' I tell her. 'The general consensus is that I am having a baby approximately the size of Danny de Vito.'

'Well,' she says, 'nothing to worry about then.'

Phew.

The lump is really very uncomfortable now. Beck has prescribed a grab-bag of different supplements for me (which she hates doing) to try to bring down my fluid retention. Vitamin E, vitamin C, dandelion-leaf tincture (all at very precisely calibrated doses or it won't work), a complicated specialist herbal mixture that tastes like a petroleum byproduct with bats' ears in it, and I'm sure if she thought it would help I would have to hang upside down every 3 hours as well. Dr Fisher just shrugged his shoulders and said he hoped it helps because he can't give me drugs.

Every now and then I forget I'm pregnant for a minute or two, and then the baby kicks or I have to move. Geoff is being very sympathetic. I can't believe I have put on 17 kilos. From behind I look like two driver's-side airbags going off.

Go and buy some 100 per cent cotton cot sheets – very hard to find. Another pregnant woman and I both put a hand on the last set. We look at each other.

She says graciously, 'You take it, you're more pregnant than me.'

Sisterhood!

'Most people,' says the shop assistant, 'don't buy 100 per cent cotton because they have to iron the sheets.'

'Iron the sheets?!' I shriek. 'Are they mad?!'

Our third childbirth class: when to come to the hospital. Melissa says to come to hospital when your contractions are five minutes apart, the waters have broken or you're overwrought, but to ring first in case they've all stepped out for a daiquiri. No, to tell them what's been happening. Once you get to the hospital a midwife will inspect you and assess your state of labour.

Here are the main points I shall have to memorise.

False contractions are irregular, don't increase in intensity and usually go away if you lie down.

The waters breaking can be a tiny trickle or 1–2 litres (1$^{3/4}$-3$^{1/2}$pt) of amniotic fluid coming out. Put on a pad. You're supposed to write down the time your waters break and note the quality and colour of the fluid. If there's a stain, or blood in the waters, tell your midwife or hospital staff immediately, by phone.

Don't ring everyone and tell them you're in labour or they'll all be round to the house or turning up at the hospital or getting times wrong and starting rumours. Don't play hockey – conserve your energy for the labour.

Everyone is on the edge of their seat. This is what we came for – a bit of a chat about the real thing. Mind you, I thought there'd be a lot more beanbag action, and a lot more practice breathing. Apparently it's out of fashion. I am so glad Melissa is not the type to say, 'Pinch your hand as hard as you can', each week to demonstrate the pain of labour.

Melissa says not to worry if you poo during labour, and you probably won't because diarrhoea is often an early sign of labour so you'll have got rid of all the poo before you deliver. Anyway, now that I've done a wee on my own floor because my pelvic-floor muscles are so hopeless, I suspect I can poo on the hospital's, no problem.

Everyone is rather surprised to learn a few things. No wonder the baby comes out with its eyes closed – otherwise the first thing it would see is its mother's . . . ahem . . . arsehole. Also, after the baby comes out there's an enormous gush of fluid: the banked-up amniotic fluid – and up to 300 millilitres (10$^{1/2}$fl oz) of blood. (A 'post-partum haemorrhage' is technically more than 500 millilitres (21fl oz.)

At that point I thought things would be pretty much all over but I'd forgotten there's the third stage – the placenta comes out. (In order to demonstrate the placenta, Melissa drops the 'baby' on the carpet, which she promises not to do if she's assisting at any of our births.) And then the midwife or doctor will do a bit of classy embroidery on any tears or cuts. Melissa gives us the hospital's March stats: four hundred and fifty deliveries, two hundred and twenty-two intact perineums. Yikes.

info

pre-eclampsia

what is it?

It used to be called pre-eclamptic toxaemia (if your mum had it, that's what it would have been called). It only ever happens in pregnancy, and it's diagnosed from a combination of signs and symptoms, including a rise in blood pressure; swelling of the ankles, feet, hands and face; sudden weight gain due to fluid retention; upper abdominal pains; visual disturbance; and protein in your wee.

Pre-eclampsia is a serious condition that affects up to 10 per cent of pregnant women, usually in the late stages of pregnancy, though it can occur as early as Week 26. Occasionally the onset will coincide with labour and, rarely, it can occur after delivery. The cause has still not been established.

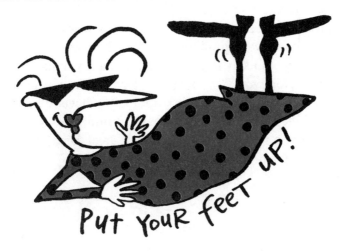

Put your feet up!

Pre-eclampsia can interfere with the blood supply to the placenta, affecting the baby's growth. It can cause the baby to come early as labour may be induced in an attempt to prevent further rise in the blood pressure. Untreated high blood pressure can damage the mother's kidneys, nervous system and blood vessels.

Sometimes pre-eclampsia can get worse very fast: symptoms (apart from fluid retention) may include persistent headaches, blurred vision, 'seeing' flashing lights, upper or mid abdominal pain, irritability, nausea and vomiting. Women being treated for pre-eclampsia, if not hospitalised, should get emergency medical treatment at the onset of any of these symptoms.

Severe pre-eclampsia can escalate into eclampsia, which is a life-threatening condition for mother and foetus, but is now extremely rare because of better medical monitoring. Eclampsia can cause convulsions, kidney failure and coma. Blood vessels in the uterus go into spasm and cut down the blood supply to the baby.

checks

Early detection and treatment mean pre-eclampsia is better checked for and managed, though it can't be prevented. Your urine and blood pressure are checked at each antenatal visit, and you should tell your pregnancy carer about any puffiness or swelling, headaches or gastric pain. (Having only one of the pre-eclampsia symptoms, such as fluid retention, doesn't mean you have pre-eclampsia.) As pre-eclampsia can occur at any time from 26 weeks it is important to seek help if you suffer from any of the symptoms mentioned above. Visit your midwife or GP and if you still do not feel well, speak to the staff at the maternity unit.

You're more likely to get pre-eclampsia if you had high blood pressure before you were pregnant; have a family history of pre-eclampsia or high blood pressure; had or have kidney disease; have diabetes; have had or are having a multiple pregnancy; had pre-eclampsia in a previous pregnancy; are a teenager or an older mum; or if the pregnancy is your first.

treatment

Treatment for very mild pre-eclampsia may include bed rest at home or in hospital and careful monitoring of you and your baby. Tests may include blood and urine checks, monitoring of the foetal heart rate, and ultrasound scans to check the weight of the baby and measure the blood flow to the placenta.

If the condition progresses or is advanced when diagnosed, you'll need to go to hospital. You may need medication to wrestle

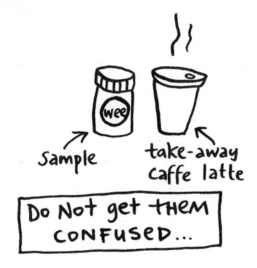

Sample

take-away
caffe latte

Do Not get them
CONFused...

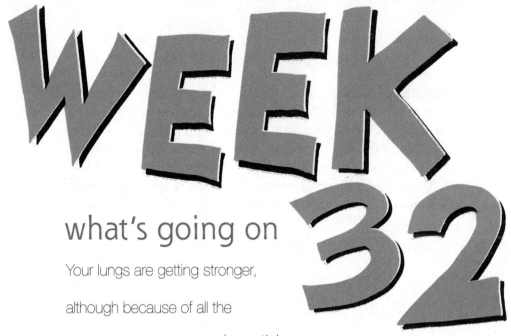

WEEK 32

what's going on

Your lungs are getting stronger, although because of all the pressure you may feel breathless if you overdo it. You may be starting to get a bit sick of the whole pregnancy thing. It's uncomfortable being this big, you're running out of outfits and as for sleeping well – ha!

The baby's lungs are stronger too, but not fully ready to go yet. The baby is filling out with fat, although it still looks a bit on the skinny side. It might be upside down in readiness for the lunge to the outside world. This is pretty much your complete baby item, covered in vernix. If the baby was born now it would open its eyes and take a peek at the world (except it can't focus on much at this age and will look endearingly cross-eyed). Weight: about 1.7 kilos (3lb 12oz).

cm   1   2   3   4   5   6   7   8   9   10   11   12   13   14

OH MY GOD MY BABY'S going to Be A SCORPIO!

sorry Munchy

Average approximate baby length this week from head to bum

15 16 17 18 19 20 21 22 23 24 25 26 27 28 29

DIARY

I walk into Anne's Midwives' Examination Room.
'You look tired and bloated,' she says.
Charmed, I'm sure.

She says the insomniac sore legs when lying
down are probably due to the fluid retention. She listens to the
baby's heartbeat, asks if the baby's moving (is it ever: the Chelsea
bun does all-night salsa), and measures the length of the uterus.

'The baby's doing beautifully – you're doing brilliantly well,'
she says.

It's very kind the way she does this sort of positive bit after
telling me that I look like shit (in the nicest possible way).

There are no safe drugs for fluid retention during pregnancy,
she explains.

'Why can't I take diuretics?' I whine.

'Two reasons. They reduce placental blood flow, and they can
mask the symptoms of pre-eclampsia.'

Oh all right, smartypants.

She takes a couple of vials of blood to check if there's a high
level of uric acid and to check if my platelets are at all 'deranged'
– both signs that I might be susceptible to pre-eclampsia. I quite
like the idea of my platelets being deranged. I'm so responsible
these days there should be some part of me acting like an idiot,
but on second thoughts I can definitely do without pre-eclampsia.
I have to come again next week because I'm retaining so much
fluid Anne wants to keep an eye on it.

Week 4 of the childbirth class: Melissa's potted version of
stuff that might happen that isn't your ideal plan. Forceps might
be used if you're too tired to push any more, the baby seems to
be staying put, you've been pushing for too long (1–2 hours), or
there are signs of foetal distress. Usually you'll get an epidural
first. I can see why when Melissa holds up a pair of forceps. They
look like very upmarket, Italian, oversized salad servers from one
of those designer shops full of stuff that people don't really need
but has 'Alessi' written all over it. There are three types: rotator
forceps (also known as Kiellands forceps), Wrigley forceps and
Neville Barnes forceps. I hope nobody ever says, 'This is a job for

Neville.' It never ceases to amaze me what men will name after themselves.

Then there's the rather sophisticated-sounding ventouse, a vacuum cup that they can stick on the baby's head and, well, pull it out. (It's a vacuum in the sense of the plumber's mate, not the type you do the carpet with.) Melissa sits there absent-mindedly playing with the soft-toy baby on her lap. So far she's folded it in half and is waving one of its feet past its ear.

Emergency caesareans are performed when a large baby is stuck, the cervix just isn't getting any wider or the baby is really distressed. Usually you'll get an epidural or a spinal block to numb the lower half of your body. After a caesarean you get morphine or pethidine – 'Hi baby! Mummy's reeeeally stoned!' Usually you're on a drip and have a catheter for weeing for up to twelve hours. The baby feeds as normal, and the dad, another helper or a staff member does the nappy changes and baths and stuff.

And then there's the bizarre-sounding 'induction'. A hospital obstetrician may bring on ('induce') labour if you're more than one to two weeks overdue; if your little bub isn't growing well; or if you have pre-eclampsia. Melissa says she knows of a doctor who induced a baby because its mother didn't want a Scorpio, and another one who refused to induce a baby on the fourth of July for an American couple.

Then Melissa talks about stillbirth. Everyone in the room goes very quiet. She says she doesn't want to talk about it, but she has to because it does still happen rarely that a baby is born dead, or is born with so many problems that it slips away from life a few days later. She says that in the case of a stillbirth, the baby often hasn't moved for a day or two before the labour. So always call your midwife if you haven't felt the baby move for 12 hours. Usually the baby's fine and just quiet, getting ready for labour, and the midwife will play you its heartbeat for reassurance.

If a baby is stillborn, the hospital organises to have photos taken and inked footprints on a card done, even if you don't want these mementoes at the time. (One bereaved mum called after three years to get her's.) Melissa's eyes fill with tears as she talks, and so do mine.

info

birth plan

what is it?

You write down all the things you want to happen during your labour. It's not a legal contract, but rather a memo of understanding between you and your midwives and other birth attendants: it can cover everything from what pain relief you want to who's going to hold the baby first.

It's also a starting point for discussion with your midwives or obstetrician about their usual procedure and about the policies of the hospital or birth centre, and about things such as playing the music of your choice during labour, family and friends being able to visit straight after the birth, and so on. You may not be able to have your own way on everything – this is the time to find out.

Discuss your birth plan with the midwives or obstetrician early on, so that you're not still negotiating as the baby's coming out. The birth plan is usually incorporated in the antenatal notes as a page for you to write on. Tuck a copy away in your handbag.

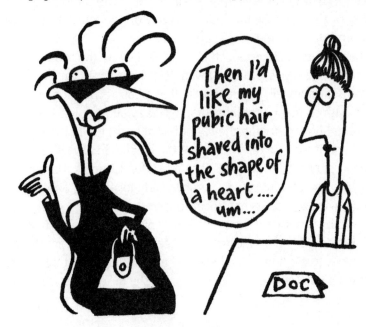

what's in it?

Most birth plans represent a best-case scenario, but what if there are unexpected difficulties (induced labour, forceps delivery, emergency caesarean)? For example, if you have a caesarean you will probably want to keep the baby with you, not have it whisked away immediately for weighing and measuring, as this time can be very important for bonding with your baby. You will need your birth attendants to agree, so it's good to have it in your plan.

Your birth plan may be a long and detailed list of what you want to happen at every stage of your labour or just a memo letter to your midwife or obstetrician saying what you want. You might want to include:

⊚ Who will be at the birth (with any phone numbers).

⊚ What you'd like to have around you to help you feel more comfortable and relaxed, such as music, massage oils and photos.

⊚ What clothes you would like to wear during the birth (hats and gloves are passé, and don't forget that anything that goes lower than your hips is likely to come off very second best in the stain department).

⊚ Whether you want a tape recording, photos or a video of the birth, and who will be taking these.

⊚ How, and how often, you would like to be monitored – some foetal monitors inhibit walking around.

⊚ Whether you would like to be able to eat in the early stages and drink (any preferences) through the labour.

⊚ What your preferred pain relief options are.

⊚ What delivery position you'd prefer – squatting, sitting or on all fours perhaps.

⊚ Whether you object to an episiotomy (a cut made at the entrance to the vagina to pre-empt any tearing).

⊚ Who you would you like to cut the umbilical cord?

⊚ Whether you want your baby placed on your chest for the first hour after birth. This skin to skin contact has many advantages for you and your baby and most hospitals have a 'baby-friendly' charter that includes this as a policy.

⊚ Whether you would accept drugs to speed up the normal delivery of the placenta.

pain relief options

Way before you're due, the following people will give you advice on pain relief: your obstetrician, your midwife, your partner; plenty of people who haven't had a baby; plenty who have; and a large man called Trevor who you meet at a bus stop.

The final decision rests with you. In your birth plan, you can choose the pain relief you'd like for an ideal delivery, but accept that you may have to resort to, say, a caesarean. Having a back-up plan means that you won't have to make any spur of the moment decisions about pain relief during labour, if for example it lasts longer or is more painful than you ever expected.

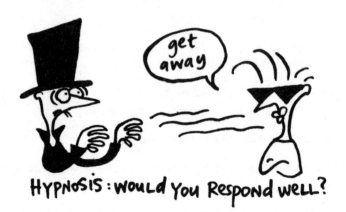

HYPNOSIS: WOULD YOU RESPOND WELL?

non-drug methods

The following non-drug methods of pain relief are often suggested (for each of these, faith in the method will help – if you're sceptical now, you may be a lot more so when you're yelling):

⑥ Acupuncture.

⑥ Reflexology (a form of acupressure massage of the feet).

⑥ Aromatherapy – this is *not* pain relief, it's just dickering with the atmosphere.

⑥ Breathing and meditation techniques – these need to be learnt and practised before labour.

⑥ Massage – this also needs to be practised before labour by the person who will give it.

⑥ Moving around – keeping mobile can help take pressure off your back, as well as distract you from the pain; some women find that standing or forward-leaning positions are much more comfortable during contractions and childbirth. Belly dancing – well, a kind of hip-swaying movement – works well for some women during contractions.

⑥ Hydrotherapy – a warm shower or bath will help to relax you; sitting in water can provide pain relief by supporting the abdominal wall and decreasing the pressure on muscles during contractions. Many hospitals and birth centres have warm birthing pools which tend to be used more frequently for labouring mothers rather than at the time of birth. They can also be hired by your midwife if you are planning a home birth. (Just be sure your floor/ceiling can take the weight!)

⑥ Localised heat – hot towels and heat packs can help mask pain and reduce muscle cramps and spasms.

⑥ Vocalisation – groaning, chanting or singing to 'release' pain, otherwise known as Just. Plain. Yelling.

⑥ TENS (transcutaneous electrical nerve stimulation) – a TENS machine delivers a very low electric current to stimulate the skin through pads attached to either side of the spine, creating a tingling sensation. This current can block the pain signals coming from the uterus and also has the effect of increasing the production of the endorphins – your natural pain relief. TENS machines only offer slight pain relief, but some women find it is enough. It can be used safely throughout labour but needs to be started very early in labour for the effects to work. Some hospitals offer TENS machines to mothers in labour but you may need to hire one for a hospital (or home) birth.

⑥ Music – more dickering with the atmosphere, and be warned: a lot of people make elaborate birth tapes and end up throwing them across the labour room.

the hard stuff

Gas Entonox, also known as inhalation analgesia, is a mixture of nitrous oxide (laughing gas) and oxygen, inhaled during contractions through a mask or mouthpiece. It is generally accepted that it eases perception of pain, but doesn't provide a complete block. Many women like it because it's easy to use and you control it yourself. The gas takes 15 to 20 seconds to work, so you breathe it in just as a contraction begins. Entonox can be used safely throughout labour and appears to have very little effect on the baby. Some mothers find that it makes them feel sick and light-headed. If this happens you can simply stop using it.

Pethidine and other painkillers Pethidine is the most common painkilling drug on offer. Painkilling drugs, usually given as injections during the first stage of labour, dull the sensation of pain by stimulating opiate receptors in the brain and spinal cord. A pethidine injection takes about 20 minutes to work and lasts from one to three hours. The amount of pethidine given depends on the stage of labour and the size of the mother. It is very relaxing and some women find that this lessens the pain. However, it has certain side effects such as making you feel 'woozy', light-headed or sick. It is often given with another drug which stops the sickness. If given close to the time of birth, it may make the baby sleepy and affect its breathing – this is usually remedied by giving the baby a little oxygen or a drug called Narcan after the birth, to reverse the effects. Pethidine can be given by midwives.

Epidural and spinal block Many women request an epidural as this is the only way to completely numb the pain of labour yet allow you to stay conscious. The epidural numbs all sensation in the abdomen and, in the past, used to also affect the nerves in the legs and bladder (making it neccessary to insert a catheter in your bladder as you wouldn't know when you were weeing). However, epidurals that don't numb the legs and bladder are now routine in most large maternity units. They must be performed by an experienced anaesthetist and are therefore only available for a hospital birth. A spinal block injection is similar to an epidural but goes direct to the spinal fluid and works almost immediately. It is often used for caesarean delivery.

With an epidural, a local anaesthetic is first injected into your back. Next, a fine, hollow needle is inserted between two vertebrae in your lower back, then a catheter is inserted via the needle into the epidural space and anaesthetic is injected into it. The needle is then taken out and the plastic catheter remains, strapped to your back and over your shoulder. The filter at the end of the catheter allows epidural drugs to be replaced in the right spot in the back to block pain, and allows further painkillers to be given throughout labour and delivery if needed. The procedure usually takes about ten minutes and the anaesthetic takes effect within a few minutes.

Epidural anaesthetic is often used when women are in great pain, if the baby is in an awkward position (such as breech – bum not head down), if it's a multiple birth, or with a forceps or suction delivery. An epidural can sometimes make it difficult for you to push because you can't feel the strong second-stage contractions; but your doctor or midwife should be able to tell you when to push. Some people choose to let the anaesthetic wear off a little towards the end so that they can feel the contractions again.

There is very little risk involved with having an epidural or a spinal block administered by an experienced anaesthetist. Occasionally an epidural only blocks pain in part of your abdomen, but the anaesthetist can often fix that. Less than 1 per cent of women who have had an epidural report having a headache lasting up to a few days. Having an epidural or spinal block in itself won't affect your baby.

Local anaesthesia The two most common forms of local anaesthesia given during labour are a pudendal nerve block, which involves an injection to numb the lower vagina and perineum before forceps or a vacuum instrument is used to pull the baby out; and perineal anaesthesia, injected into the perineum to reduce discomfort or, most commonly, to perform an episiotomy (a cut to the vagina). Both types of anaesthetic take effect within a few minutes. Minimum doses are used so as not to affect the baby.

General anaesthetic This is almost never used during labour, but is sometimes necessary or preferred for caesareans, especially in an emergency. Except in special circumstances, an epidural or spinal block is safer and better for mother and baby during a caesarean.

more info on labour and pain relief

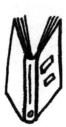

All the pregnancy books reviewed in 'Week 2' have information on labour, birth and pain relief. If you want a book on natural pain relief, try:

Labor Pain: A Natural Approach to Easing Delivery by Nicky Wesson, Healing Arts Press, US, 2000.

your record

✳Jot down the main points of your birth plan – how would you like your labour to go? (After you've had your baby, you can compare and contrast reality with Plan A).

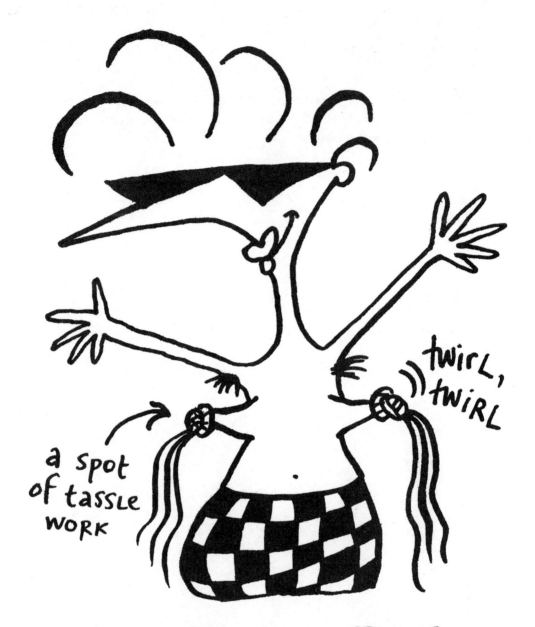

twirl,
twirl

a spot
of tassle
work

How can you prepare
for
BREASTFEEDING?

15		17	18	19	20	21	22	23	24	25	26	27	28	29

Average approximate baby length this week from head to bum

WEEK 33

what's going on You feel like there's not another thing that could be fitted inside you, not even a Mars Bar. Well, maybe a Mars Bar. Your navel is probably sticking out. All the baby really needs now is more surfactant to coat its lungs and some more fat. It has an excellent chance of survival if it comes out now. As well as blinking, the baby is starting to learn to focus its eyes on close things like its own extremities and the umbilical cord. Weight: about 1.9 kilos (4 lb 3oz).

DiARy I've been reading even more lists in books and pamphlets about what to take to hospital: pillows, hot water bottle, TENS machine (if you think it might work); sanitary towels the size of the Isle of Wight; clothes for the baby, including babygro with legs, vests, socks, baby-blankets, bootees (get out), and a baby seat for the trip home; cameras for still photos and videos (no thanks); a mobile phone to ring people up (will I remember to switch this off?); your admission forms for hospital already filled in; books and magazines; your address book; oh, and possibly some occasional furniture and a kayak.

I've checked the hospital's policy on giving out info about the birth: they refuse to tell anyone anything. Having confirmed her presence with the switchboard, the parents of my friend Peggy drove straight to the hospital when she was in labour and tried to force their way into the delivery room while she was yelling at them to go away. Most unseemly. And I won't be leaving a message on the answering machine saying we've gone to the hospital. In fact I'm going to leave a message saying, 'I haven't gone to the hospital, I'm just not answering the phone. Do not call the hospital. Repeat, and this means you Aunt Julie, do not call the hospital. Leave a message.'

Another fluid-retention vigilance visit to the midwife clinic to have blood pressure checked. The waiting room is an endless parade offering excellent people-watching opportunities. Today there is a couple who look straight out of the pages of Italian Vogue. Her: full, heavy make-up, hair done by the caring hands of a professional in the last 5 hours, Manolo Blahnik shoes, Armani suit, gold jewellery and diamonds the size of small mammals. Him: full-length suede overcoat, tailored suit, silk tie, designer specs, carefully cultivated two-day growth. Not a hair out of place, not a piece of lint. I can't imagine what they would do with a baby. Put it in a vase, maybe.

When it's my turn, I climb up on the bed thing, which is so narrow it always reminds me of being on a ship (especially when I was feeling sick). Anne gets out her tape to measure the uterus and feels my stomach and starts laughing.

'My, it's a whopper,' she says.

Now, don't get me wrong. If the boss was telling me about a pay rise, or an Italian sailor was taking off his strides in a sexual fantasy, the words 'My, it's a whopper' could be exceedingly welcome. When the phrase refers, however, to something that has to come out of your vagina, sometimes referred to amusingly as the birth canal in a pathetic attempt to make it sound bigger, well, it is a different kettle of episiotomies entirely.

Anne's approach to the big-baby question is basically to wait and see what happens during labour. She says that ultrasounds have proven notoriously unreliable in judging whether a baby's head will fit through the middle of its mum's pelvis. I suppose I had better read a bit more about caesareans, just in case.

Anne says I could get my GP to refer me to a skin specialist who can remove the moles and skin tags that have gone berserk, but advises waiting until three months after the baby is born because they often disappear by themselves. (The moles, that is.) However, it is the fluid retention that is really getting me down. I'm from a generation that has been taught (wrongly as it happens) that you can be somehow in control of your body – even change its essential shape by diet and exercise, or surgery. The feeling of being totally OUT of control – along for the ride, part of a biology experiment – is deeply disconcerting. I have reached the point with the fluid retention where even the disgusting-tasting dandelion-leaf tincture I'm taking only goes so far towards keeping me distinguishable from a hot-air balloon. Now I just have to put up with it. Unless my blood pressure goes up as well, there's no danger to the baby.

An uneasy feeling grows that David Attenborough is outside my house with a film crew, waiting to breathlessly narrate the next bit of my life. 'And now the Pregnant Woman has only six weeks to go,' he whispers to the camera, as he crouches behind the camellias. 'Inside, she is groaning and puffing every time she lifts her enormous weight from the couch. She is now totally demented about getting the nursery set up, and if her mate does not perform the act of clearing his things out of this room by the agreed deadline of thirty-five weeks, she will eat his head.'

My dreams are getting weirder and weirder. The night before last I dreamt that Geoff left me and took the furniture, and I forgot to ask him if he was interested in seeing the baby after it was born. Then last night I dreamt I had given birth and then one of the nurses (who were all dressed in pastel French maids' uniforms – a very sartorially satisfactory dream) said, 'There was another cord hanging out so we followed it back in, and it was attached to another baby, which has been hiding behind the uterus the whole time. So now you've got two.'

Week 5 of childbirth classes: Melissa devotes the evening to breastfeeding. I must admit I had kind of blanked out the idea of breastfeeding. After Melissa wipes the floor with my illusions and gives us all a new pack of expectations, I fully realise that if I breastfeed I must accept that for several months I won't be able to (a) sleep, (b) work, (c) speak, (d) twirl tassels in opposite directions while they are attached to my nipples.

It's just that apparently you have to feed the little blighters at least every 4 hours in the early days, and apparently you're supposed to be awake while that happens. I can't imagine who designed this system. No wonder women in some other cultures aren't allowed to do any work or housework or even get out of bed for the first few weeks after childbirth. And apparently for the full benefits that everyone raves about (boosting the baby's immune system, annoying old fuddy-duddies who simply go gaga at the sight of a publicly bared bosom, etc), you need to breastfeed for a minimum of six months.

Melissa drops a few hints: go to the loo and wash your hands before you breastfeed, and have a set-up next to your chair with a glass of water, phone, etc on it. It seems that you can't actually pop out of a long office meeting and whack the baby on a gland for, say, 7 minutes before handing it to a passer-by and rushing back in. Indeed, some babies can stay on for up to half an hour each side! And sometimes they want it and sometimes they don't! And it might not be the 7 minutes you choose! And you can't just fill them up when it suits you because it takes 2–3 hours to 'fill up' the breasts with milk again! Dear, oh dear, oh dear.

There are an awful lot of instructions about breastfeeding, but at least everyone now admits it can be really difficult. Plus Melissa is pretty sure that most of the midwives and breastfeeding counsellors (bet that looks good on a passport) at our local hospital have their story straight, and we won't be plagued by seven different recommended methods while we're learning. Eventually, she assures us, we should be able to whack a baby on our bosoms upside down in the dark while riding a horse backwards side-saddle. But in the beginning it can be all rather laborious and it doesn't always work out for everyone.

The first stage does not sound like fun. During the day or two after you give birth, your breasts get engorged temporarily due to an excessive blood supply and become really big and hard and painful. This is when you need to get some savoy cabbage leaves (really) out of the fridge and put one in each bra cup. Nobody really knows why it works, but I'd like to meet the person who worked it out.

The idea of expressing breast milk – pumping it out and putting it in bottles – which I'll have to do if I go back to work (or even leave the baby alone with Geoff for a few hours), seems even more weird. I can vaguely remember as a child seeing rows and rows of dairy cows being milked and I am starting to have visions of myself that are along the same lines.

Back home, mulling over this, I can't find my Fat Boots. In the vague frame of mind I'm in, they'll probably turn up in the toaster. I specialise in sentences that are in search of an endi . . .

info

what to organise before hospital

ⓖ Go to antenatal classes, and do your reading. Labour and delivery are unpredictable, and it is very helpful if you and your partner or labour support person at least have *some vague idea* of what you might be in for.

⑥ Write your birth plan (see info in 'Week 32').

⑥ If you have another child, organise child care well in advance: this may need to be available at a moment's notice – even in the middle of the night – so it's a good idea to have a first choice and a back-up. Make sure they are well briefed on the plan so they are not freaked out to find both parents gone. Having a sibling is quite enough trauma in itself.

⑥ Plan your transport to hospital; don't drive yourself. If your birth partner will be driving, then make sure they know where to park (and have a permit lined up, if needs be). Collecting a car from the pound is not the perfect prelude to taking a baby home.

⑥ Try to have nursery items and baby clothes organised by about now, just in case.

⑥ Have a freezer stocked full of easy food, ready for the first few weeks at home. You could prepare soups, pasta sauces, quiches, pies, lasagnes or casseroles. Put it this way – you won't want to be plucking any chickens. When you go home your priorities will be (a) baby care, (b) sleep and (c) – there is no c.

⑥ Have some light, nutritious early-labour food, such as home-made chicken stock, beef broth or pureed fruit, in the freezer.

⑥ If you can afford it, arrange for a cleaner (friend, relative or agency) for the first few weeks at home, especially if you know you're having a caesarean.

⑥ If you plan to use it, order a nappy-wash service. They generally only need a day's warning, but you may as well make a call putting them on notice while you have time.

⑥ Fit the baby seat in the car, and practise buckling and unbuckling with a teddy bear. You'll need the seat to take the baby home so stash it in the boot, ready for action.

Find out what labour aids your hospital maternity section or birth centre can provide during labour and what you might need to bring in yourself – does it provide tape players and aromatherapy burners, for instance? Always double-check, when ringing to say you're coming in, that whatever you need is still available just in case it's been booked by someone else. If you plan to use a TENS machine during your labour you need to book it now. Some hospitals provide them (sometimes for a small fee). Otherwise Boots and Lloyds chemists rent them.

⑥ When the time comes, phone your midwife, hospital or birth centre to tell them you're in labour and ask about when you should come in.

⑥ If you are planning a home birth you need to prepare the things advised by midwives to protect home furnishings. The midwives will usually give you a home birth pack with the pieces of equipment that they might need at the time of birth.

what to take to hospital

Your hospital or birth centre will give you a list in advance of what it recommends you bring in for yourself and the baby.

bag for labour

⑥ Labour aids might include: a music tape or CD; massage oil; birth ball; massage roller (or tennis ball); a water-spray (many women rate this their #1 aid); lip cream; food and drink for your labour support person and sustaining snacks for yourself; warm socks with non-slip bottoms; glucose sweets or sugar-free lollipops; aromatherapy oils.

⑥ Take something to wear such as a large T-shirt, giant-sized cotton shirt or cotton nightie. If you want to keep some semblance of being covered up during labour, go for a front-buttoning shirt (or back-to-front hospital gown) so you can have easy skin-to-skin contact and breastfeed your baby after delivery. You might also need a couple of pairs of dark undies and some pads to absorb leaking amniotic fluid while you're in labour.

⑥ Pack toiletries – soap, shampoo, conditioner, toothbrush and toothpaste, moisturiser, hair elastics, hairbrush, shower cap – plus ear plugs and an eye mask for a bit of sleep in the ward, and make-up if you want to joosh up a bit for visitors. You will probably need a bath towel, and some hospitals ask you to provide your own pillows.

⑥ The support person's clothes should be comfortable, not too warm, and easy to wash. If your support person is likely to be, for instance, giving you pain relief massage in a birthing pool, they might also want to pack a swimming costume; hospitals do try to restrict the number of people running around in the nude.

Apparently some people who are into 'creative visualisation' look at a photo of their dog. Of course they're obviously insane.

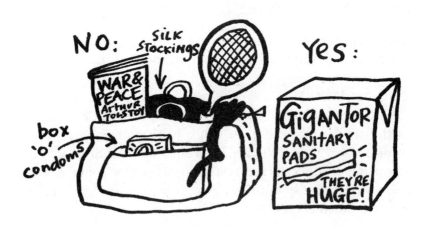

a bigger bag for the hospital stay
⑥ Take a few packs of super-soaker sanitary pads – these are sold as maternity pads.

⑥ Include a few front-opening nighties, a dressing-gown, slippers, six pairs of dark cotton undies. (It would be nice to have a clean nightie each morning and each night, and plenty of cotton undies – it's a leaky old time – so pack according to your helper's washing plans. Will the washing be done every couple of days, or not until you all get home?) You can wear regular day clothes in hospital, but the combination of a sore, tender and tired body, the high temperatures at which hospitals are generally kept and the number of times you'll need access to the business end makes cotton nighties a practical choice.

⊚ Take at least two very firm nursing bras for supporting tight, engorged breasts, and nursing pads to soak up the leaking breast milk when it 'comes in'.

⊚ Pack going-home clothes for you (probably maternity clothes because your tummy will still be big); and for the baby – include a hat and a warm blanket if the weather's cold. New babies love to be wrapped up firmly because it's more womblike.

⊚ Pack a few snacks for you. Waking in the early hours to feed your newborn baby brings on the munchies and you may feel a bit of a nuisance asking the staff to prepare toast and marmalade. Having some crackers, crispbreads, biscuits or bananas in your bag is ideal for a midnight snack. (If you want to watch your weight at this point then crispbreads are ideal snacks as they are high in carbohydrates but low in fats and sugars – as opposed to chocolate biscuits!)

⊚ If you have a toddler or young child, a wrapped present for them is a good investment, so they feel central to the action when they come to visit for the first time. This is the beginning of a difficult time for them, and they may just see the new baby in a better light if they think it's brought them a special present.

WEEK 34

WANDERING HANDS

cm 1 2 3 4 5 6 7 8 9 10 11 12 13 14

what's going on

From now on your baby will hog all available space and squash up anything silly enough to get in the way, like your lungs. If you find yourself breathless, sitting or standing up straight will help. So will taking it easy. If you're interested in going to childbirth classes but haven't organised this yet, you'd better make that phone call now. And lay in the baby clothes. It's for real.

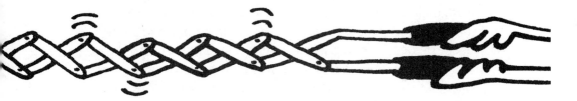

Your body is starting to put the final touches to the baby: it's the finishing-school stage. From now on your bub is pretty busy practising sucking, breathing, blinking, turning its head, grabbing things (such as its other hand or the umbilical cord) and stretching out its legs. But there's not quite enough room to actually do that, hence the jarring kicks you may feel. The baby's skin is becoming smoother and less translucent – more like the final skin colour. Weight: about 2.1 kilos (4lb 9oz).

Average approximate baby length this week from head to bum

5 16 17 18 19 20 21 22 23 24 25 26 27 28 29

DiARY

It's really hard to find comfy positions. If I lean back, I get heartburn. If I lean forward, I'm not resting, I'm listing. If I lie down, I can't get anything done. If I don't lie down, the fluid retention reaches epic proportions. If I walk around, I aggravate an ache in my groin. At the start of the day my face is all puffy. By the end of the day my ankles are all puffy. I skitter between nausea and indigestion and faintness and wondering if that weird feeling could be hunger.

I try to imagine what the Chelsea bun will be like when it comes out but am finding it hard to get past the thoughts of labour itself, and how on earth I can get all my work finished.

Geoff finally cleans up his room but leaves all his footie trophies on the mantelpiece. There is a rather tension-ridden scene with me trying to be diplomatic ('How would you feel if we put them up in the sitting room?') and Geoff looking grumpy. Perhaps it is some deep-seated male displacement thing going on. Poor Geoff. He gets his own back by putting a load of new baby things in the washing machine (to make sure there are no manufacturing chemicals left on them) and waving a very tiny sock at me, which he knows perfectly well will reduce me to tears.

Aunt Julie, meanwhile, has heard something on the radio about asthma and is now obsessed about dustmites in the baby's room. 'It's thoroughly dusted and vacuumed once a week,' I lie. Then when I say I am looking for a woollen blanket to wrap the baby in when it's cold, she starts on about that. 'Nobody I know wraps a baby in a wool rug,' she says. 'They might throw one onto the pram, but it's not for wrapping up.'

'Yes, okay,' I snap. 'I'll just throw it on the pram, then.'

Oops. Just remembered we don't have a pram. Must get Geoff to ring his friends Luke and Sita to claim theirs.

Buy some extra-large pyjamas to take to the hospital. Start to pack hospital bag. The top of the pyjamas doesn't even look like it will fit me now, and as they were mail order I didn't realise they were going to say 'Brand New Mum' on the pocket. How embarrassing. And I think that will be fairly obvious without anyone having to read my pyjama pocket.

The gum nodule thing just above my front teeth seems to be getting worse. It bleeds profusely every time I give them a brush and is clearly visible as a kind of bulge between two teeth. I have started to spit blood like a prize-fighter. The only book that mentions it is *What to Expect When You're Expecting*, which says it's called a pyogenic granuloma, or in the usual deeply reassuring doctor language a 'pregnancy tumour', which is actually completely harmless and will go away right after the baby's born. Which is not what my dentist says.

My dentist says (after inquiring whether the baby's father is my boyfriend or my husband, a question obviously essential to dental hygiene): 'It won't go away. I can just slice it off. It will bleed for an hour or so and then be all right.'

Call me crazy, but I'm going to wait and see.*

The last childbirth class: by this stage all the people in the class who were going to loosen up have loosened up. Only two couples haven't lost their quiet, stunned-mullet approach to everything. One woman keeps looking at her partner as if he's a ghastly apparition and she's suddenly realised she's tied to him for the rest of her life.

The picture I'll take with me is of women bulging in the middle, with their hands crossed over their lump and their male partner leaning towards them. The woman who wanted her birth on the Internet, and her husband, the filthy show-offs, arrive halfway through the class, with their baby! It came two weeks early, on the weekend, and they're still high. Melissa confides that she doesn't let parents come if they've hit the baby-blues. You don't want a brand-new mother sobbing in a class, I suppose.

Melissa shows us two videos of couples with new babies. The men all work away from home and the women at home. The couples talk about lack of privacy and personal space, their relationship as a couple, tiredness, guilt, coping with a distressed and needy baby (the gist seems to be that 'this too shall pass'). And there's footage of a woman with twins: she looks a bit like someone has hit her on the back of the head with a rubber cricket bat. You would, wouldn't you?

* The book was right.

Melissa talks about having an unsettled baby. New ones sleep 16 hours a day, but after a few weeks or months they can cry for a few hours a day no matter how well fed and clean and cuddled they are. This is often in the early evening.

We gallop through some different things to settle the baby, how not to expect much from your sex life until at least after the six-week check-up (one man mishears and shouts 'Six years?!'), contraception (twelve condoms at once, thank you), services available if you get into trouble with feeding, sleeping or crying, and baby safety.

Revelation: one woman in the class asks, 'Shouldn't you have the baby checked out by a paediatrician before it goes home?' Melissa says yes, this happens routinely with a hospital birth and you'll have a GP visit after a home birth. I hadn't got so far as thinking beyond an obstetrician. But I guess they are mother and foetus specialists, not baby specialists.

labour

You might or might not notice the early signs of labour. If you do, rest and eat – labour could start at any time and you need to conserve your energy, though the Real Thing may still be up to a few days or even weeks away.

When your contractions start, they may be 'pre-labour', sometimes called 'false' contractions. These are quite bearable – more uncomfortable than painful – and irregular, and go away if you move around, lie down or have a bath. It's often difficult to tell the difference between 'pre-labour' and the 'latent phase' of the first stage of labour (during which the cervix dilates 1–3 centimetres), so don't hesitate to telephone your midwife, the hospital or birth centre to describe what's happening and to find out whether to stay at home or go straight to the hospital or centre, or, if you're having a home birth, whether you need your midwives NOW.

Call your hospital immediately if:

⑥ When your waters break, you notice a green or dark stain in the amniotic fluid; this is meconium – the baby's first poo – which can be a sign of foetal distress.

⑥ You have bright red bleeding, which may indicate a problem with the placenta.

⑥ You feel or see the umbilical cord in your vagina. This is called cord prolapse and is very rare (especially in a first birth). But it is an emergency. Ring for an ambulance, open the door, then kneel down with your bottom in the air and head and shoulders down – this takes pressure off the cord. Stay in this position even on the way to hospital and do not touch the cord. Don't panic; you have time, though you will probably need a ceasarean on arrival.

When contractions start in earnest, they will usually:

⑥ Be regular.

⑥ Get stronger.

⑥ Last for longer.

⑥ Come closer together.

⑥ Be increasingly tough to cope with.

Time their length and frequency and give this information to your midwife, or the hospital or birth centre.

The 'average' labour *for a first-timer* goes something like this:

⑥ First stage – the latent stage when the cervix dilates from 1–3cm and then the active stage when the cervix dilates fully to 10cm (average 10 hours).

⑥ Second stage – build-up to pushing, then the baby is born (average 2 hours).

⑥ Third stage – the placenta and any other bits no longer needed are expelled (about 10 minutes after the birth if oxytocin is given, up to an hour if delivered naturally).

Gosh, that sounds neat. In reality your experience might be radically different. The latent stage can be long and drawn out for some mothers and although you will probably be at home as you don't need constant care from a midwife you will need company from your birth partner. The active phase is more intense and it is then when you may think of going to the hospital.

When you arrive at the hospital or birth centre, or when the midwife or doctor arrives at your home birth, you'll have a medical examination, which will probably involve:

⊚ Checking your blood pressure.

⊚ Checking a urine sample.

⊚ Checking your temperature and pulse.

⊚ A feel up your vagina to see how dilated your cervix is.

⊚ The baby's heartbeat will be checked with either a handheld doppler (an ultrasound device) or a pinard (midwife's stethoscope). A continous electronic recording may be made of the baby's heartbeat if there are any concerns. This is usually done by placing two belts around your tummy, attached by wires to a machine, and a printout is made of the contractions and the heartbeat.

Make sure the midwife makes a note of your relevant health details or special needs. Ideally things will now proceed according to your birth plan. But any unpredictable turns will have to be dealt with as they arise.

All the following advice may fly out of your head, so get your birth support person to read it, too, so that they can remind you.

first stage

For some women the latent phase of first-stage labour – the first 3cm dilation – is barely perceptible; others experience intense backache and painful contractions. For some it happens quietly over a long time; for others it may all happen in just a couple of hours of full-on labour. Contractions may last 30–35 seconds, and could be regular or irregular – anywhere from five to twenty minutes apart. You'll probably be at home and may even be able to sleep through some of this phase. Rest as much as possible and have some of the light snacks you have ready in the freezer. It can help to have warm baths, and you should keep timing your contractions. It is not too early to use a TENS machine.

By the time you're well into the first stage, you'll probably be in hospital and looking to your coping strategies: massage, TENS machine, relaxation techniques, breathing techniques. Not to mention drugs. Remember to wee frequently: the area is feeling such intense sensations from labour that you mightn't notice you need to wee. Stay as mobile and upright as possible. Try out different labouring positions for greatest comfort. Stay hydrated, taking ice chips, juice cubes or sips of water.

Try to rest completely and relax between contractions, and not expend energy anticipating the next one. Use positive visualisation and psyching techniques ('stay focused', as Bruce Lee might say). You might perhaps concentrate on a mental picture of a flower opening; or focus on the positive goal of seeing your baby; or chant something ('This will end'), whatever. Clenching everything up can hinder the progress of labour, so with your partner or labour support person's help use whatever it takes to go with the flow. If you can't stand the pain, or if this phase has gone on for a long time and you've had it, feel free to yell 'DRUGS!' around about now.

transition

This is generally considered to be the most challenging time of labour. It happens at the very end of the first stage of labour. For some mothers this phase may last no more that five minutes but for others it can be longer. Contractions are strong and getting stronger, lasting longer – 60–90 seconds – and coming at shorter intervals. Sometimes there's no time to rest between them, and you're probably exhausted. You may feel hot or shivering and cold, or alternate between temperature extremes. You may be nauseated or vomiting, and feeling overwhelmed or unable to cope. You may feel totally pissed off with everyone around you. (Foul and abusive language is common and entirely acceptable).

At the end of this phase your cervix will be fully dilated, and you'll be ready to start pushing. If you've hung in there without drugs, your support person can remind you that you are nearly there, that you'll have your baby very soon, and you can hit your support person. If you have the urge to push during this phase, before the cervix is fully dilated, you may be advised to blow or pant instead.

second stage – pushing and delivery

About a third of labouring women have a resting, or 'latent', phase at this point before their body starts urging them to push the baby out – the active phase of the second stage. The go during this phase is to listen to your body when it comes to pushing. Contractions will still be 60–90 seconds long, but may be further apart (2–5 minutes), so you can rest between them. No need to pop the capillaries in your eyeballs or hold your breath beyond the point of comfort or turning purple. Using lots of shorter moments of bearing down with each contraction is less stressful to the baby, and makes it easier for the pelvic floor to relax, than one big, breath-holding push, like the ones you see in the movies.

This more relaxed approach may make the second stage a bit longer than if you use the PUSH approach, but is probably less stressful for you as well as the baby. During this phase you might be making some deep guttural grunts and moans, which many other pregnancy books seem to think will embarrass you. You'll be far too busy to be embarrassed. You might also push out a poo during this phase. No big deal.

Don't worry about your baby not being able to breathe while it's in the vagina. Nature designed things so it's still getting oxygen from the placenta during this stage.

Actual, honest-to-goodness birth There's more panting as the baby's head pushes against the perineum. You'll be asked by your midwife to try not to push but instead to relax the pelvic floor, aiming to slow down the last bit to avoid tearing (or the need for an episiotomy). You may be offered a bird's-eye view of proceedings with the help of a mirror: this is a fascinating prospect for some, horrifying for others. You choose.

Mums often describe the sensation of the baby's head emerging as stinging, burning or intense pressure. A midwife may 'support' the perineum and anus (apply pressure from the outside to counter the bulging). This can help make it less painful. After the head emerges, the baby rotates so that its shoulders line up with the widest part of your pelvis and the little body slithers out. Hello there! Finally meeting and holding your baby is an indescribably awe-inspiring, emotional and happy time. (Or not, of which more later.)

Complications in the second stage If there are complications in the second stage of labour the midwife will call the obstetrician to help to deliver the baby with either forceps or a ventouse. This may be:

◎ To assist in the delivery of a breech birth.

◎ To help a baby who is in an awkward position.

◎ To assist a mother who is exhausted and can push no more.

◎ To help speed the birth of a baby showing signs of distress.

The mother will need some form of local anaesthetic in the vagina if her delivery is to be assisted. The obstetrican will then decide which instrument to use. Forceps are like a pair of salad servers that are placed around the baby's head over the ears so that when the mother gives a push the baby can be gently guided down the vagina. A ventouse or vacuum extractor is a soft rubber cup which can be placed on the back of the baby's head, attached by suction and then used to turn and deliver the baby. The ventouse is usually the first choice when deciding what instrument to use partly because an episiotomy often does not need to be performed as a routine and it is easier to apply to the baby's head.

The baby will be marked by both choices of instrument. These marks are not permanent but look quite dramatic at birth. The ventouse leaves the baby with a swollen and sometimes bruised mark at the back of the head. The swelling settles after a few hours and the bruise will take a few days. The forceps sometimes leave the baby with a red indentation over the cheek bones, but this too nearly always fades after a few hours.

third stage:
the placenta and membranes expelled

You may be so engrossed in your new baby, you don't notice the third stage. The uterus continues to contract, causing the placenta to come away from the wall, taking with it what's left of the amniotic sac as it detaches; further contractions will push the placenta into the vagina, from where it can be pulled out, or pushed out with another contraction. The contraction of the muscles of your truly amazing uterus also seals off the blood vessels at the site of detachment. The placenta comes out more quickly if an injection of oxytocin is given to speed up contractions.

The placenta is rather like a large piece of liver – quite a shock if you had been thinking purely about delivering a baby. After you've expelled it, it's inspected to make sure it has been delivered whole and the hospital may retain it to do pathology tests, or more likely simply dispose of it. Some mothers plan to bury their placenta in the garden, or even cook and eat part of it. (There's a theory that this can help recovery and combat the blues. Some animals eat their placenta but I reckon that's just because they don't have any vitamin B6 tablets handy.) If you'd like to take your placenta home, check with your midwives that they'll hand it over. You can also ask whether your hospital would like to donate your umbilical cord for cells to be used in treating leukaemia.

After the placenta is expelled, you'll be checked to make sure you don't have post-partum haemorrhage ('post-partum' means after delivery). It's diagnosed when the blood loss is 500 millilitres or more; the usual loss is less than 300 millilitres. It happens to about 5 per cent of mothers.

The 'fourth stage', hardly ever mentioned in the textbooks, is stabilisation and getting acquainted with your baby, enjoying skin-to-skin contact, keeping your baby warm, the baby having a red-hot go and first drink at your breast, the standard reflex and observation tests on the baby done by a doctor or midwife, clamping of the umbilical cord, and any sewing up of the perineum.

your record

✳ Where are your childbirth classes? Who takes them? What has stuck with you the most from the classes?

You May Need Bigger Shoes

WEEK 35

what's going on

That baby is taking up stomach space – smaller meals more often are easier to digest. You're probably finding it hard to get your shoes on and off. Wear slip-on shoes unless you need the ankle support of lace-ups. You've probably gone up a shoe size as well, especially in width, maybe permanently. Try to walk a bit every day until the baby arrives. To reduce the swelling in your feet and ankles, stand on your head a lot. Or at the very least sit down or, preferably, lie down and put your feet above the level of your heart as much as possible. (This can be especially effective in getting yourself extra room on public transport, particularly if you shout obscenities as well.) Toenails are in. The fingernails may be poking over the end of the fingers. Your baby would fail that test they do at the start of netball games, and can scratch itself. Weight: about 2.3 kilos (5 lb).

Average approximate baby length this week from head to bum

DiARY

Help, it's going too fast. I'm not ready but I'm sick of being pregnant. Rosie, who does the accounts at work, says she lost 15 kilos at the birth, including the weight of the baby, and I must say THAT'S an attractive proposition. I'm wondering how long my legs will carry me. I'm terrified of getting on the scales.

I take an inventory of stretch marks. Several red-purple stripes on the underside of each breast, and on each hip a bunch of marks that looks as if a hand held me too hard on each fleshy part. Nothing on the tummy itself, which has stretched more than anything. What gives? Me.

Yet another visit to the midwives for the fluid-retention check. Anne (I really hope she'll be on at my birth) measures the height of the baby, gives it a feel and says, 'Oh God.' First 'My, it's a whopper' and now 'Oh God'. For some reason I feel resigned rather than horrified. I suspect this tactic is to soften me up and get me used to the idea of a boombah bambino.

I show her the birth plan and she reacts to each point.

Will the hospital induce at the due date? (No. We let you go ten, even fourteen, days over.)

Ideally I would like to avoid either a vaginal birth or a caesarean. However, there do not seem to be many other options. (Ha ha. By hook or by crook the baby will come out.)

At the labour I want to have my partner, Geoff, and my herbalist friend, Miss Beck, who will probably prescribe herbs and supplements after the birth. (Fine.)

I would like to be kept informed of what's happening. (Yep.)

I would like to avoid monitoring that might 'tether' me to the bed, and avoid an epidural, if possible. Geoff is particularly concerned about the possible side effects of an epidural, but understands it might not be avoidable. Anyway it's my decision. (It certainly is.)

I would like to avoid an episiotomy, but would rather be cut than tear if necessary. (Although sometimes an episiotomy is unavoidable, we will try to avoid it. Actually it's better to tear naturally unless it looks like you're going to tear down to the bowel or up to the clitoris.) (Me: That's quite enough. Fine. That's quite enough chat about torn clitorises for one day.)

I don't want gas, would rather take pethidine. (You should try the gas, and see if it works.) (Me: No way – haven't you seen that movie *Blue Velvet?*, where Dennis Hopper has this mask on and . . .) (No.)

My Major Fears, in order, are:

1 possible neurological damage from epidural. (About the same chance as getting hit by a jumbo jet, unless you already have a history of trouble, such as multiple sclerosis.)

2 episiotomy. (We'll try hard not to. Whatever it takes to get a healthy baby out with the least amount of damage possible all round – that's our mission.)

While Anne is checking my blood pressure, I remark that it doesn't seem to be within the laws of physics, but I appear to have put on another 4 kilos. This means I have put on 20 kilos!!! And I'm not eating crap – in fact I'm not eating a lot at all. Anne says don't worry, I'll probably put on another 5 kilos before I give birth. I am absolutely flabbergasted.

'It's not humanly possible,' I say.

'Don't forget,' she says, 'you can lose 12 kilos just at the birth, and all the fluid over the next couple of days. Of course you can actually puff up after the birth as well. But you'll lose it. It's easier to lose the weight that's not junk food.'

I don't tell her I have at least three Magnums a week.

Susanne has given me a book of baby names that someone sent her from the States. It's kind of fascinating and depressing (surely we can think of names ourselves) in equal measure. Geoff refuses to open it but, spurred by my babel of odd names and their historic and literary associations – Hezekiah, Ringo, Heathcliffe (I think not) – he presents me with two alternative volumes, *Crystal Palace FC, Player by Player* and *The Rough Guide to Jazz*. The jazz book is actually Very Cool for picking babynames and before too long we're both at it. Art, Miles, Roscoe, Cannonball seem promising for a boy. And the girls are just as good: I mean Billie Holiday, Blossom Dearie – they're pretty hard to beat.

Palace turn out to be strong on Andys, Nigels, Robs and indeed Geoffs. Geoff says footballers need a name that can end in -y, -sy, or -o, as in 'Giggsy' or 'Keano'. But didn't they play for Man United, I ask innocently. They're just examples, he growls. I think we better stick to the jazz book, which is formally accorded prime reading space by the loo. However, it's the American book which comes up with Chelsea bun's new name – Oofty Goofty, after a Texan circus clown.

info

caesarean delivery

A caesarean section operation is a surgical procedure to take the baby out of the uterus through your abdomen. It's usually called just 'a caesarean' or 'a caesar'. A standard caesarean is considered to be a very safe procedure when performed by a specialist in a good hospital. But it is not a walk in the park. A caesarean is major surgery. (The way some people blithely refer to it, you'd think the baby just came out of a handy zipper.)

how common is it?
Depending on several factors, your chance of having a caesarean might be a lot greater than you think. Getting on for twenty-five percent of babies end up being delivered this way in the UK. Read up on it because it might happen to you, even if you've had a 'perfect' pregnancy.

what happens?

During a standard caesarean, you'll have the top half of your pubic hair trimmed or shaved, and you may be fitted for some very glamorous anti-embolism stockings. These help prevent the occurance of a deep vein thrombosis. Then you'll be taken to the operating room. In this very brightly lit room all the medical staff will wear shower caps, face masks and blue theatre clothes, and so will your support person. An intravenous (IV) drip will be put into your arm, then the anaesthetist will give you an epidural injection (or spinal-block injection if speed is necessary) to numb the lower half of your body (see 'Week 32'). As well, a catheter tube will be put into your urethra for the wee to flow into a bag. A screen will be put up between you and your tummy; it can be lowered at the time of the birth for you to see your baby being born.

The lower part of your tummy will then be swabbed with antiseptic and your obstetrician will make an incision just above your pubic hairline, usually horizontal and about 10 centimetres long. Then the obstetrician will cut through layers of fat and muscle to the uterus wall, cut open the uterus and pull the baby out. You may have some sensation of pulling or pressure but should feel no pain.

It all happens very quickly: the baby is generally born 5 to 10 minutes after the first incision. The baby will be shown to you and then will be fully examined by a paediatrician standing by in the room. If the baby doesn't need to be taken away for special care, you will have time for a long cuddle. You often feel a little uncomfortable balancing the baby on your chest because of the numbness of the local anaesthetic, and this is where the birth partner is so useful in being able to cuddle the baby next to you during the remainder of the operation. Measuring or baths are not important enough reasons to separate you and your baby at this crucial time, so insist on this time together.

You might be too preoccupied to notice what happens next, but usually you'll hear some gurgling, slurping noises when the amniotic fluid is suctioned out. The placenta and membranes, and the swabs, are removed, then you are stitched up. This can take quite a while because it's not just one row of stitches, it's several different wounds to be sewn, including layers of skin, fat, muscle, and the inner and outer walls of the uterus.

why would you need one?

A caesarean can be elective: you 'elect' to have one on the advice of your obstetrician and make a hospital appointment. Or it can be emergency surgery performed unexpectedly and suddenly when a problem develops during labour. In the case of an elective caesarean, you have to weigh the pros and cons of setting a date rather than waiting for the spontaneous onset of labour before having the operation. These can be discussed with your obstetrician and midwife.

If you want to avoid having a caesarean, talk to your obstetrician, but remember that there's never a guarantee you won't have one. The basic criterion is whether a caesarean will be less of a risk to the mother and baby than a vaginal birth. In some cases the decision is clear cut, in others it's more open to interpretation. Some reasons why you might end up needing a caesarean are:

◎ Placenta praevia (the placenta is positioned over the cervix).

◎ Placental abruption (the placenta comes away too early).

◎ You have a medical condition such as pre-eclampsia or eclampsia (see info in 'Week 31').

◎ The umbilical cord is 'prolapsed' – coming down into the vagina, possibly cutting off the baby's circulation if the baby's head is against the cervix.

◎ The baby is in an awkward position – perhaps sideways, which is known as the 'transverse lie', or bum not head down, which is called the 'breech position' (though many obstetricians will agree to try first to deliver a breech baby in the normal way).

◎ The baby's head seems to be too big to fit through its mum's pelvis; this is technically called cephalo-pelvic disproportion (CPD). Labour fails to progress and the cervix does not open and the head remains high in the pelvis.

⑥ Active genital herpes in your vagina (the baby may catch the herpes from sores as it is born).

⑥ The baby is sick or isn't growing properly.

⑥ The baby's lowered or erratic heartbeat during labour indicates it is distressed or in danger and/or the samples of blood the obstetrican takes from the baby during labour show signs of oxygen deprivation.

recovery from the surgery

Probably the first thing you'll notice when you're in the recovery room or back in your own hospital room is that you're still hooked up to the IV drip and doing wee into a bag through a tube, which will continue for up to a day. There will be a very nice drug coming through the IV drip, probably morphine or pethidine, or you might have been given a Voltarol suppository in theatre which gives you several hours of pain-free time. You might be hungry, but you won't be allowed to eat anything until your bowel shows signs of post-operative activity (okay, farting), at which time your IV can be removed. You will be given some sips of iced water to start with.

Your baby will be tucked into bed with you as soon as you leave the theatre for you to have some of that special skin-to-skin time together. If you are planning to breastfeed then the baby usually feeds now. If your baby has had to go to the neonatal unit for some special observations or care then your birth partner will be encouraged to go too and a photograph will be given to you until you are able to visit your baby or your baby is well enough to be returned to your bedside.

Over the next week your pain relief is likely to be reduced in strength. Don't skimp on relief – it is important to have regular analgesia even before the pain returns. The idea is to keep one step ahead of it so ask the midwives for it if they miss your due time. The analgesia prescribed will be safe for breastfeeding.

Try to move and get up as soon as possible. As soon as you can feel your legs again, start flexing and rotating your feet, and doing leg bends in bed. Get out of bed and go for a walk as soon as you're allowed to. It'll be just a small shuffle round the bed, first time, but soon you'll be going down the corridor and back. Don't go on your own because you'll be a bit woozy. Early mobility will help to avoid complications such as pain from gas, difficulty weeing, and blood clots in the legs. And it's amazing how quickly you start to feel better once you are mobile. But DON'T OVERDO IT. Do only half as much as you feel you can, even if you're sure you can walk around the whole block on day four. Discipline yourself to increase the exercise a *little* bit each day, otherwise you'll set back your recovery.

Laughing, coughing and sneezing in bed are less painful if you bend your knees and support your scar with a pillow. If you're standing up, bend over and put your hands over the scar. Avoid constipation, as it will be painful. If it gets to dire proportions (say, four days without a poo) your midwife can prescribe an anal suppository. Your tummy will look as if it's in the earlier stages of pregnancy for a while and will be sore. But on the plus side there will be no stitches in your fanny and you can sit without pain.

Your hospital stay will be longer than for a vaginal delivery – four or five days, depending on hospital policy and how you feel. Don't be swayed by friends or staff – if you want to go earlier or stay longer, discuss it with your midwife and do the best thing for you, not for some bureaucrat's government policy guidelines on bed allocation based on funding cuts. After you go home, you will be visited by a midwife who will check your caesarean scar and healing. The skin stitch is usually removed before you go home, if it hasn't already dissolved.

Full recovery is longer than for most vaginal deliveries – it's about six weeks until everything is healed up and several more weeks before you're up to full pre-pregnancy exercise capabilities. And of course it is harder to look after a baby and recover from major abdominal surgery at the same time. You will be very tired, and your body will be in shock for longer. Go easy on yourself.

The double burden of looking after a baby and recovering from surgery can lead to feelings of depression and some women believe they are 'failures' because they have not had a natural birth. Having a caesar, though, doesn't necessarily mean you'll have negative feelings about the birth – not least because it may have saved your life or the baby's.

You're usually told not to drive until your six-week check-up (mainly because it hurts to brake so you may brake more slowly than usual), although some doctors believe it is safe after about four weeks; if you do drive before six weeks, check with your insurance company that you are covered. You're also usually told not to reach above your head to get things down from shelves or do any similar activity, or lift anything heavier than your baby, before the six-week check-up.

more info on caesareans

 Caesarian Birth: Your Questions Answered by Lowdon Barlow, NCT/Derrick, 2004.
Good practical tips and sound advice based on a wealth of research evidence.

your record

✳ List your possible names for a girl a boy or either.

what's going

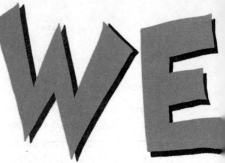

on You're tired. You've probably got sore feet, fluid retention causing swollen everything, and tingling fingers; and you could be breathless or dizzy. If you're really lucky you might even faint. You'll be having a weekly antenatal check from now on. You may get stabbing pelvic pains or aches – like a 'stitch' – which are probably the pelvic ligaments loosening up. The baby's head may be down low in the pelvis and can bounce up and down on your cervix giving you 'shocks', particularly if you sit down too quickly. This doesn't necessarily mean that the baby is 'engaged' (in position and ready to come out head first). You should begin to feel movements every day, even if it's only a little leg wave.

Those new lungs are still not completely finished. The baby has put on lots of fat. If it hasn't turned upside down already, it may be about to. (If it's still the wrong way up by the time labour starts, you may have a breech birth – meaning bum first instead of head.) Weight: about 2.5 kilos (5lb 7$^{1}/_{2}$ oz).

EK 36

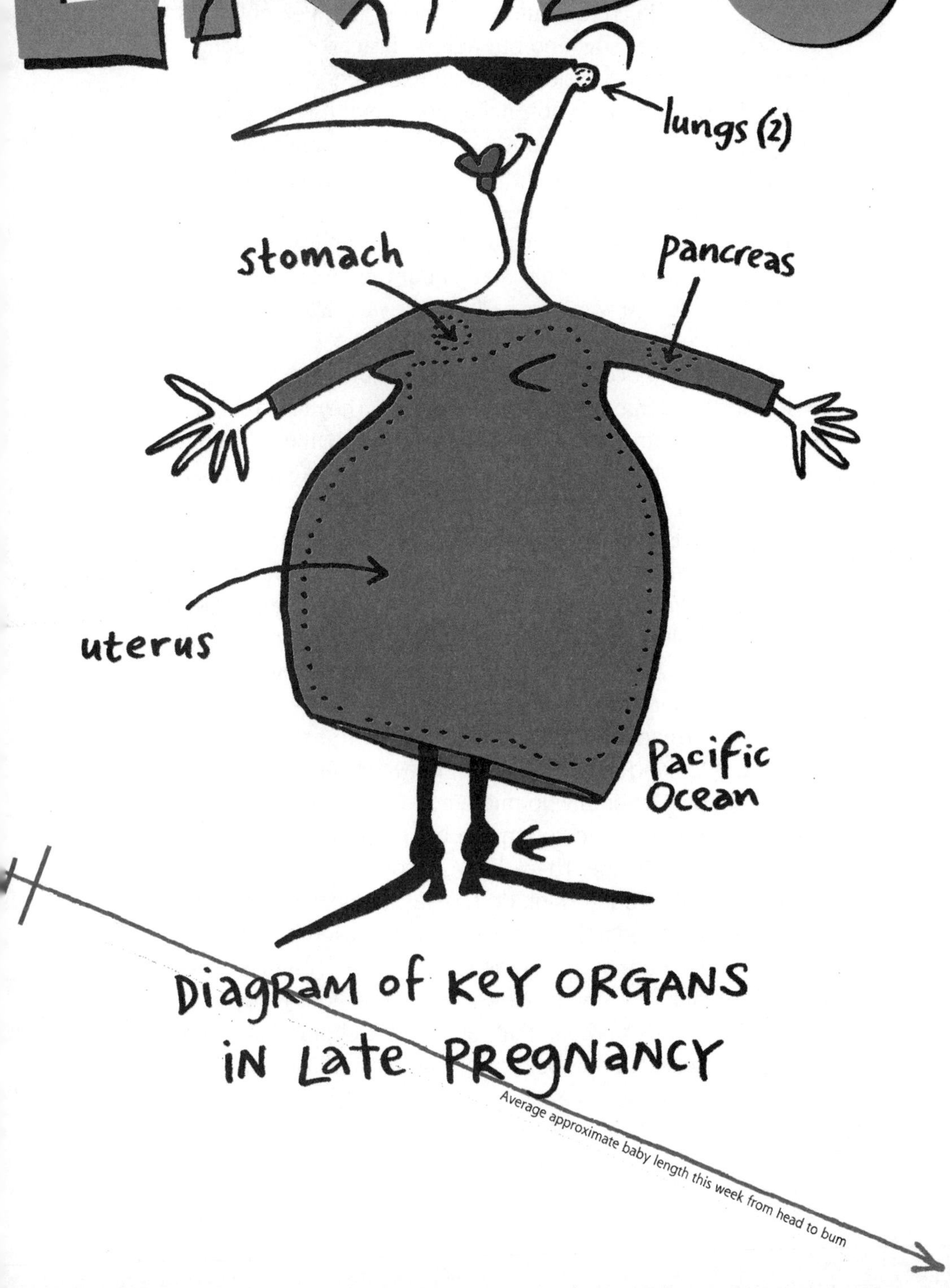

lungs (2)

stomach

pancreas

uterus

Pacific
Ocean

DIAGRAM OF KEY ORGANS
IN LATE PREGNANCY

Average approximate baby length this week from head to bum

DiARY

Wish I had given up work. The boss wants me to fly to Glasgow for a business meeting. Fat chance. Ha. That would be a hollow laugh except that I feel anything but hollow. Instead of waddling, I now lurch from side to side like a drunken Yeti.

On the way up to my hospital appointment (I have to go every fortnight in the last month), a woman in the lift tells me she had a one-hour labour and not to worry, it doesn't even hurt. I think she might have been at the pethidine cabinet. The obstetrician sees me with Anne and says I'm still 'carrying high' so it won't be soon, but I should read about caesareans just in case.

'I'd bet that you won't go early,' Anne says. She reminds me I'll probably put on another 5 kilos.

The lumps that come and go in my armpit have nothing to do with deodorant, the obstetrician says. They're actually breast tissue getting over-excited about soon having to produce milk, and are called 'breast tails'. Which sounds like a stripper's speciality to me.

Aunt Julie is making cushions (don't ask me why). Uncle Mike is ringing up to see how I'm going. Just had a horrible vision of Aurelia and Aunt Julie meeting over the head of the new baby in the hospital. Must warn Mike to keep Aurelia away until we come home. Keeping Aunt Julie away would be possible only with a very cunning plan and some Semtex.

Finally surrendering to the inevitable, Geoff is sleeping on the couch, and looking rather well on it, I have to say.

My old pal Deborah who migrated to the country with her toddler has sent us a pink bunny rabbit, home knitted by one of the ladies in the village. Thank heavens some people are keeping up the old skills. I don't think I'd have a clue how to begin knitting a rabbit myself. Deborah, bless her, has also taken it upon herself to create a database of all my friends, all ready for a mass email of the birth announcement. We've got two versions ready to go, one that says Eddy and one that says Pearl. Deborah made a bid for Dean instead of Eddy but lost on the recount. Anyway, I think that's all the options covered.

I've been thinking about the pros and cons of having a boy or a girl. Boy: won't be so bombarded with 'you're ugly' messages from advertising and film and TV. Girl: will probably find it easier to talk about emotions and be slightly less likely to play war games on the roof. Although, truth be told, it's impossible to really imagine what it will be like when this baby is OUT. The baby-being-IN thing and the getting-the-baby-out thing just take up so much brain space.

The worst thing about being this pregnant, except for being uncomfortable and increasingly nervous (could be any time from now), is that if you have someone to cuddle it's an exercise in geometry. It's impossible to get really close with a third person stuck way out there in the middle.

late babies

why are babies late?

Your baby is not likely to arrive at precisely midnight on the 266th day of pregnancy. So if it isn't early, it's going to be ... late. We don't know exactly what makes a woman's body go into labour, but it's believed that the baby, when ready to be born, somehow releases hormones or prostaglandins or some signal that doctors don't know about yet. This triggers the softening of the cervix, ready for it to dilate and let the baby through, and sets off the contractions of the uterus.

Only about 5 per cent of babies are born on their given 'due date'. Of the rest, roughly half are 'early' and half 'late'. First pregnancies are more likely to be 'overdue' and subsequent bubs more likely to come early. If you go beyond 2 weeks over, the doctor will probably induce the birth. (Incidentally, in France, a pregnancy is counted as 41 weeks – a more relaxed schedule.)

how long can you go?

All the research evidence indicates that if all is well with your pregnancy and the baby there is no need to think about inducing the labour. It is not until you go beyond forty-two weeks, that slight risks to the baby's health during labour and at birth occur. This could be an increased risk of the baby becoming distressed during labour because the placenta is not working as efficently, and the risk of the baby having a poo and then inhaling it at birth causing a nasty pnuemonia.

With careful monitoring you could go up to forty-four weeks, although most obstetricians and midwives don't like to leave it that long and will probably suggest an induction around the forty-second week of pregnancy.

Some of the most common methods of checking that an overdue baby is okay are:

⑥ You keep a 'kick chart' to monitor how much the baby is moving.

⑥ Electronic monitoring of the baby's heart rate to make sure it is not distressed.

⑥ An ultrasound to help estimate the baby's size and the amount of surrounding amniotic fluid.

induction methods
Membrane Sweep
This is usually the first thing offered as a gentle way of increasing the chances of labour starting naturally. Membrane sweeping involves your midwife or doctor placing a finger just inside your cervix and making a circular, sweeping movement to separate the membranes from the cervix. It can be uncomfortable and may cause a small amount of bleeding, but it will not cause any harm to your baby and has been shown to reduce the need for other methods of induction.

Prostaglandin Prostaglandins (which are like hormones) are found naturally in the uterus; some prostaglandins stimulate contractions at the beginning of labour. A synthetic prostaglandin gel or pessary (like a large pill) put next to the cervix can ripen it and trigger labour. It usually takes a number of doses, sometimes spaced over more than one day, before labour starts, but it is one of the least intrusive methods of induction.

Artificial rupture of the membranes (amniotomy) A plastic hook called an amnihook (sort of like a crochet hook) is used to break the membranes of the amniotic sac. Often it is enough just to brush the hook against the membranes, but sometimes it will have to be inserted to make a small hole. It usually doesn't hurt at all. Once the membranes have been broken, labour usually follows quickly as the baby's head is no longer cushioned by amniotic fluid so descends, putting pressure on the ripe cervix and encouraging it to widen. Breaking the membranes also triggers the release of prostaglandins, which help to speed up the labour process.

Artificial rupture of the membranes is a very effective method of induction on its own if the cervix is ripe. Amniotomy is often used during an otherwise normal labour to speed things up, and also if an electrode needs to be attached to your baby's scalp to monitor its heartbeat.

Oxytocin A synthetic form of oxytocin (the hormone that causes the uterus to contract) is given through a drip to increase the strength and regularity of contractions. The membranes will probably be ruptured as well. Contractions brought on by oxytocin are usually stronger, longer and more painful than normal, so pain-relief drugs are often used during labour.

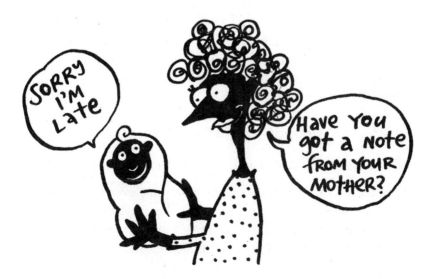

Other methods:

◎ Acupuncture or acupressure – often a course of a few treatments over a few days – which must be performed by a trained specialist.

◎ Some homeopathic remedies can be used to help ripen the cervix – again these must be prescribed by a homeopath experienced in pregnancy care.

◎ Nipple massage – gently massaging one nipple at a time (massaging both nipples at once has been shown to cause foetal distress), either by hand or with a warm, moist cloth, alternating nipples every 15 minutes for three periods of up to an hour each day, can stimulate uterine contractions and ripen the cervix.

◎ Semen is rich in prostaglandins, which ripen the cervix – the easiest way to 'administer' it is by having sex with, ermm, a man.

◎ Orgasm results in several strong uterine contractions; it is thought that these, combined with sexual arousal, can stimulate prostaglandin production.

◎ Keeping moving – keeping upright and moving allows a little extra pressure to be exerted on your cervix by your baby's head, which may stimulate ripening, but remember not to overdo it.

◎ Visualisation – some people believe that the power of suggestion can affect the body. If you're good at this sort of thing, try to relax and visualise the birth (leaving out any bits that make you anxious). Some women have found that watching films of babies being born triggers labour (remember all those stories about *Three Men and a Baby*?).

characteristic features of late babies

◎ Late babies often look a bit different from those born on time.

◎ They are sometimes described as looking 'overcooked' because during their extra time in the uterus they lose fat from all over their body, and their skin becomes red and wrinkly and may 'crack' as the waxy coating of vernix disappears.

⊚ They tend to have longer fingernails and more hair.

⊚ Although often skinnier, they keep growing in the uterus so they are larger all over than babies born earlier.

⊚ They are generally more alert than babies born earlier.

your record

❋ What labour issues do you feel really strongly about?

❋ How do you feel about medical intervention?
    What if it becomes necessary?

❋ What have you included in your birth plan?

what's going on Your bosoms may have developed a mind of their own and be leaking for no apparent reason or when a baby cries. (Any old baby will do.) The stuff is the colostrum, which will give your newborn baby protein and antibodies in the few days before your milk 'comes in'. The baby can't tumble around so much because it's run out of room, but the kicking and whacking can have a real force when they do happen. From here on in, try to be strict about getting as much rest and sleep as you can. Labour and recovery are much easier if you are well rested.

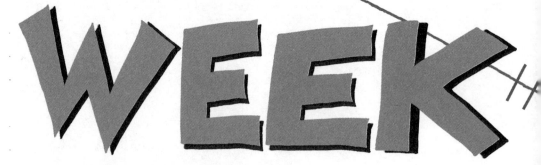

The baby isn't doing much except putting on more weight. The tiny lungs are getting ready to work on their own. The baby has a firm hand grip and is swallowing about 750 millilitres (26 fl oz) of amniotic fluid a day.

Weight: about 2.7 kilos (5lb 14 oz).

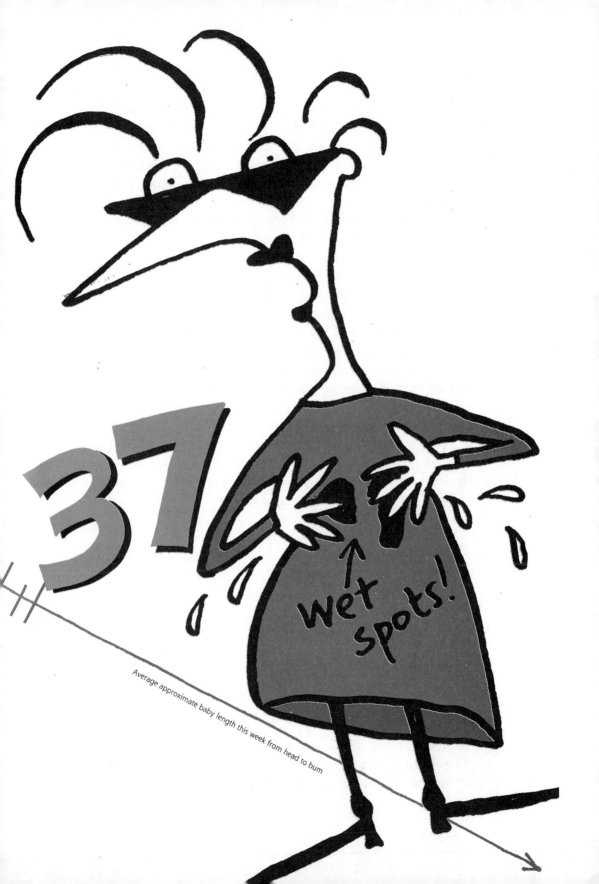

Average approximate baby length this week from head to bum

Wet spots!

37

DiARY

I hit the wall and give up work. I had planned to work until the first contractions, but something has happened to my brain. I was working too hard for contemplation, and my mind was demanding space. So of course what always happens when you stop working? I get a stinker of a cold.

At the midwives' clinic, Anne says, 'Don't have the baby on Saturday.' She is going for her motorbike licence. She says her helmet is very black and racy. I say if I do go into labour she'll have to come, but she can wear her helmet.

'It's part of my mid-life crisis,' she says cheerily.

I have been overcome by an ineluctable torpor. In other words I lie on the couch and watch 'The Bold and the Beautiful', and, I feel pretty strange just writing this, 'Fifteen to One' and 'Countdown'. But it is pointless to try doing otherwise. My priorities are all changing. Work is a distant memory within a couple of days and I feel utterly consumed by sloth hormones. I can't even seem to call people back on the phone.

I buy some lollies to put in the labour bag for energy and eat them all by 3 o'clock. I have written down the phone numbers of the hospital and Geoff's work and Beck's mobile, but if I don't pin them to the inside of my underpants I'll probably lose the lot.

info

your newborn baby

Newborn babies can look pretty weird. Yours might have the following:

◎ Blood and creamy vernix all over it (premature babies have more, late babies may have hardly any).

◎ Puffy, bruised or squinty-looking eyes.

◎ A head that looks elongated from being squeezed through the pelvis and vagina. This will normalise, often within hours, although it can take up to a couple of weeks; the bones have spaces between them so that they can squish up during birth; these harden within a few months to become one thick skull.

⑥ A swollen lump on the head, caused by the ventouse vacuum.

⑥ Temporary indentations on the face or head, or a pointy-headed look from use of the forceps.

⑥ Lanugo on the body – the downy hair is often across the shoulders, on the back, and on the face around the hairline (with more if the baby is premature). It usually rubs off within a few weeks.

⑥ Small white spots, like pimples, on the face. These are called milia and caused by temporary blockages of the sebaceous glands.

⑥ Red blotches – often called 'stork marks' because they look as if a stork has held the baby in its bill (yeah, right) – on the back of the neck at the base of the skull, the forehead and/or the eyelids. These are caused by little veins close to the skin – they will disappear after a year or so and only reappear with heat and stress, such as tantrums, during childhood.

⑥ 'Mongolian spots' – bluish-grey patches on the back, the buttocks and sometimes the arms and thighs. These are more common in Asian and darker-skinned babies; the spots will fade away.

⑥ Other birthmarks (see a paediatrician if you're concerned about a birthmark).

⑥ Big, swollen baby genitals and swollen breasts, even some spotting of blood from the baby vagina, due to a temporary oversupply of oestrogen.

⑥ Testicles that may not yet have 'descended' (more common in babies born before 36 weeks).

⑥ A bruised bum and very swollen genitals, if it's a breech-birth.

⑥ Jaundice – more than half of all newborn babies become 'jaundiced' (yellow) about three to four days after birth, but the baby's liver soon deals with this pigment, caused by the breaking down of unneeded red cells, and only a very small percentage of babies need treatment with sun or ultraviolet lights to come good.

routine medical stuff

The APGAR test will be performed to assess the baby's health. Named after its originator, Dr Virginia Apgar (oh my God, something's named after a woman), it's also an acronym for the check:

⊚ **Appearance** (colour).

⊚ **Pulse** (heartbeat).

⊚ **Grimace** (reflex).

⊚ **Activity** (muscle tone).

⊚ **Respiration** (breathing).

In each category 0, 1 or 2 points are given, and a score of 7 or more is considered to be good. The test is conducted 1 minute after birth and again 5 minutes after birth. A very low score will mean emergency medical care is needed.

It is common to suggest that all babies be given a vitamin K injection very soon after the birth as a preventative measure against haemorrhagic disease of the newborn (HDN). (If you're having a homebirth, check whether the midwife will give it.) It can be given orally but it is not so well absorbed into the body this way and will need repeat doses at one and two months.

A full weigh, measurement of length and medical check will include the test for congenital dislocation of the hip (CDH), which can be corrected during the first three months using braces or a harness to stabilise the legs while the hip joint develops.

The Guthrie or PKU test, routinely done a week after birth, involves a blood sample being taken from the baby's heel and is a screening test for the disorders of phenylketonuria and hypothyroidism, both of which are best caught early for treatment.

hearing tests

Most hospitals now do hearing tests on newborn babies – ask if you can get one before you go home. Ear experts say that, to give kids the best chance of learning language and to speak, deafness should be detected as early as possible: ideally in the first weeks, but certainly within six months. If you can't get a newborn test at the hospital, check with your GP or midwife to find out when and where you can have your baby's hearing tested.

things you mightn't know

⊚ Some newborn babies don't have tears when they cry until they are 1–3 months old.

⊚ The eye colour a baby's born with may change before they're a year old. Despite what many people say, not all babies are born with blue eyes, especially dark-skinned ones.

⊚ Newborn babies often develop sucking blisters in the centre of their top lip.

⊚ Newborn babies can't focus very well and are not good on colours. But they can see at a distance of 12 inches (30cm), or the distance from the breast to your smiling face. At two days old they can recognise their mother's face.

⊚ The first poo, meconium, is like something out of a horror movie; thick and sticky, it looks like extruded, green-tinged tar, but once your milk 'comes in' it gives way to the characteristic little-baby poo: yellowish and liquidy, with curds. This can come out at speed and you soon learn to be ready at nappy change time to intercept a stream. (Baby-boy wee can also travel quite a distance at short notice, in a large arc.)

⊚ The stump of the umbilical cord drops off in about a week or two, and the hospital midwives will show you how to take care of it in the meantime.

⊚ Soft sounds and listening to melodic voices is one of their favourite pastimes and they are able to recognise their parents' voices within the first week.

⊚ Almost all parents who decide to circumcise boys do so for religious reasons. It is now understood that there is no medical or hygiene reason to do so.

what's going on

The nesting urge is likely to be at fever pitch. Many women find themselves scrubbing underneath shelves and may have to be restrained. Don't do anything that involves standing on a chair or a ladder, no matter how much you feel that dusting the curtain rail is crucial to life as we know it. You might have aches and pains caused by your ginormous uterus. A gentle walk should help.

The baby is technically 'full term' – that is, fully developed – as it enters this week, although most doctors say forty weeks is full term too because that's the typical length of a pregnancy. Most of the lanugo has fallen out, but the baby's still covered in vernix. About 14 grams ($^1/_2$ oz) of fat is laid down each day from now on. The baby probably has a bowel full of meconium in a rather disgusting-looking hard rope of greeny-black stuff. Once the baby's out and starts on milk, the poo will be much more liquid. The baby still moves every day, but not very far. Weight: about 2.9 kilos (6lb 5oz).

WEEK 38

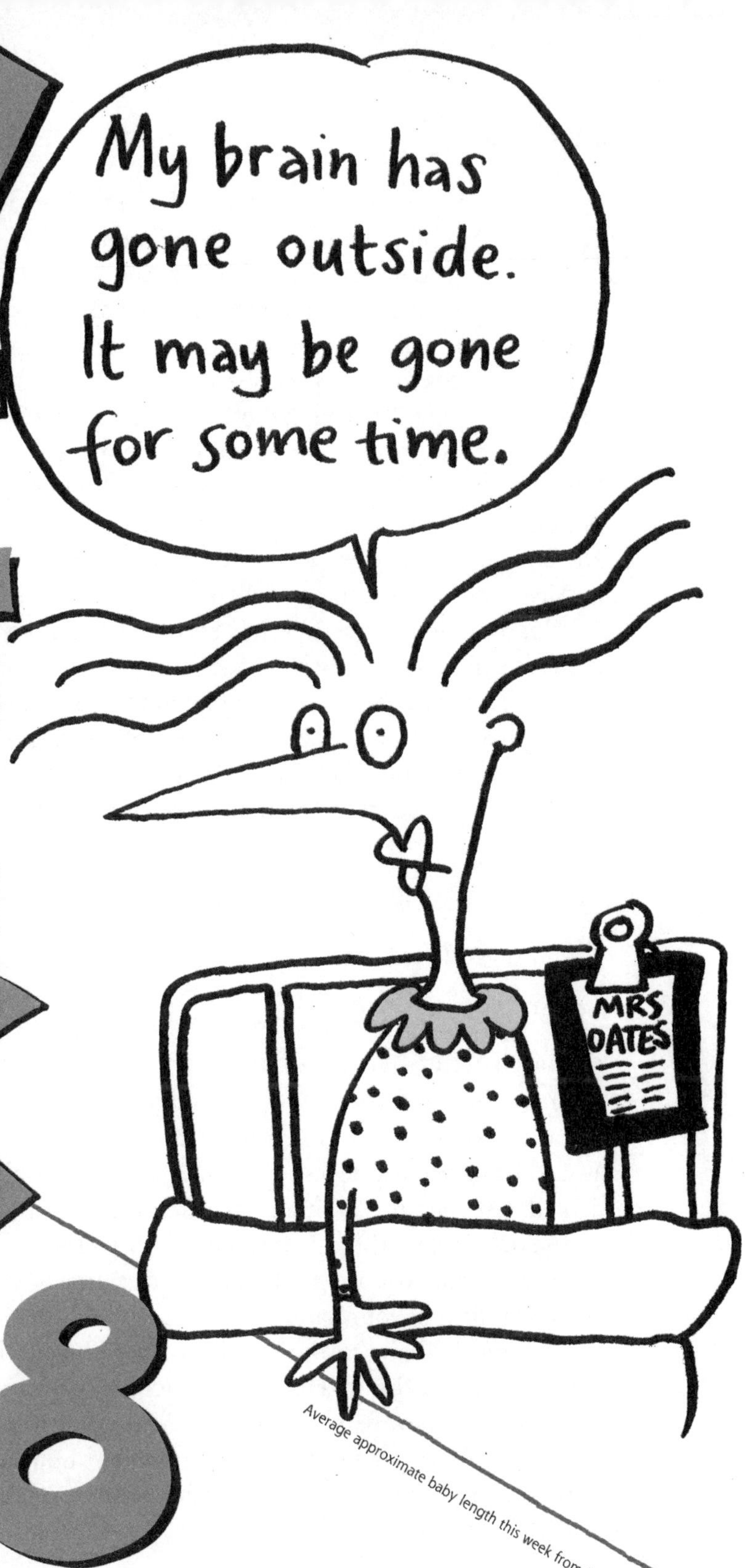
My brain has gone outside. It may be gone for some time.
MRS OATES
Average approximate baby length this week from head to bum

DiARY

Geoff comes along with me to the midwife appointment, where we spend the session talking giant babies with Anne. She says reassuring things about giant babes not necessarily being a problem as their mums pelvises can cope. Some of them simply pop out of their mothers singing a sea shanty, I'm sure. But she says they (the hospital, not the giant babes) will induce ten days or so after the due date if I'm still lying around doing my walrus impressions. I inquire politely about which weekends she's not on call, and promise to keep my legs crossed until she comes back on duty. The only time I can sleep properly is between 8am and noon. Luckily I don't have to be anywhere.

Not returning phone calls has become standard and I have taken to living in my dressing-gown. I'm all nested out. The house is getting untidy again, but I can't be bothered cleaning it. At least I know that Geoff will make the house spotless before I bring the baby home because otherwise he knows I would have him killed.

Wish I hadn't agreed to go into work once a week.

info

your body after the birth

immediately afterwards

After the birth of your baby, you might feel shivery and shaky, ecstatic, exhausted, sore, empty, blank, numb, sleepy or wide awake: whatever you feel is okay, and certainly won't be unprecedented. (At least one woman has taken the first look at her baby and said, 'Where did that come from?'.) If you've had an epidural, (or a caesarean) you may still have a wee catheter in your urethra and an IV drip in your hand.

Putting the baby to the breast as soon as possible after birth helps stimulate the uterus to contract and to squeeze out the placenta. Your new baby might not be hungry yet, but it's nice to meet a nipple anyway and feeding in the first hour after the birth is usually the best time for breastfeeding to be a success.

in the following days

You will get help and support from many professionals: your midwives, the hospital doctor and obstetric physiotherapist (who will remind you about your pelvic floor), and your local health visitor. When you go home from hospital the midwife visits you to help with the baby, answer any queries and give you her tips on breastfeeding and how to enjoy those early days of parenthood. When the midwife stops her visits (after around two weeks) a health visitor will take over. Health visitors are specialists in child health and development. Their role is to follow the baby through the first few years ensuring that it meets all the appropriate milestones at the right age, and offering you all sorts of advice from feeding to weaning and childhood immunisations.

Beyond any doubt, you will also get a lot of advice from people who visit you – much of it conflicting as there are so many ways of doing things and no particularly hard and fast rules. You and your baby need to find what works for you. Eventually you will have your own set of rules and practices and will be just as good at telling other new parents exactly what they should do.

Here are some of the basics you should know about during the first few weeks:

Bleeding (the lochia)   The lochia – the discharge of blood, mucus and tissue from the uterus – will continue for two to six weeks after the birth. It is kind of like having a period at first, with some clots. It changes to a pink or brownish colour and ends as a yellow-white discharge.

ⓖ Have plenty of maternity pads. (Because the cervix takes a while to close and tampons can cause infection, you can't use them until your first real period after the birth, and that could be months away if you're breastfeeding.) You can use the new, ultra-absorbent, thin pads if you like, but the extra padding of the thicker maternity pads might make sitting more comfy.

ⓖ Tell your midwife if you have very heavy bleeding, or if the discharge has a yukky smell or the bleeding suddenly gets bright red. Also tell the midwife straight away if you haven't bled at all since giving birth.

'Afterpains' 'Afterpains' usually occur for a few days (or more) after you have given birth, as your uterus contracts back towards its normal size. It's quite common to feel afterpains during breast-feeding. Taking mild pain relief like Paracetamol is safe whilst breastfeeding.

Haemorrhoids and constipation Labour and delivery can give you haemorrhoids, a distension of the blood vessels at the entrance to your anus. Try not to strain when having a poo, even if you're constipated, because it will make the haemorrhoids worse. Some people don't poo for a few days, especially after a caesarean, and you might need to ask for a mild laxative to help.

⑥ If you have haemorrhoids, ask your obstetrician, midwife or the nursing staff about icepacks and ointment for relief.

⑥ You may also need to eat more fruit, vegetables and cereals for fibre, and drink lots of water. See the hints on how to avoid consti-pation in the info in 'Week 8'.

Your poor sore fanny There will usually be 'some level of discom-fort in the perineal area', as doctors say, after a vaginal delivery, ranging from bearable to excruciating; you may need some pain relief for a day or two after delivery. If you've had an episiotomy or tear, the midwives in hospital will show you how to look after the stitched area so that it heals up well, and will regularly check the site to ensure that it is.

⑥ Regular baths with *very diluted* (10 drops per bath) tea-tree oil and lavender can help the healing process.

⑥ Wash stitches gently, even just with water, two or three times each day. Dry the area well after bathing and give yourself some pants-off airing time if possible. Don't dry stitches with a hairdryer unless you have a cool setting – some people numb the area with ice or drugs and then scorch themselves with a hairdryer that's too hot or too close. It might be better to wave a paper fan or a handy copy of *Hello!*

◎ Try leaning forward (with your hands reaching towards the floor) when you wee so that wee doesn't get onto the stitches.

◎ Splash out (so to speak) on some thick, soft toilet paper.

◎ While having a poo in the first couple of days post-delivery, support the perineal area firmly with a pad or wad of toilet paper.

◎ Avoid constipation by keeping your fibre intake up and drinking plenty of water.

◎ Try sitting on a rolled-up towel or with a pillow under each buttock or hire a Valley cushion from your local NCT branch representative. Don't sit on a rubber ring – it will direct more blood to the area, creating more pressure.

◎ Ask your doctor to prescribe anti-inflammatories or pain-killers that won't be transferred to the baby in breast milk.

◎ Take vitamin C for healing.

◎ Pelvic-floor exercises will stimulate circulation in the area and assist in the healing process. The first few times the area will feel very tired and trembly, and you may have some numbness, but do as many as you can as soon as you can.

◎ Most doctors say no bonking until the six-week check-up at least – possibly *after* the six-week check-up would be better (*during* might be considered a little inconsiderate). Invest in a tube of KY jelly especially if you are breastfeeding as the hormones that help to keep your milk supply going have a very drying effect in the vagina no matter how aroused you feel.

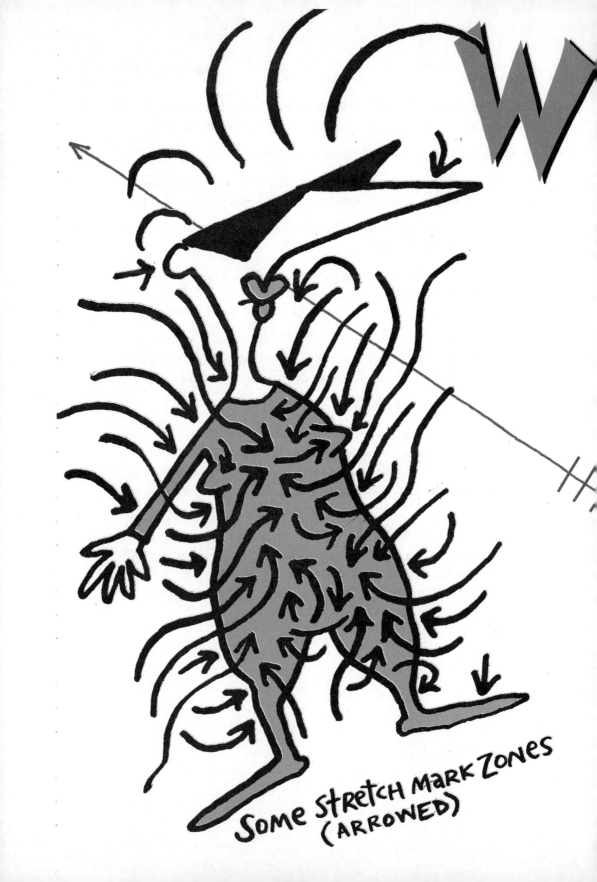

SOME STRETCH MARK ZONES (ARROWED)

EEK 39

what's going on The cervix gets softer and thinner, ready to open wide enough for a baby's head to come through. Any time from now it could release the mucus plug, which will end up on your knickers and is a sign that labour could start in the next few days (or even hours). The uterus is still practising contractions; in fact that pesky Mrs Braxton Hicks may be visiting rather too often and possibly confusing you about whether it's actually labour or not. You are probably completely fed up with being pregnant and have forgotten what your feet look like.

Your baby's genitals at this point have been over-excited by all your extra hormones and will be very large indeed in comparison to the rest of the body. They will return to a more seemly size a few days after the birth. Overall, the baby's growth slows down this week in preparation for birth. Weight: about 3.2 kilos (7 lb).

Average approximate baby length this week from head to bum

DiARY Latest inventory of body changes: gigantic, veiny knockers with brown nipples; new, brown, flat moles on them, and heaps of skin tags under each one; huuuge tummy; purple, stripey stretch marks on bosoms and hips. And I can't see my legs or pubic hair. For all I know they've been stolen. I know why whales beach themselves. THEY JUST CAN'T BE BOTHERED ANY MORE.

Having a baby is a preposterous proposition. How can this huge, hard thing possibly come out of a vagina? I hear about a woman whose first words after labour were 'What a completely shocking thing to happen.' I've also heard so many stories about people looking blankly at their newborn baby and wondering what on earth to do with it. I'm determined not to panic if I don't bond straight away.

I ask Susanne, 'Is it like an out-of-body experience?'

'No,' she says. 'It's a get-out-of-my-body experience.'

I still can't tell what my body wants – am I hungry, tired, nauseous, getting a cold? I have no idea. Walking is hard now, the damn groin pain never goes away: those ligaments must be under so much strain the anchor points are constantly stressed.

At this week's midwife visit, Anne looks exhausted – she's been up all night delivering babies. I didn't sleep much either.

'Is anything worrying you? Is there anything you want to ask?'

'No. Except don't go off duty, and did you get your motorcycle licence?'

Turns out she didn't do it a fortnight ago, so now she's going for the test this Saturday. I'll have to get that across to Oofty Goofty so she-he doesn't turn up at the weekend.

People are so different about babies. Attitudes range from the clucky to the disbelieving, through to distaste and secrecy.

I told my accountant, 'I feel stupid and tired.'

She was horrified I'd said it aloud. 'Don't tell anyone!'

There is a conspiracy of working mothers to hide the effects of pregnancy and motherhood so as not to be discriminated against.

I look up 'pregnant ladies' on the Internet and the first eleven matches are hardcore porn sites.

info

feeding your new baby

You may as well read this now because you won't feel like reading it straight after your baby's born! It's hard to think past labour at the moment, but when it's over you'll be preoccupied with your bosoms.

Breastfeeding is the best way to feed because breast milk is perfectly designed to nourish your baby with all the right nutrients and supply antibodies to boost the baby's immune system, which formula milk can't deliver.

In the past, babies were weaned onto plain old cow's milk, which wasn't very good for them, being designed for calves, not human babies, but now infant formulas are specially designed to give as many of the nutrients in breast milk as possible. Formula still runs second, but it's a much better second than it used to be.

breastfeeding in the first days

◎ For the first few days after birth the baby will be drinking the golden yellow pre-milk, colostrum, which is specially designed to nourish a baby and provide it with antibodies before it gets the milk. Most babies will lose a bit of weight until the milk 'comes in', and then start to gain again.

◎ At first breastfeeding might be painful, especially if your baby is having trouble latching on properly (latching on is often called 'attachment') and chomps on the nipple or can't seem to stay 'on' and suck. The baby needs to take most of the areola as well as the nipple in its mouth and the nipple goes to the back of the mouth. Different mothers and babies find different feeding positions suit them best. Use your time in hospital to get as much help and advice from the staff as you need. Your midwife will give you advice and help if you have had a home birth.

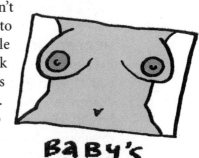

BaBy's fAvouRite View

⑥ If you're having problems breastfeeding and feel that the midwives have done all they can to help you, ask to speak to the breastfeeding counsellor – most hospital maternity units have someone in this role. Or you can contact an NCT breastfeeding counsellor (see 'Help', p.403 for contact details).

⑥ When your milk comes in (usually after three or four days), you can expect your breasts to feel full and hard. Your midwife will be able to give you advice on how to ease this, such as expressing a little milk before each feed and applying hot cloths or cold savoy cabbage leaves.

⑥ If your nipples are sore then you might need a cream to apply: breastfeeding counsellors recommend different things, from pure lanolin, which you don't have to wipe off before the baby drinks, to a camomile-flower ointment called Kamilosan. Often breast milk itself is the best treatment and squeezing a little milk onto the nipple after a feed keeps them protected from cracking and soreness. You don't need 'tough' nipples, you want pliable ones.

⑥ If you can, try to let your nipples dry in the air after feeding. Exposing them to very mild sunlight for short periods (3–5 minutes) will dry any excess moisture, and the ultraviolet light helps them to heal.

⑥ You might be asked if you can feel your milk 'coming in'. This is like a shiver, a prickle or even a stabbing pain in each breast, though sometimes you don't feel it for days or even weeks after the birth – or ever – but the 'let down' of your milk will happen at each and every breastfeed.

hooray for bosoms

Because breast milk is so fabulous for babies, because it helps you to bond with your baby, and because it's on tap and free of charge, it's really worth persevering if you have initial trouble breastfeeding: very few babies and mothers can get their act together straight away. The crucial thing is to try to relax (which is hard when you've got a hungry, crying baby and you can't get it

BREASTFEEDING BASICS

Sit comfortably with a drink to hand (preferably non-alcoholic), answering machine on or phone off the hook, and take a deep breath and lower your shoulders ...

⑥ Rest the baby on a pillow so that it can come up to the breast and make eye contact with you.

⑥ The baby should be lying on its side facing you (you can remember this as 'tummy to mummy').

⑥ The baby's nose should be in line with your nipple ('nose to nipple').

⑥ Support your breast by placing your fingers flat on your ribs at the junction of your breast and the ribs, keeping your thumb uppermost.

⑥ Support the baby's head and shoulders in such a way that its head is free to extend slightly as it is brought to the breast – so that its chin and lower jaw reach the breast first.

⑥ Move the baby towards the breast so that its nose and upper lip touches the nipple causing its mouth to gape wide open.

⑥ When the baby's mouth is wide open, move the baby quickly to your breast and aim your nipple towards the top of the back of its mouth. Its lower lip should be as far from the nipple as possible.

⑥ The baby is then ready and with a wide mouth and a strong tongue it will suck rhymically taking short breaks every so often but still remaining attached.

If the connection is painful, break the suction the baby has on your nipple gently, by first sliding your little finger into the baby's mouth next to your nipple, and then pulling the baby off gently. Otherwise it will be very hard on your nipples.

to 'attach' properly). Most mums and babies take a while to learn breastfeeding together, perfecting it over time.

A middle road could be expressing your milk and putting it in a bottle to give your nipples a rest. You can also supplement a low supply with formula. Even managing one week or better still one month of breastfeeding is a big bonus for your baby. And if it really doesn't work, you have a fine back-up with formula: your baby will not starve. So give it another go.

It's more convenient to get the feeding sorted out before you leave hospital, than at home. Though when you go home you do get visits from a midwife which is some help. Ask to watch another mother feeding her baby if you like. Quite often, you'll get conflicting advice from midwives about how to hold the baby, how to position yourself while you feed and how often to feed for how long. If it's all putting your head in a whirl (you'll be madly sleep deprived, which doesn't help), choose to listen to ONE of them – or call in the breastfeeding counsellor – and don't be swayed from their advice if it's working. Choose someone who clearly likes babies, is encouraging and gentle, and takes the time to help you, sit with you, watch your technique and try different ways to help. (Don't choose anyone who grabs your breast in one hand, the baby in the other and brings them together like a clash of cymbals.)

not breastfeeding

If you find you can't breastfeed your baby, or breastfeeding is not for you, it's nowhere near the end of the world. The way people go on about it, you'd think not breastfeeding was the equivalent of making the baby drink gin and wheeling it across motorways during blizzards in a war zone. Look at the adults around you. Look at the kids around you. Can you tell who was bottle-fed? Course you can't. Many other factors affect a child's development and immune system, including the amount of chemicals in an environment, access to fresh, healthy food, and exposure and building up a resistance to germs.

Instead, you can enjoy the relaxed feeling of bottle-feeding your baby while making eye contact, and the freedom it gives you because you can always get somebody else to feed the baby if you'd like to go out for an hour or so and have an affair with a couple of firemen. Now crank up the steriliser, tweak those teats on the bottle. And get on with it.

Your midwife or health visitor can help you with all the stuff you need to know about sterilising equipment and storing and heating bottles.

Stuff to tell nosy people

'I have an illness controlled by medication, which mustn't be passed through breast milk to my baby.'

'Both my nipples blew off during a wind storm.'

'It's easier to get the gin into a bottle.'

'I can't breastfeed, and I don't want to talk about it. Gosh, that's a lovely blouse.'

'My husband has engaged a wet nurse.'

'Oh, just BUGGER OFF.'

 See Breastfeeding in 'Help' (p.403).

your record

* What are your feelings about breastfeeding?

* How long would you like to breastfeed for?

what's going on This is the magic week when your baby is 'due', unless somebody has cocked up the dates. But this is based on averages, so don't expect to give birth on the due date. If you do, it is simply showing off.

The baby is rounder and fatter and probably ready to be born. It is now about 200 times heavier than it was at twelve weeks. Boys are often bigger than girls.

Weight: about 3.5 kilos (7lb 10oz).

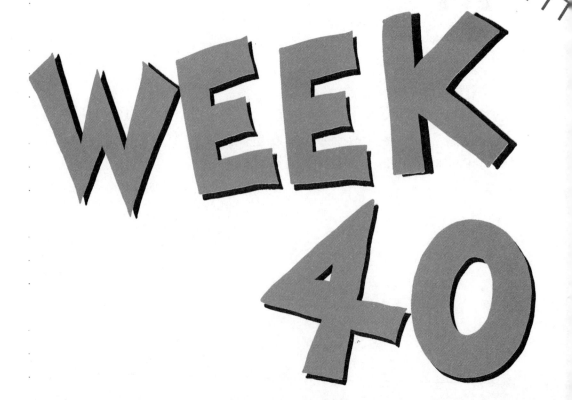

WEEK 40

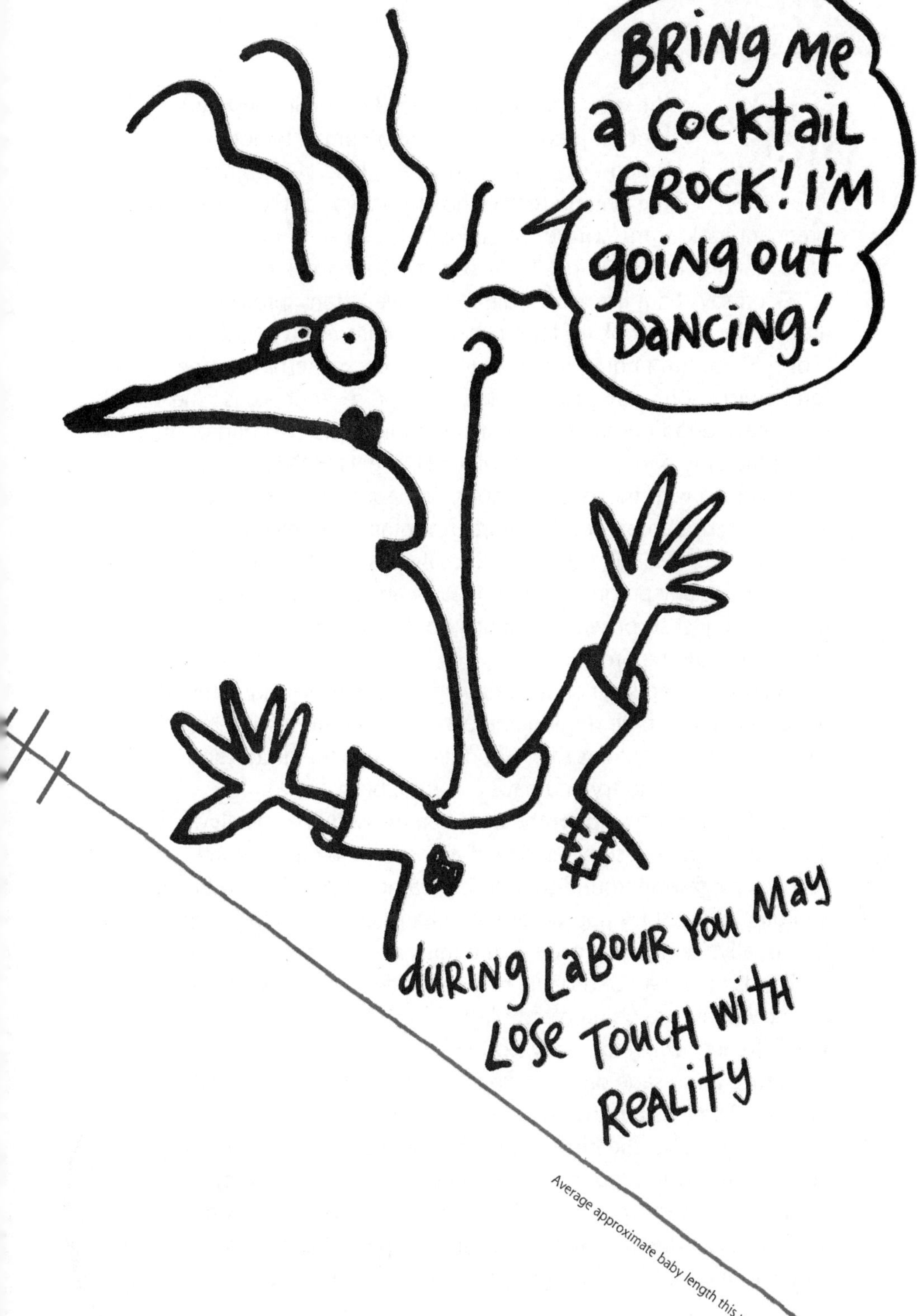
BRING ME A COCKTAIL FROCK! I'M going out DANCING!
during LaBour You May Lose Touch with Reality
Average approximate baby length this week from head to bum

DiARY

I'm due. It's official. The end of the longest and biggest pregnancy known to human biology. When I go to the midwives' clinic, the women in the waiting room who are only a couple of months pregnant look at me with expressions between contemplation and panic: 'Surely I couldn't get THAT big', they are thinking.

Geoff says I am like a cat waiting to have kittens, prowling around the house looking for a good cupboard to give birth in – or tidy up. I'm finding it harder to drink Beck's herbal uterine tonic concoction – I'm just sick of it, but I persevere because she says I have good uterine tone, which I am immensely proud of, it being the only part of my body which HAS ANY TONE.

Obsessed with the idea of labour. Someone tells me of Kathy Lette's description of a post-caesarean vagina as 'honeymoon fresh'. If I didn't laugh I'd sob m'self silly. It's also becoming clear to me how many pregnant women worry about pooing during labour. I'm just surprised your lungs don't come out your bum considering all the pressure.

Have left a message on the answering machine saying nothing's happened yet. People ringing and asking all the time. All the ones who are already mothers say, 'Good luck', 'Take the drugs' and 'You're not going to try and have a natural birth are you?'

Uncle Mike turns up on the doorstep dressed like a Hollywood B-movie costume designer's idea of a part-time pimp: opaque, yellow-lensed wraparound sunglasses, leather jacket, heeled boots and grey beard. I try not to stare. Aurelia is always waiting in the car, usually taking advantage of the mirror on the passenger visor. He hands me a bag of organic mangos and remarks casually that he and Aurelia are going off to Glastonbury. 'So', I venture, 'you won't be here when the baby's born?'

'Leave a message on my mobile!' he cries gaily as he heads for the gate. Family support. What would you do without it?

I dream about the birth: I am lying on a sexy, pink satin-quilted four-poster bed reading a magazine full of photos of gorgeous clothes I could afford that would look quite nice on me (I *said* it was a dream) when a man in a leopard-skin suit comes past with a cocktail trolley on wheels full of excellent cakes, bottles of attractively coloured alcohol, an icebucket and some syringes. 'Martini?' he inquires politely.' Or perhaps an epidural?' Just at that moment a perfectly charming baby pops out of my vagina. 'Ow,' I remark, absent-mindedly. 'Why, thank you, I'll take a gin and lime. And a small colostrum for my new young friend.'

Just in case this doesn't happen, Anne has arranged with the hospital doctors for me to have an induction. I am scheduled to go into the maternity hospital next Monday at 5pm to have my cervix annointed with a prostaglandin that mimics the one in the body that basically says, 'Lady, start your engines for labour.' I have to stay in hospital, and they might put some more in the next morning. Then I should be able to start on my own without the oxytocin drip, although in some cases the membranes have to be broken by the midwife if the waters don't break by themselves. All quite scary.

Beck's given me acupuncture twice to try to move the baby along a bit, and I've taken some tiny homeopathic pills. The baby finally 'engages' (goes into firing position) after two days of this. So TIRED. Some anxiety attacks, but mostly sort of numb.

Everyone is ringing up saying, 'Has anything happened?'

'NO!'

info

your hospital stay/early days

Midwives will be assigned to you in hospital (or at home, if you've had a home birth). Their job is to take care of you as you recover from the birth and they are also there to help you learn how to feed and look after your baby. Ask them anything you want to know, and take full advantage of their time and knowledge. Most women spend 24–36 hours in hospital after giving birth (or three nights, following a caesarean). You can go home sooner if both you and the baby are doing well and you feel ready to go home.

If you feel you need more time in hospital – either because you're still not feeling a hundred per cent or because you don't feel ready to cope with the baby on your own – talk to your midwife and explain that you need to stay a couple of extra days.

exercise

If your hospital offers postnatal exercise or physio classes, try to get along. It's a good way to get into an exercise routine that you will hopefully continue in the weeks after you get home; it will help your body recover; and moving about should help you to feel less stiff and sore. The emphasis tends to be the pelvic floor and stomach toning exercises. Even if you hardly take part, it's good to know how to do these.

Once home, you probably won't have the time or energy for exercises for a while, beyond a bit of pelvic floor and stomach toning. Even if you feel buzzing with energy (in your dreams), it is advisable to wait until after the six-week postnatal check up with your GP before returning to the gym or aerobic exercise classes. Once there, be sure to tell the gym staff or instructor that you are a postnatal mother because you still need to take care of your back and other joints. The body is not producing the relaxin hormone any more but it continues to affect the joints until the baby is about four months old. Avoid running and high impact exercises for these few months.

You could try a specialised postnatal exercise class. They tend to be better paced and you will be in the company of other mothers also trying to regain their fitness level.

food

⊚ Nutrition and beating hunger are important issues for breast-feeding. Ask your midwife or health visitor for suggestions.

⊚ It may be nutritionally sound, but hospital food is usually, at best, pathetically boring and portions are small. Get friends to bring you decent food such as fresh fruit. Most wards have a fridge and access to a microwave so you can have a stash of your own.

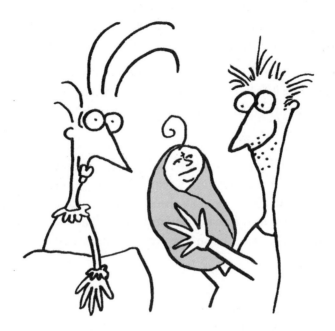

visitors

◎ Don't feel obliged to see everyone who wants to check out the baby while you're in hospital (or in your early days at home). In hospital, make the most of this time when your meals, cleaning and other needs are being taken care of by other people to recover from the birth and to prepare yourself for when you go home. You may actually want to ban all but a few close friends and family from visiting for the first few days so you can rest and spend time with your baby.

◎ Hospital visiting hours are not as strict as they used to be, but you can pretend that they are, and if you don't want people dropping in outside the set hours, enlist the help of the midwives and ward staff, they can be appropriately officious.

◎ Ask people to phone your partner or the hospital before they come to visit. If you're too tired or don't feel up to seeing anyone, don't hesitate to say so. You're not on stage. Get your partner to tell people how long they should stay for, and to usher them out ('it's time for your rest'). People often have no idea when to go.

If flowers get in the way or cause allergies, ask people who are coming to visit you not to bring them. Instead have one or two close friends bring you a small bunch to brighten things up.

paperwork

Registering the birth   You have a legal duty to register the birth of your baby in the first six weeks of its life, unless you live in Scotland where you have only three weeks. At some hospitals the registrar comes to the maternity unit on a daily basis so that you can register the baby before you go home (assuming you have

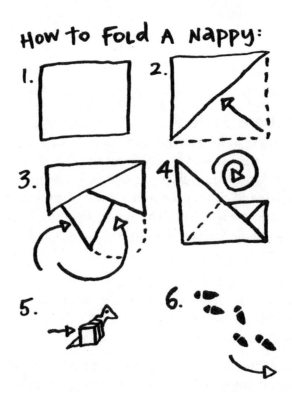

thought of a name that is). In other areas you have to make an appointment at the local registry office and go along in person. If you are not married and wish to put both the parents' names on the birth certificate you must both attend together. If you are married only one partner need go.

Once your baby is registered you will be given their birth certificate. This is a short form stating the chid's name and sex, and the date and place of birth. If you want a copy of the full certificate (a nice paper job with details in writing rather than computer printed) you need to pay a small fee. Your baby will also be issued with a National Health Service number. You are then able to register your baby with a doctor.

Registering for benefits You need the birth certificiate to claim for the benefits that are due to you. You can obtain a form for the child benefit payment from you local Social Security Office. This is paid either weekly or monthly directly into your bank account or by a book of orders to cash at the post office if you prefer.

If you haven't already, call your nearest Benefits office about any government benefits you may be entitled to, such as the single parent's benefit or the Surestart program that sets out to assist disadvantaged families around the time of birth.

Health cover If you have private family health insurance, you will have to add the baby to your policy. Usually you have about eight weeks to do this after the birth, but check to make sure your baby will be covered.

Birth notice You might want to write a paragraph for the classifieds in the newspaper and keep that edition for the baby when they grow up.

what's going on If your pregnancy has been

'average' (forty weeks long), your baby is out in the world and

perhaps sleeping off the shock. After your baby is born

a whole bunch of hormonal activities happen, quite suddenly.

Your body expels the placenta, which has been pumping out

huge quantities of hormones. Suddenly you're bereft of the

'happy hormones' and getting a boost of hormones such

as prolactin to help breastfeeding. Your body looks less

pregnant, but your tummy is still very big. You're bleeding from

the vagina as the body expels all that nice uterine surface the

baby needed. Your body is recovering from the massive

shock of childbirth – whether natural or surgical. Give yourself a

break. Don't do anything but recover and be with your baby.

The baby may have some characteristic newborn

marks, such as 'stork marks' (red, rashlike shapes on the

forehead, eyelids and/or back of the neck) or temporary marks

from forceps. More than half of all newborn babies develop a

yellowy tinge to the skin and eyeballs, called jaundice – it's no big deal. Your baby is sucking colostrum because your

milk probably won't come in until day 3 or 4. The bub will be

down a bit from its birth weight before the breast milk kicks in.

Don't worry about this: too much scientific measuring and talk

of weight-loss percentages can be freaky – lost weight in those

first few days is expected in all babies and the loss can be

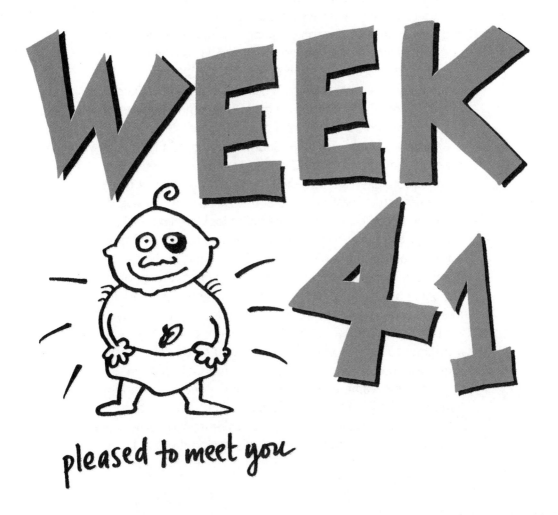

WEEK 41

pleased to meet you

It's time. We drive to the hospital primed for the prostaglandin-near-the-cervix induction, with the bag neatly packed with all the things we'll need for labour, feeling nervous but excited. Luckily Maternity isn't busy so I get my own room. It all seems a bit dreamy. I'll have the induction, sleep a bit, then in the morning, when contractions will probably start, ring Beck and tell her to come in sporting her best midwifery hat.

DiARY

Anne comes into our room wearing a lovely suit and some Issey Miyake perfume on her way to a movie, and puts the gel on my cervix. What a charming bedside manner she has – she chats away about something else and one could almost be at a dinner party if she didn't have her hand up your fanny.

A second midwife arrives in a white jacket and navy pants and puts a piece of electronic equipment on wheels next to the bed and attaches a belt around my tummy. This is the monitor. It continually rolls out a graph of any contractions and a graph of the baby's heartbeat, which is usually up around 150 beats a minute. Geoff and I start to play cards, pretending that we can keep our mind on Snap! instead of all the machinery.

A long time later I write this: Suddenly I noticed that the baby's heartbeat had dropped to 80 beats a minute, and then it went down to 60 beats. And so began the worst two hours of my life.

Geoff tried to reassure me that it was probably normal, but when the midwife came back she had a look on her face I never want to see again and rang for an obstetrician, who, it transpires, was just about to have his first meal in 24 hours in the canteen. Within 5 minutes he was in the room, looking at the graph. 'I'm just going outside to consult with someone, and I'll be back in a moment to tell you what we're going to do,' he said calmly.

Left alone, Geoff and I held hands and tried not to look as frightened as each other. 'He's going to do an emergency caesarean. Beck's not going to make it,' I thought suddenly.

The doctor came back in and sat on the bed, and held my hand and said – I still can't write these words without crying – 'Your baby is distressed, and if it's this distressed because of a Braxton Hicks contraction, we won't risk going through labour.'

Behind the scenes an anaesthetist, a paediatrician and another obstetrician were rushing in from elsewhere in the building. The midwife marched Geoff off to wash and mask up, while a nurse wheeled me out on one of those cold, gleaming trolleys and into the white, shining operating theatre, where there were people with blue paper masks, shower caps and gowns.

The anaesthetist put an IV drip in my left hand, and then gave me a spinal-block injection into the lower back, with me curled in a foetal position while a nurse held my hand. It was really scary staying perfectly still so he didn't get the wrong bit of the spine. As the anaesthetic started to work, Anne (who had been paged at the cinema) came in with her midwife colleague, two obstetricians, a paediatrician, and – thank God! – Geoff, who looked like he was playing an extra in 'ER'. They put up a blue fabric screen over my chest so I couldn't see my tummy. Everyone fussed around behind the screen for a moment.

'Let me know when you start,' I said to Anne.

Everybody laughed.

'We've been in for 3 minutes,' she said.

When I looked up at the huge light with the flat globe cover, I could see the reflection of my insides, yellow and pink and purple. These were the things I was thinking: 'Please let my baby be all right', 'Thank God I'm not having a home birth', and large stretches of blank that probably had something to do with shock.

'There's your baby coming out,' said the second midwife, taking a Polaroid photo.

'Is it Eddy or Pearl?' I asked.

'It's Eddy!' everyone chorused.

And suddenly Anne held up a silent, purple, slimy creature with a screwed up, tiny little face and a smudge of dark hair. A sob caught in my throat as I reached out and gently touched my baby's leg with the back of my hand. Instantly he was whipped away to a table by the paediatrician and the midwife, who gave him a rub down with a warm towel and then a few puffs of oxygen with a plastic face mask. 'He's just fine', said the paediatrican. 'He's got all the right things in all the right places.' His little body started to turn a reassuring pink colour.

And then Eddy started to cry. All the experienced people in the room broke into huge smiles. 'That's a good cry,' they said simultaneously.

Anne and the paediatrician did some tests on Eddy over in the corner of the room, on a kind of heated bed that I later found out is called a resuscitator (glad they didn't mention that). Meanwhile the two obstetricians were doing their downstairs needlework on what Geoff would later refer to as 'the tummy smile': my curved red scar. When they had finished and gone off with cheery greetings, Anne brought Eddy, wrapped in a rather fetching white swaddling cloth, for me to cuddle in bed, and showed Geoff how to hold him, with his hand supporting his head. We were both shaky and in tears and I of course was drugged out of my mind. In fact I couldn't believe any of this was happening.

After a while, Anne and a nurse wheeled me and Eddy and perhaps Geoff, too, though he may have walked, out of theatre and off to the Maternity recovery ward, where three other mothers-and-infant-Caesars were already installed. I drifted in and out of sleep while Geoff sat vigil, holding Eddy in his arms in a kind of trance. I came to wondering where on earth my pregnancy had gone, before seeing Eddy, and panicking if he was allright. I didn't feel an immediate surge of overwhelming love. Mostly relief that he was okay, and anxiety about how to get him on the breast for a snack of colostrum. Eddy just looked tired and tiny, and slept a lot. And guess what? He wasn't even a whopper: 7lb 14oz (3.6 kilos). Damn. All the rest was Magnums.

info

coping when you get home

getting organised

◎ As in hospital, insist that friends and relatives call before visiting, or set aside particular times, and continue to tell them how long to stay. Oh and make them make their own tea.

◎ If friends or relatives offer to help with cleaning, cooking or shopping, ACCEPT IMMEDIATELY!

◎ There will be days when preparing dinner will seem impossible or unbearable. Prepare for these by doing extra large batches when you do cook so that they can be frozen. If friends and relations offer to bring you meals, ACCEPT IMMEDIATELY! Keep take-away menus from a few decent local places.

◎ If you can afford it, get a cleaning service in for a few hours once or twice a week so that the basic housework, such as cleaning the bathroom and kitchen, is always done. If you can't afford it but can't stand being in a messy house, just keep one room tidy. This will give you somewhere to relax or see visitors.

◎ If you live by yourself, try to organise a roster of friends to come by each day for the first few weeks so that you can have an uninterrupted half hour to take a shower or bath, sit down without the baby or get out of the house briefly.

looking after yourself

◎ Try to get out of the house every day to help keep yourself sane. If you're going somewhere like a shopping centre, check out the parents' facilities and whether there are lifts or flat escalators. If you have to negotiate a lot of stairs, you may be better off with a baby sling than a pram.

◎ If you have a partner, make time to go out alone with them, even if it's just for coffee, while a friend looks after your baby.

⑥ Try to get time each day to do your postnatal exercises (especially the pelvic-floor ones) you'll find you have more energy for them in the mornings. If you enjoy exercising with other people, a postnatal class after a few weeks will also give you a chance to talk with other new mothers.

⑥ Use the time when your baby is sleeping during the day to have a nap or relax. Put your needs ahead of visitors, housework and other chores.

⑥ Don't pretend you're coping if you're not: share things with your partner or friends. Talk to your health visitor if you think you are getting some postnatal blues (for more on which see 'Week 42'). They are specially trained to help mothers with new babies.

a crying baby

Small babies often cry for mysterious reasons but remember, it is their only way of communicating their needs. Here are some tips to stop your baby crying if they are not hungry, tired, hot, cold, wet or in pain from wind, a dirty nappy or whatever else you've checked for:

⑥ Curl up together in bed in a warm, dark, quiet room, tummy to tummy for maximum skin contact.

⑥ Try a warm bath and baby massage (though some babies hate both until they're a few weeks old) – ask a midwife or health visitor for a demo or to recommend a local course; basically, be gentle, use any sort of oil you can eat, and stop if it makes the baby cranky.

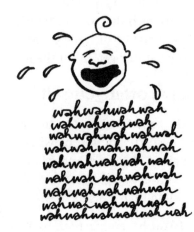

⑥ Rock with your baby in a chair.

THE GREAT DUMMY DEBATE

You'll find most baby books sternly frown on using a dummy, especially after the baby is three months old, but mother and baby sleep clinics often use them. Dummies aren't supposed to be used automatically as soon as a baby cries. But if a baby is fed, clean and burped and yet has got itself into a hideous, sobbing, can't-remember-why-I'm-crying-but-I'm-hysterical-now-and-can't-stop-yelling state, a dummy is heavenly. Take no notice of what the books say; the authors aren't there to hold the baby when you're going nuts. Wait and see if your baby is like this before buying a dummy.

If you do decide to use one, here's the huge drawback nobody tells you about. The baby may become 'addicted' to it, and if so there'll be a period when the dummy will actually make the baby cry more because when a dummy falls out the only way a young baby can get it back in is to cry for you to come and put it in – several times a night. These weeks can be just not worth it, and a good time to wean the baby off the dummy. Eventually, some time between 5 and 10 months, a baby is able to replace a dummy on its own, and so the 'addiction' will continue.

There are various types of dummies on the market, some of them claiming to be orthodontically shaped (though you'll have a hard job convincing a dentist they are good for teeth). To avoid the baby getting thrush in its mouth, replace the dummy every few weeks, and throw it out if it looks the worse for wear with wobbly or torn bits. You'll need at least two or three to rotate through the sterilising process once your baby works out how to spit the dummy – and then to cry for it after it's hit the floor.

⑥ Play soothing music (you might feel like an idiot at first, but sing to your baby – anything soothing, even if you have to make it up – and if you 'can't sing', your baby won't notice).

⑥ Walk up and down your sittingroom about 5,000 times with the baby over your shoulder.

⊚ Try to distract the baby by holding them level with your face and nodding your head, while making a (pleasant) noise or grinning – this can give them such a surprise that they forget what they were crying about.

⊚ Go about your business with the baby in a sling.

⊚ Try an approved dummy for newborns (see previous page).

⊚ Accept there's nothing you can do, and get someone else in to hold the baby while you walk around the block.

getting your baby to sleep

Try to get into a settling routine when your baby is due to go down so that they start to associate certain things with relaxing and going to sleep. You might use sounds (singing, music or even rhythmic noises like the washing machine), movements such as rocking in a chair or being carried close to your body in a baby sling, massage, a warm bath, or a ride in a pram or even a car. (A car is an expensive habit to get into and not great if you're exhausted, but it can do the trick in extremis.) For most parents the routine of a play in the bath, then a short massage before putting on bed clothes, followed by a feed in a dimly light bedroom gives the baby the right message. When they get a little older, a night-time story can be added to the routine.

⊚ Use a dimmer switch or soft lamp to feed by at night-time, and avoid stimulating the baby or they'll think it's play time.

⊚ Overtiredness is a common cause of crying, and paradoxically can make it harder for the baby to get to sleep. A baby can seem 'hyped up' when they're really overtired. Soothing methods that involve walking, rocking or singing to the baby may end up stimulating them more, so that it is harder to get them to sleep. Instead, try stroking your baby's head or tummy, patting its back rhythmically, or make soothing hushing sounds.

⊚ You don't need to be silent while your baby is sleeping. It's best for them to get used to normal noise levels.

and the rest

For all the other stuff you'll worry about such as wind, vomiting and weird-lookin' poo, see your baby health centre nurse, peruse 'Help', and always have a baby-care book on hand (see Baby-care Books in 'Week 43').

SUDDEN INFANT DEATH SYNDROME (COT DEATH)

The cause of Sudden Infant Death is not known: basically what happens is that the baby (usually in the first six months) stops breathing. Fortunately, instances of SID have been quite rare in the UK since 1991, following a health department campaign to follow key risk-reducing measures. These are:

1 Place your baby on its back to sleep.

2 Don't smoke when you're pregnant or during your baby's first year, or allow anyone to smoke in the house or car.

3 Keep your baby's head uncovered when it is sleeping and don't let your baby get too hot. Remember to remove hats and extra clothing as soon as you come indoors or enter a warm car, bus or train, even if it means waking your baby.

4 Place your baby in the 'feet to foot' position in the cot to prevent them wriggling down under the covers (they normally wriggle up, away from where their feet are).

5 Don't use bumpers or bedding such as duvets and pillows in the cot or crib and keep toys out, too, if they might pose a risk.

Sleeping with your baby can be enjoyable and makes the night feeds a little easier. But, you should be careful not to let the baby get too hot under your bedclothes, snuggled up close to your body. The SIDS Foundation advise against sleeping with your baby if you or your partner smoke or have been drinking alcohol or have taken drugs which cause drowsiness.

After about the age of 6 months, babies may stop sleeping in exactly the position you place them and put themselves into all sorts of positions (bum up in the air is a particularly entertaining one). Some older babies roll onto their tummies during sleep, and by this age they should be able to move themselves if they get into any breathing trouble.

A few younger babies who are always placed in the same position to sleep may develop a flattened or unusual head shape. In most cases this does no harm and 'fixes itself' before school starts. Current SIDS research still indicates babies should be put to sleep on their backs, but you can change the head positions for each sleep, from face turned to one side, then to the other, then to looking straight up. (If your baby always seems to turn its head to face out into the room, you can alternate putting the baby at different ends of the cot, so their head isn't always in the one position.) And if your baby's head seems to be oddly shaped or crooked, have it checked out by a paediatrician for your peace of mind.

Remember it is good for your baby to play on their front when awake and try not to let the worry of cot death stop you enjoying your baby's first few months.

See the sections on Sleep and Parenting and pregnancy help, and for SIDS, Grief and Loss, in 'Help'. The SIDS foundation website is *www.sids.org.uk*

your record

✳ Scribble down everything about your labour. I know you don't believe it now, but you will forget!

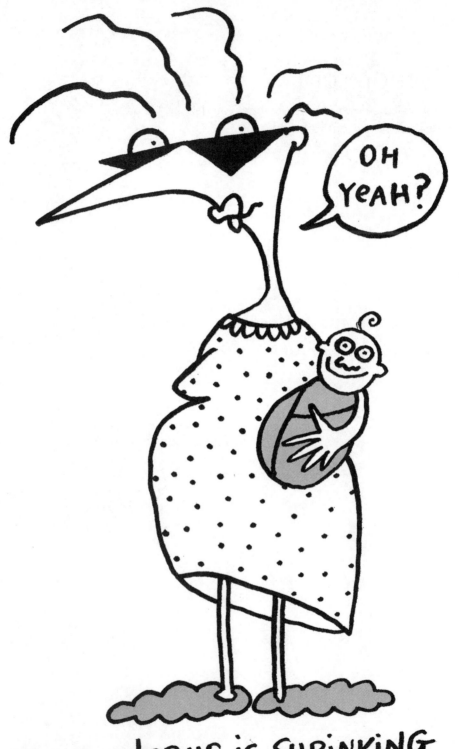

YOUR uteRUS iS SHRiNKiNG

what's going on

Your uterus is slowly shrinking, contracting each time you breastfeed – it will be back to its right size in about six weeks. Your muscles and ligaments are all adjusting to the loss of relaxin but they will remain affected for the next four months. Retained fluid may still cause puffy ankles and sore joints, especially the knees, and the problem may stick around for some weeks.

Your baby will be starting to grow at a very fast rate. Sometimes it will seem as if you can see the difference in a day. Your baby can't see very much because their eyes only focus on things within 30 centimetres (1ft), and probably isn't smiling yet: this can make a baby seem very passive and not much fun. But before you know it they'll be staring at you with eyes on full-beam, and within about five weeks you'll be seeing gorgeous gummy grins.

WEEK 42

DiARY

I'm writing all this down later, as the week after Eddy's birth was a haze of drug-addled fatigue and incomprehension. I know I'm supposed to say it was a wonderful, joyous time full of relief and laughter and sense of achievement, and that sort of palaver, but somehow it just didn't feel that way.

The caesarean and all the drugs left me in a numb state of shock, a veil of pain-killers seeming to deaden brain feelings as well as pain. Anne said I had been very unlucky and that she only sees one or two cases a year where, after induction, the heartbeat suddenly drops and stays low for more than a couple of minutes. But I just had to be that one or two. It didn't feel as if I was providing Eddy with the greatest introduction to life, lying prone on a trolley, wired up to a drip. And somehow I couldn't connect Eddy with the babe who had spent so long inside me. Maybe it was because we hadn't gone on the journey of labour together, and I hadn't felt him being born. Maybe it was the drugs or the shock, or because having a real live baby actually felt hyper-real.

Eddy, however, was doing his best to bond. He looked exactly like Geoff without the 5 o'clock shadow. He had fists that could be gently opened into small starfish, and mother-of-pearl fingernails, and a very serious expression. He was tiny and lovable, mysterious and passive.

It felt like we were constantly doing things TO him – trying to breastfeed him, changing nappies, wrapping and unwrapping him. His 'littleness' made both Geoff and I feel very protective and scared at the same time. We spent ages looking at Eddy's little face, wondering what he was thinking. 'Probably "get me another bosom",' said Geoff.

Eddy's bed was a plastic tub on a trolley next to mine. The midwives – led by Anne – would come round and lift him up and help me try to breastfeed. I hadn't realised how hard it would be. Nor how physical. The midwives would take Eddy and thrust him onto my breast, nipple to the back of his throat, as they coaxed him into snaffling a few drops of colostrum. He seemed to be getting something from me but I needed help from a midwife each time. On my own, we just flounced about, unconnected.

After about three or four days of Eddy waking up to be breastfed every 4 hours, a feed which would take about an hour or more each time, I hadn't had more than 2 hours or so of sleep in a row. And as a person who needs 9 or 10 hours' sleep a day, this was taking its toll. I did what I always do when I'm tired. I cried and cried.

It just felt like I couldn't cope, couldn't function with the immobility and pain and feeding, if I didn't get some proper sleep. And my attempts at feeding were still pitiful and painful, with razor-painful nipples (one had a crack nobody could see except me). Things only really got better when Anne brought round a breastfeeding counsellor, who stayed for an hour, said breastfeeding was almost always like this before the milk comes in, and to persevere, Eddy wouldn't starve, and she COULD see the nipple crack.

I rang Beck every day I was in hospital to tell her how tired and incompetent I felt. She sent in vitamin B, herbal tonics and stern instructions to get out into the fresh air. Eddy just lay wrapped up in a blanket looking at everything as if he were trying to memorise it. 'I'll get better at this caper,' I promised him, Eddy presumably was thinking 'I'd like some more of that bosom business, if it's all the same to you, Leaky.'

info

postnatal depression

what is it?

Most women experience what is known as the 'baby blues' – feeling weepy and sad – often on about day four after giving birth when the 'happy hormones' go and the prolactin kicks in for real milk production. For most women these blues only last a few hours, or at most a couple of days, but some find that the depression stays, or returns, and gets worse.

Sometimes it's hard to decide where the baby blues end and postnatal depression (PND) begins. PND is a real and unpleasant illness that affects perhaps one in ten of all new mums. Recently there has been some research into the incidence of PND in the partners of new mothers, which suggest that it could affect some men in the same way.

what causes it?

No one knows why PND affects some women more than others, but hormones seem to be the main culprits. Oestrogen and progesterone levels drop rapidly after childbirth, which may trigger depression in a similar way to fluctuating hormone levels causing PMS (pre-menstrual syndrome). There's some evidence that it runs in families.

The following are all recognised as contributing factors in PND and logical reasons why you may feel down.

ⓖ Exhaustion – childbirth wears you out; so do visitors and trying to follow any kind of schedule once you have a baby. One of the reasons for exhaustion is that your volume of blood has suddenly been cut by 30 per cent so a lesser volume is reaching your muscles than they have become used to, making them tire easily and feel weak. It takes a few weeks for your body to readjust to this. Sleep is one of the first things to suffer once the baby is born, and if you are depressed you can suffer from insomnia so you're unable to take advantage of even the ludicrously short sleep periods available to you.

ⓖ A traumatic birth – this can cause shock and disappointment.

ⓖ Frustrating or bad hospital experiences – you might feel you need to get away from all the prodding, the unfamiliar cramped surroundings and the artificial air.

ⓖ Anxiety about coping – going home can seem overwhelming and terrifying when you think about how much you have to do, especially if you have other children to look after.

⑥ A sense of failure – this can arise from feeling unable to cope with all the things you think you 'have' to do to be a good mother; disappointment if the birth didn't go according to plan; or feeling that you have somehow failed as a woman if you are having problems feeding and settling your baby. In reality, almost EVERYONE has a problem at some point.

⑥ A health problem – most new mothers will suffer from at least one of the following: backache, fatigue, mastitis (infection of the milk ducts), painful episiotomy stitches, major sleep deprivation. Feeling physically unwell adds to depression.

⑥ Ennui – after spending nine months on a high of anticipating seeing your baby for the first time, you may find yourself feeling underwhelmed. It is quite common to find your baby less than scintillating company until you have had time to bond emotionally. Tiny, new babies are very passive – there's none of the cooing, extended eye contact and sticking their heads up out of flower pots we associate with babies (and greeting cards) for a few weeks or months yet. The guilt you experience when you feel bored by or distant from your baby only adds to the depression.

⑥ Loss of individual identity – before the birth, everyone is focused on the pregnant woman and how she is feeling, and afterwards many women feel that they are less important to their family and friends as all attention is on the baby. You may feel as if people have stopped seeing you as an individual and now see you only as a 'mother'.

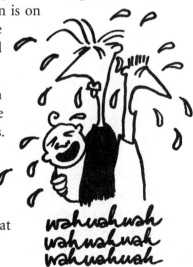

⑥ Perfectionist or anxious approach to life – PND appears more in people who tend to worry or are perfectionists. Many women feel disappointed in themselves if they have always dealt with things to exacting standards in their professional and social lives and suddenly feel unable to reach that level of 'perfection' in motherhood.

wahwahwah
wahwahwah
wahwahwah

◎ Subsequent pregnancies – PND is more common in women who already have children. Having to look after older children as well as a new baby is likely to place even tighter constraints on the time you have to yourself and to get enough rest. It can be scary wondering how you'll cope.

◎ Loneliness – if everyone you know is busy with their own lives and yours revolves around the baby, you may feel as though you are missing out on 'life'.

◎ A feeling of being trapped in this lifestyle for the rest of your days – 'Why on earth did I have a baby?'

signs and symptoms

◎ The blues and the feelings listed above persist for more than a couple of weeks.

◎ Sleeplessness and/or lack of appetite.

◎ Low self-esteem.

◎ Confusion (even over simple taks) and/or panic attacks.

◎ Extreme anxiety about the baby and yourself.

◎ Feeling 'flat' and despondent.

◎ Feeling angry or aggressive towards yourself or your baby.

◎ Feeling wildly out of your depth.

what can be done?

If your depression lasts longer than a few days you should discuss your feelings with your partner, health visitor and GP. If possible take your partner to see the GP with you. Before you go, write down a list of all the symptoms that you are suffering from. Do not go on suffering depression in the hope that it will go away. Postnatal depression is an illness and it can be treated successfully with anti-depressant drugs (some women also find oestrogen or progesterone supplements useful).

These drugs are not addictive. They make the unpleasant symptoms fade until they go completely. Indeed, it is important to

CHILD HEALTH CLINICS

Somewhere near you is a child health clinic. You may not have noticed it, but it's about to become a part of your life. Depending on where you live, it may be found at your local Health Centre, or attached to your GP practice or it may be a completely separate building just down your road.

The health visitors are based at the child health clinics and are required to visit you when the baby is eleven days old. They usually ring and make an appointment to visit you at home. Your hospital or home midwife will have notified them of your birth.

After that first home visit, you will go regularly to the clinic for appointments with the health visitor to check on your baby's general progress (and how you're doing yourself), to weigh and measure your baby, and to ask a ton of questions about baby care.

You should be able to contact your health visitor at any time during the day and they are generally supportive and helpful with any problems or queries you have and are trained to pick up any problems you may not have noticed. If you have a personality clash or a problem with one particular health visitor ask to see one of their colleagues. They'll probably be as relieved as you.

Child health clinics usually run new parent postnatal programs, and can put you in touch with parents' groups, mothers' groups and playgroups. They are good places to find pamphlets or posters about local toy libraries, babies' and children's activity groups, and other services, and they often have noticeboards for people to advertise baby clothes or equipment and babysitting.

remember that all mothers recover from postnatal depression. As the recovery proceeds, the bad days get fewer and less upsetting and the good days become more numerous. Gradually the bad days disappear completely.

You can also develop your own strategies to help counteract PND, or extended baby blues. For example:

⑥ Begin by confiding in someone – your partner, a sympathetic member of your family, or a friend. Then set up a support network of family, friends and professionals. Accept help from others rather than feeling as if you have to prove you're capable by doing it all yourself. Remember that in sensible cultures babies are looked after by an extended family or even a whole tribe of people from the moment they're born. We weren't meant to do it alone.

⑥ Look after yourself – use the time when your baby sleeps to rest instead of catching up on all the things you think you should have done such as the housework; treat yourself to things that help you feel pampered and relaxed, such as a massage or haircut.

⑥ Get some fresh air – gentle exercise such as walking or yoga, with or without the baby, is calming and releases energy. Try to spend a little time each day realising it IS day, and not just sleeping, eating and feeding the baby in a twilight, indoor world.

⑥ Get together with other new mums – contact the women in your antenatal class or join a postnatal exercise class; or ask the local health visitor what times the new-mothers' group meets: this will give you a chance to talk with women experiencing the same things, and will help you feel part of something, rather than excluded.

⑥ Ask someone you trust to look after your baby while you do something relaxing such as going for a walk or seeing a friend.

⑥ Be aware that your partner, if you have one, might also have the blues. They might benefit from counselling or special help as well, and it's a good step for the baby's sake too.

⑥ Ask your GP to rule out (or in) a thyroid problem that could cause similar symptoms to PND.

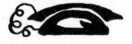 See Postnatal depression in 'Help'.

your record

✳ Write down your first impressions of your baby: who the baby resembles, colouring, characteristics, temperament, whatever.

✳ Who came to visit you in the first week? Did they give anything special to the baby?

what's going on You're tired. You're still trying to get breastfeeding to be smooth and easy for both of you. Your body has started to heal. You're trying to cope with visitors as well as looking after the baby. You're in a dreamworld. FORGET THE BLOODY HOUSEWORK.

You'll find the tiny outfits that fitted in the first week of birth start to get too small (the baby's outfits, not yours). Your baby's eye colour may be changing, and the baby hair might be falling out, to be slowly replaced by a new lot. After another couple of weeks the shrivelled, stumpy bit of umbilical cord will come away from the navel and you'll see what your baby's tummy button looks like. The hands will stay curled in fists for a few weeks yet. Length and weight? Oh who cares. Forget the statistics for a minute. Every day your baby's

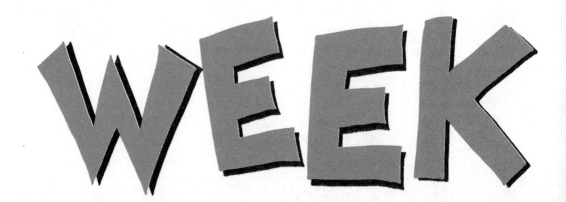

WEEK

getting closer to becoming a social being
who sleeps more and doesn't cry so much
(although the amount of crying reaches
a peak at about six weeks old). So every
day you're getting closer to the time when
you can get some more sleep. Live in the
moment, as babies do. Forget about
what you have to do tomorrow or next
week. Take it one day, even one hour,
at a time, sister.

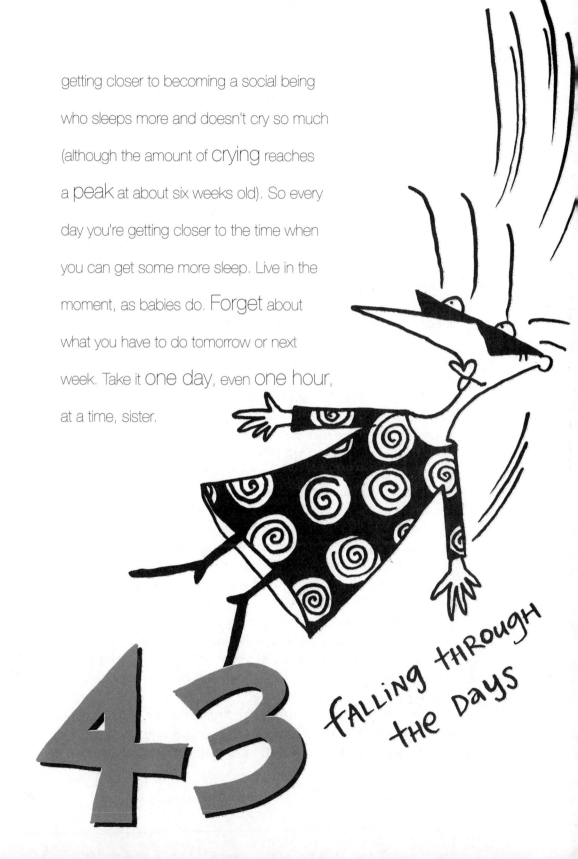

43

falling through
the days

$DiARY$ The thing that really helped me to get a grip on the blues was getting home into an environment with fresh air, and the chance to sit outside even if I felt like a zombie and was not at all sure what to do with a tiny baby. It was kind of comforting having the hospital midwives nearby, but nothing like being at home. Besides, I was visited by Anne each day.

I was so tired in those early days I thought it would never end. I cried towards the end of every day when fatigue started to overwhelm me. We discouraged visitors because rather than offering help, so many seemed to need attention. Even the flowers people sent seemed demanding. The visitors who were really helpful were the ones who would pick up the baby or otherwise make themselves useful around the house.

Aunt Julie hadn't got hold of me until I was 3 months old, when Mum died – so she was a bit at sea with a small bundle and convinced that every snuffle meant cot death or convulsions. Geoff tried to limit her visits but she came all the same every day, bustling around the kitchen, scrubbing the bathroom. We came to appreciate her more than we'd ever imagined.

All at once, though, I felt lonely. I was too tired to make the effort to reach out to friends and it seemed like I was living in a fog of fatigue, robotically waking, feeding the baby and trying to sleep again; like some kind of wet nurse on Valium. Beck told Geoff to make me go outside for a walk in the afternoons so at least I would feel like I knew which was day and which was night, and that there was an outside world. This helped a lot.

Every time I think about how I told everyone I'd start work part-time in eight weeks, I'm overwhelmed with stress and anxiety. I've got to try to go with the flow. Eddy is waking up every 4 hours, which is not too bad compared with some babies, but I am still absolutely knackered from lack of sleep. Not only do you have to live day by day, but sometimes hour by hour, without looking forward or back. Susanne described the first few weeks as 'falling through the day', and she had her sister and mother to help.

Geoff and I seem absurdly busy and occupied, just with looking after a baby who spends most of the time asleep. We're lucky if one of us has had a shower by nightfall and somebody can make the dinner. The washing machine and dryer seem to be going all day long and there are mountains of nappies . . .

Then we crack. We swap to disposable nappies and begin using the cloth ones as essential, all-purpose shoulder drapes, wipes, bum cleaners and soft surfaces for the change table. Eddy sleeps up to an extra hour or two at night with a disposable nappy on, and I decide he might as well be more comfortable in the daytime as well.

There is a certain guilt in this, and we expect to be raided by the Baby Police at any moment. I listen to a caller who rings up a radio station and says that women who use formula baby milk and disposable nappies are 'lazy'. About 100 people ring and say they'd like to kill her. Hurrah! I do feel guilty about the environment, though, so I've joined Greenpeace in Eddy's name.

Breastfeeding is easier than it was at the beginning, but Eddy still has a lot of trouble attaching, especially to the left nipple (which is odd because it has always been his father's favourite). The scar and pain from the caesarean make everything harder, including finding a good position for breastfeeding. I need two pillows to balance him on, and how to feed him insouciantly and – arrgghhh – in public is a complete mystery to me.

Eddy has 'wind' and he cries and cries inconsolably after all the daytime feeds, really screaaaaaaming in the ear of whichever parent is holding him: it's extraordinary how loud a baby can yell. It's so hard not being able to take the pain away, and hard to remain patient with the crying. Yesterday I found myself raising my voice in frustration and saying angrily, 'Shut up!', which is about as useful as saying, 'Act your age', and as soothing as a lovely death-metal song. Luckily I get hold of myself, stop raising my voice, and just end up crying as well. I read the Crying Baby leaflet that Melissa gave us at the antenatal class, and check out the other pregnancy books' advice. But nothing really helps. I just have to keep saying, 'This will end, this will end.'

I ring the breastfeeding counsellor from hospital and ask, 'How do I tell, when the baby cries three hours after a feed, whether he's hungry or there's something else wrong?'

'Just feed him when he cries,' she says.

'But it may be too soon and he isn't hungry,' I reply, knowing from experience that if I feed Eddy after 2 hours he'll projectile vomit. Which, by the way, is such an extremely shocking moment it makes you draw your breath in and open your eyes really wide like Kate Bush singing ;Wuthering Heights'.

'Some babies feed every hour,' she says. 'You can't overfeed a baby on breastmilk. If they don't want milk, they won't suck. You and Eddy'll get your balance before long. Hang on in there!'

And so it goes. Cry. Feed. Sleep. Nappy. The endless cycle. I'm supposed to be doing exercises to help the post-caesarean body in my spare moments, but I might as well be told to read a couple of novels a day – there is just no time at all. And when there is, I'm afraid I need to be horizontal, usually with ear plugs in, my head under the pillow, an eye mask on, dreaming of getting stuck into a bottle of whisky.

early outings

Baby excursions in the first few weeks can be a tad gruelling, and you should never feel you have to go anywhere. It's good just to take your time at home, gradually getting to know your baby, apart from going for short walks in the fresh air, or sitting in the park.

One of the worst things about early forays out the front door is that you are giving your first public performances as a new parent. Heaps of new mums cry with frustration the first few times they try to collapse that damn new pram into the car or get off a bus with a baby AND some shopping. After a few days they can do it backwards and upside down in the dark with one foot. It's just a matter of practice.

If you're still getting the hang of changing nappies, breastfeeding and working out why the hell your baby is crying, going out can be a bit stressful. Also, the virtually full-time nature of new-baby care doesn't change just because you're out. Your baby will still need to feed, be burped, have their nappy and maybe clothes changed, be settled down to sleep, feed some more, sleep – or whatever happens at home – while you're trying to have a cup of tea, stay awake and sound intelligible, or get home before dark.

Don't worry: it gets easier every time.

so what's in the bag?

The big bag that all parents haul about with them contains whatever you need to change and feed the baby. Its exact contents alter as the baby grows older, reaching peak capacity during toddler years, when it includes all nappy-changing equipment plus sundry snacks, drinks, security blankets and can't-leave-the-house-without-Binky-type toys.

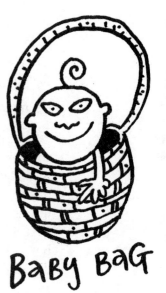

BaBy BaG

The newborn-baby bag will need to contain:

⑥ Spare nappies – you need at least two even for an afternoon jaunt. If you are using cloth nappies, you may find it more convenient to use disposable nappies and baby wipes for excursions.

⑥ A change of outfit in case the going-out clothes get poo on them (which is more likely if you have cloth nappies).

⑥ A surface to change the nappies on – some bags have a built-in change pad; if yours doesn't, a waterproof-backed changing sheet on the floor works just as well.

⑥ Whatever you use to clean your baby's bottom at change time: a small container of water or small bottle of nappy-change lotion, and some cotton balls, or a packet of baby wipes. Nappy-rash cream, which forms a barrier between wee and skin, if needed.

⑥ A few plastic bags to bring dirty nappies and clothes home in – re-using supermarket bags is ideal, but check they're not ripped, and tie a knot or two in them for safety until you use them (then tie them up firmly again) in case another baby or a toddler gets hold of them.

⑥ A couple of clean muslin squares to drape over the shoulder of anyone holding the baby as a vomit guard or chin wiper.

⑥ Sun hat if it's hot, cap or hat if it's cold.

⑥ A couple of toys – newborn babies see mostly contrasts rather than colours for the first six months, so black and white toys are good, and they also like those plastic rings in a chain that you see dangling on prams.

⑥ Bibs if you are already using them.

⑥ Sterilised bottles of freshly made up but cold formula milk with protective sterilised caps if you are bottle-feeding, kept in an insulated bottle carrier. Better still, take the right measurement of cooled boiled water in a sterilised bottle (with a sterilised cap on) and add formula from a sachet to it while you are out, then heat it up. This prevents bacteria forming. Never take bottles of hot formula out and never try to keep them hot. Bottles should be drunk within an hour of being heated.

The main thing about the big bag is this: have it packed and ready to go at all times. Getting around sleeping, feeding and changing times and actually out of the house is a finely tuned exercise in time management. There is no time for delay while you hunt about looking for things to put in the bag (except, of course, freshly prepared bottles if you are bottle feeding).

To have the bag ready, you need duplicates of nappy change lotion, or wipes and barrier cream – probably in smaller, more portable-sized containers or packages than you would buy for use at home. You also need to remember to restock the bag when you get home from an outing. Get used to bringing it in every single time in case the car goes away with it, or you need to restock before you go out in the car again.

As well as the big bag, you may need somewhere portable for the baby to sleep. You can take a carricot (the body of some prams converts to a carricot, which is handy for visiting), or a quilted baby bag, or a lambsfleece, or a moses basket. You can let the baby sleep in the pram if you keep an eye on it all the time. If it's a short visit, newborn babies can be just as comfortable sleeping in their car seat or parents' arms. Be very aware of other people's toddlers and pets as a potential danger: they may not be used to babies or take any notice of warnings.

You can wear your baby in a sling as a charming fashion accessory, with optional vomiting feature, so long as the baby is not going to be in a smoky environment, and someone can help you when the baby gets too heavy.

Leaving the house gets easier when feeding and sleeping turn into something resembling a routine. About when they're asking for their first pocket money, maybe.

and by the way . . .

⑥ If a certain book or person is making you feel guilty, avoid them. (I burnt one nameless book in the back garden when I read in it that a 'clever' mother shouldn't have to get up more than once a night if she juggles the times of feeds and anticipates her baby's crying at night. You may think it feels bad and wicked to burn a book. It felt FANTASTIC.)

⑥ After a few weeks your bosoms will stop being so hard and full before each feed, and stay much floppier, but they are actually producing more and more milk for your growing baby. Don't assume you're running out because your bosoms are softer between feeds: your body's just getting more efficient. And it's common for one breast to produce more milk than the other – or be easier for the baby to 'draw on'.

⑥ If you have committed yourself to other projects and you find that looking after a baby is harder than you thought, try to get out of everything you can, if possible without damaging your work prospects, or decide which prospects you're prepared to sacrifice. Or find ways to get more help with the baby.

⊚ Show friends and family how they can help. Many people, and not only men, will be feeling inexperienced and tentative, and scared of hurting a small baby. Show them the way, and everyone will have a better time.

⊚ If your baby screams blue murder when you do the bath thing, avoid the stress. It can be much more restful to get in the big bath together and cuddle while you wash, or to just wash bits of your baby with a flannel. And you don't have to do it every day.

⊚ Say it loud and say it proud: IF THE CHOICE IS BETWEEN SLEEPING AND THE HOUSEWORK, SLEEP.

IMMUNISATION

Immunisation means giving vaccines by mouth or injection to make a child resistant to a particular virus or bacteria. Vaccines work by stimulating the immune system to produce antibodies to the infection. The diseases that your child will be immunised against are all infectious and unpleasant; some are fatal, while others cause permanent disability. Many of these infections are now rare, thanks to vaccines.

There are routine childhood vaccinations for Polio, Diptheria, Tetanus, Whooping cough, Hib (haemophilus influenzae b), Meningitis C, Measles, Mumps, Rubella and in areas where tuberculosis (TB) is common, newborn babies are also given a BCG immunisation.

Immunisation schedule You can check your schedule with your GP or health visitor but in practice you will be sent an appointment inviting you to attend for each immunisation. If your child can't make an appointment, don't worry – you can arrange a new date. Usually there are injections or oral vaccines, including vital booster shots, scheduled for when the child is 2 months, 3 months, 4 months, 1 year, 15 months and just before starting primary school, with a final top-up of some things at abour 15 years old or before they leave school.

Helping your baby through it A baby should not be immunised during a feverish illness. It's best to postpone it until your baby is completely recovered. Also talk to your GP or health visitor before the immunisation if: your child has had a serious reaction to a previous injection; has a severe egg allergy; has had a fit or convulsion; is having treatment for cancer; or has (or has a family history of) any disease that affects the immune system.

Side effects Find out from your GP or health visitor what side effects to look out for after the injections and check that it's safe to give infant Paracetamol about 15 minutes before the injection. In case of a raised temperature afterwards (a temperature over 37°C) giving another dose of Paracetamol is recommended. Make sure you ask the best way for you to take your baby's temperature. (The sugar-free version of baby Paracetamol is recommended and babies like its taste).

Your choice Having children immunised is a parental choice and can be a difficult decision to take when there are controversies about certain vaccines (notably the combined Measles, Mumps and Rubella – MMR). However, vaccination has been one of the great health promotion successes, and many diseases that were once common are now rarely seen. Indeed, that's why we are as concerned about the possible risks of vaccines as the morbidity and mortality of these diseases.

 Ask your GP or health visitor for all the information and leaflets that are available, and see Immunisation in 'Help'.

BABY-CARE BOOKS

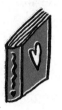

Kidwrangling: Caring for Babies, Toddlers and Preschoolers by Kaz Cooke (yes that's me), Michael Joseph, UK, 2004.

A whopper sequel to this very book you're reading, that covers everything from the first day at home with a newborn to the first day of schools, stopping all stations at crying, sleeping, your post-baby body, bosoms, bottles, illnesses, clothes, tantrums, vaccinations, childcare, parties and travel. And banana in your hair.

The Rough Guide to Babies by Miranda Levy, Rough Guides, UK, 2006.

Rough Guides navigate Planet Baby, where life is different. There are detailed chapters on everything from getting through your first days at home and making the right feeding decisions to keeping an eye on your baby's development and coping with family relationships. And throughout the book, there are personal and professional anecdotes from new mothers and fathers, health visitors, paediatric nutritionists and many others.

Complete Baby and Child Care by Dr Miriam Stoppard, Dorling Kindersley, UK, updated 2006

This is a well designed, exhaustively illustrated tome (so that's what a nappy looks like), covering the first five years of your child's life. It can be a little regimental in its stance, but it's an excellent resource.

Your Baby and Child: The Essential Guide for Every Parent by Penelope Leach, Penguin, updated 2003.

Penelope Leach, a UK-based research psychologist and mother, became a kind of new Dr Spock when this liberal, child-centred handbook was first published in the 1980s. It's a meticulous account of what to expect during a child's development – and your part in it. What can cloy, however, is the Leach vision of a happy parent and child cooking together and constantly and merrily playing useful and fun games . . . a vision that seems unattainable for busy parents, especially if they have other children, or anything else to do. But as one stay-at-home dad says, it can be good to know what's the best thing from the toddler's point of view, even if you can't always deliver.

What to Expect the First Year by Arlene Eisenberg, Heidi E. Murkoff and Sandee E. Hathaway, Simon & Schuster, UK, updated 2004.

The American trio again with the sequel to *What to Expect When You're Expecting*. It's a perhaps even more valuable book, arranged as a month-to-month guide to issues and developmental stages, and including a reassuring range of experiences presented as anecdotes. As with the pregnancy book, it has been (more or less) adapted for the UK. When you're finished with it, you can use it as a doorstop . . . and move on to the equally gripping *What To Expect From the Toddler Years*.

Minus Nine To One by Jools Oliver, Michael Joseph, UK, 2005.

As the cover says, a 'diary of an honest mum' – through pregnancy and the first year. It's oddly like having a friend who's married to a celebrity chef telling you everything she's going through, and giving advice along the way. And as you might expect, it's got some tasty recipes for kid's food.

HEALTH CARE

Baby and Child Health Care by Dr Miriam Stoppard, Dorling Kindersley, UK, 1997.

Dr Miriam again – and this really is a book you will want to have on your shelf, hopefully little used and read. The core of the book is an A–Z of common and not so common complaints, first-aid crises (Nose, foreign body in), and childhood illnesses: how to spot the symptoms, what should you do first, when should you consult the doctor and what will the doctor do.

Safe Natural Remedies for Babies and Children by Amanda Cochrane, HarperCollins, UK, 1997.

NOT designed to be used instead of going to the doctor, this is a natural approach to baby massage and massage oils, nappy-rash treatments, insect repellents for toddlers, soothing aromatherapy, and natural approaches to the less serious baby and childhood complaints. If the condition doesn't respond quickly, as they say in the classics, seek medical advice.

BABY BEHAVIOUR BOOKS

All of the main baby-care books include advice on behavioural patterns for babies: in particular on establishing patterns for feeding and sleep. These have changed massively over recent decades. In the 1950s, parents guided by Truby King fed only every four hours, however much a child cried. Then along came Dr Spock, and later Penelope Leach and the baby and child's demands became central. Recently, there seems to have been a shift back to strict parent-decreed routines . . .

The Contented Little Baby Book by Gina Ford, Vermilion, UK, updated 2002

Check out the reviews of this on Amazon and you will think you've come across a new religion. Gina Ford, an experienced, old-style British nursery nurse believes strongly in routine and a firm hand, which she reckons babies and children appreciate. She is particularly rigorous on establishing fixed feeding and sleeping routines (the idea being to get babies sleeping through the night by the time they are 10 weeks old), which could be a step too far for your household, or not. Committed users will probably want to graduate to Ford-2, *From Contented Baby to Confident Child.*

The Good Behaviour Book: How to Have a Better Behaved Child by William Sears MD and Martha Sears MD, Harper Thorsons, UK, updated 2005.

In the US, William Sears seems to have taken on the Spock mantle (his Web site modestly proclaims him 'America's Paediatrician').

His philosophy is actually far from disciplinarian: he's known as the 'attachment' doctor (three-in-a-bed, slings, etc). In this very child-centred book, the Sears describe a variety of parenting styles, help you identify your own parenting tendencies, offer advice on how to read your children's cues, and show how to manage a variety of situations and behavioural problems that may arise (without screaming).

See 'Help' sections for specific books on breastfeeding, feeding, grief & loss, immunisation, postnatal depression, and sleep problems.
A number of months down the track I look back at those first

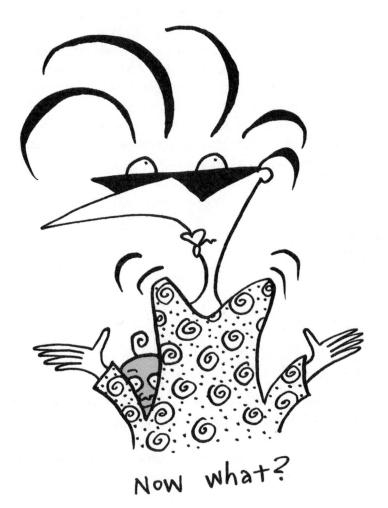

Now what?

forever after... (diary)

weeks and wonder how anyone does it without going completely mad. Before I had Eddy, when people used to talk about 'lack of sleep' I thought of it as an inconvenience – like staying up too late and having a bit of a hangover. Now I can see why they use sleep deprivation as a method of torture. Good old Ed is finally sleeping for eight hours straight a night.

I can't remember a thing about being pregnant but I still look about six months 'gone'. You know how they say you automatically lose weight when you breastfeed? Nope. And you know how they say you'll lose it when you stop breastfeeding, instead? Not me. Took me about nine months to feel robust again after the caesarean.

I breastfed for three months, then my endometriosis problem started again and I had to go on the Pill. And the Pill goes through into breast milk and that's no good for Ed. Sadly, he no longer regards my bosoms as something special, but don't get between him and a bottle of formula. He loves the stuff, and he's thriving on it. He also likes to 'chew' rice cereal, severely distressed parsnip and the tags on all his soft toys.

Some friends have disappeared over the horizon, but I've made new ones among my old NCT classmates (Geoff and I even attended an NCT 'sleep school' where we learnt what a routine was) and among other mums. Thank God for the childless pals who still ring and ask me out. I've hired someone to come and look after Eddy when I'm working part-time from home. Eddy chats away happily in baby language to himself and everyone else, and we've weathered our first ear infection (which crept up and king-hit us while we were waiting for the much-warned-about teething that happened later than most people expect). I'm afraid gummy old Ed is a little backward in the teeth department. And he's a champion dribbler, I'll have you know.

Sometimes I just want to stop the clock and have a week off. Sometimes it's fascinating, sometimes it's dead boring. Sometimes I yearn for a few hours just to myself and yet sometimes it's so lonely. And then there's that moment when he smiles and laughs and reaches out for a cuddle and I think it's the most gorgeous feeling I've ever had.

I suppose the next thing I know Eddy'll be crawling, and going to school, and designing a titanium spaceship, or cooking a dinner party for six. But until then there's a lot of cardboard books about fluffy duckies to be read, a lot of ludicrous baby hats to be worn, a lot of walks in the park to be had, and a lot of hurtling round the garden being a fairy-seeking missile. And there's a little indent on the back of his neck that's just perfect for kissing, and if you whisper 'Oofty Goofty' in his ear he might giggle again. So. If you'll excuse me . . .

The End. (And just the beginning . . .)

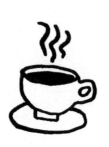

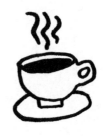

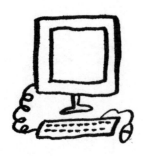

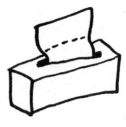

HeLP

These contact addresses and book reviews are intended as a supplement to information contained in the week-by-week sections. For specific problems, check the index.

ACTIVE BIRTH ——————

'Active Birth' is a philosophical approach to labour and birth that says we should follow our own instincts and the logic of our bodies (in essence, do what feels right). Yoga is also emphasised as a preparation for labour. Along with such organisations as the National Childbirth Trust (NCT), the Active Birth movement has helped to bring about major changes in British hospital birth practices.

The Active Birth Centre
www.activebirthcentre.com
mail@activebirthcentre.com
25 Bickerton Road, London N19 5JT
Tel: 020 7281 6760

Founded by Janet Balaskas, the pioneer of the Active Birth movement, and author of several birthing books, the Active Birth Centre offers preparation classes for expectant parents and trains Active Birth yoga teachers for a network of classes across the UK. They also have a mail order service for aromatherapy oils, baby-care products, books, etc, and hire birthing pools.

—————————

New Active Birth: A Concise Guide to Natural Childbirth by Janet Balaskas, Harper Collins, UK, 1990.
Here's the theory and practice of Active Birth, with lots of yoga exercises. For a full review (and a rundown of other birth books) see 'Week 2'.

BABIES' HEALTH PROBLEMS ——————

Many babies are born with health problems, ranging from a routine, temporary problem to a serious and dangerous one requiring intensive care and very hard decisions. Immediately there is a problem, take notes or bring a friend to take notes of your conversations with doctors and other relevant people – it can be a time when shock causes everything to go in one ear and out the other. Keep pushing until you feel satisfied that everything that can and needs to be done is being done.

In the UK (and on the Internet, if you find it easier), you can find parent support groups for specific conditions such as Down's syndrome, spina bifida, cleft lip and palate, and cystic fibrosis. Ask your GP, health visitor or paediatrician for suggestions, or try the Patient UK Web site (www.patient.co.uk) which maintains a comprehensive directory of reputable and reliable UK health/illness Web sites.

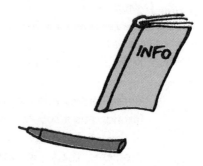

Down's Syndrome Association
www.downs-syndrome.org.uk
info@downs-syndrome.org.uk

Main UK Office: Langdon Down
Centre, 2a Langdon Park,
Teddington TW11 9PS
Tel: 0845 230 0372 (Tues–Thurs
10am–4pm)

Northern Ireland: Graham House,
Knockbracken Healthcare Park,
Saintfield Rd, Belfast BT8 8BH;
Tel: 028 9070 4606

Association for Spina Bifida and Hydrocephalus (ASBAH)
www.asbah.org
42 Park Road, Peterborough PE1 2UQ
Tel: 01733 555988

See also Screening and blood tests.

BREASTFEEDING

There are several organisations
who offer support to breastfeeding
mothers without charge. They may
run workshops for parents to attend
in the antenatal period and they
also lend electric breast pumps for
parents in special circumstances.

National Childbirth Trust (NCT)
See Parenting and pregnancy (p.409)
www.nct-online.org.uk
Breastfeeding Helpline: 0870 444 8708

NCT Breastfeeding Councellors are
trained, committed mothers who
will give advice over the phone or, if
needed, visit your home. You don't
have to be a member of the NCT
to get help: just call the Helpline

(above) and you will be connected
with a local counsellor.

La Leche League
www.laleche.org.uk
PO Box 29, West Bridgford,
Nottingham, NG2 7NP
Breastfeeding Helpline: 0845 120 2918

The Milk League exists to promote
breastfeeding and, like the NCT,
provides breastfeeding information
help and support through a network
of trained counsellors. Its helpline
(above) is staffed 24 hours a day, every
day. It can also provide tapes and
pamphlets, and for specific problems,
access to research and professional
advisors.

Association of Breastfeeding Mothers
www.abm.me.uk
PO Box 207, Bridgwater, Somerset,
TA6 7YT
24-hour helpline: 0870 401 7711

A similar service to the league,
with advice, information, and local
breastfeeding counsellors.

Jane's Breastfeeding and Childbirth Resources
www.breastfeeding.co.uk
Helpline 9am-9pm: 0870 900 8787

Jane Neesam is a founder member
of the charity Breastfeeding Network
and provides information, research
and advice on the Internet. Her site
has exhaustive links and a helpful
Frequently Asked Questions section
with good advice on breastfeeding
technique and weaning.

The National Childbirth Trust Book of Breastfeeding by Mary Smale, Vermilon, UK, 2002.

A sensitively written guide to the practical and emotional aspects of breastfeeding, with useful advice on positioning, latching-on time and successful weaning.

CRYING

See also Sleep (p.411).

If your baby's crying is driving you crazy, don't go crazy alone – contact your health visitor, GP or local hospital and ask for help.

CRY-SIS
www.cry-sis.org.uk
Helpline: 08451 228 669
(9am–10pm every day)

Cry-Sis is a charity that offers support for families with excessively crying, sleepless and demanding babies and/or young children. They operate a national telephone helpline and train local volunteers (who have experienced problems like yours) to offer ongoing support. They also produce very good information.

The National Childbirth Trust Book of Crying Baby by Anna McGrail, HarperCollins, UK, 1999.

Why babies cry, simple ideas to help, and what to try if they don't work out.

EMPLOYMENT

ACAS 'Tiger'
www.tiger.gov.uk

Maternity rights for employers and employees and an interactive calendar to help with planning leave.

Department of Trade and Industry
www.dti.gov.uk

Another site to check your maternity leave entitlement before speaking to your employer.

EXERCISE

See also Active Birth for yoga (p.402).

The Guild of Postnatal Exercise Teachers
megwalker@pnex.freeserve.co.uk
www.postnatalexercise.co.uk

The guild trains teachers and has a list of qualified teachers across the UK.

YMCA
112 Great Russell St, London WC1B 3NQ; Tel: 020 7343 1850.

The YMCA train fitness teachers for pregnancy and produce a good DVD called 'The Y Plan Before and After Pregnancy'.

FEEDING (SOLIDS)

It may seem as if your baby will never be big enough to eat solids but in six months' time you'll be mashing up stuff for the little tyke to shove in their mouth/ear/nose.

Each book on baby-care has a different opinion on what to feed the kid first and when you can introduce certain foods, and whether to offer solids before, during or after a bottle. So choose one direction and stick to it unless it doesn't work, and in that case, be flexible. (For example, cross your fingers and try the opposite.) In the meantime don't worry – your baby won't starve to death if they miss a few solid feeds. Milk is still the most important thing at this stage.

Feeding Your Baby and Toddler by Annabel Karmel, Dorling Kindersley, UK, 2004.
An excellent book with a great layout as well as user-friendly, simple and realistic recipes that should hopefully bring a little harmony to meal times.

The New Vegetarian Baby by Sharon Yntema, McBooks Press, UK, 1999.
Following on from Yntema's *Vegetarian Pregnancy* title (see 'Week 2'), this book guides you through the special developmental needs that have to be met in giving a baby a vegetarian diet, and offers loads of essential nutritional advice and useful recipes.

FERTILITY

Many fertility clinics incorporate hi-tech and low-tech investigation and treatment for both partners.

The latter may include nutritional advice and lifestyle discussions, to complement the clinic's investigations of ovulation and sperm counts. There is evidence to support the advice that smoking and alcohol decrease fertility. (There is no scientific evidence to back up the use of acupuncture or reflexology, though many people swear by it). Clinics can also recommend specialist counsellors.

British Infertility Counselling Association
www.bica.net info@bica.net
69 Division Street, Sheffield S1 4GE
Tel: 01744 750660

If you are having trouble conceiving, it can be useful to see a specialist infertility counsellor.

Foresight (Association for the Promotion of Pre-conceptual Care
www.foresight-preconception.org.uk

Foresight help fertility by optimising nutrition. Hair analysis determine deficient vitamins and minerals so supplements can be prescribed.

The National Infertility Support Network
www.infertilitynetworkuk.com
Charter House, 3 St Leonards Rd, Bexhill on Sea, East Sussex TN40 1JA
Tel: 08701 188088

Offers factsheets and a stock of recent and helpful books for sale.

Infertility, the Last Secret by Anna McGrail, Bloomsbury, UK, 1999.

A compassionate blend of facts and case studies that explains the common causes of infertility, what to expect from tests, other ways to build a family, and scenarios involving conception and not conceiving. Also includes a good list of support contacts.

Taking Charge of Your Fertility: The Definitive Guide to Natural Birth Control and Pregnancy Achievement by Toni Weschler, Vermillion, UK, 2003.

Alternative Infertility Treatments by Nicky Wesson, Vermillion, UK, 1997.

The Fertility Plan by Helen Caton, Gaia Books, UK, 2000.

These three books are especially useful for those who want to explore options other than IVF and are worth looking at if you have time to try a few options, or haven't yet started to 'try' to get pregnant and would like to optimise your chances.

GRIEF AND LOSS ——————
See also Sudden Death Syndrome (p.371).

It is rare, but some babies die in the last weeks of pregnancy and are induced stillborn. Some babies die soon after birth, or in the following weeks. Often you can't remember what you've been told by medical staff because of the shock and grief. During these terrible times there are many professionals who may be able to offer you a great deal of help, including:

> midwives and doctors
> health visitors
> hospital social workers
> counsellors

A friend or relative who can take notes of what is said by these people can be invaluable.

There are support groups for parents and siblings affected by the death of a baby, or those trying to deal with a baby who has special needs. Ask your hospital to put you in touch with them.

Grief counsellors can help a couple or a whole family, including brothers and sisters, understand what has happened. Your hospital or GP should be able to help you find one who specialises in the loss of a baby (that's important).

SANDS (Stillbirth and Neonatal Death Society)
www.uk-sands.org
support@uk-sands.org
28 Portland Place, London WIB 1LY
Helpline: 020 7436 5881 (Mon-Fri 9.30am-5.30pm)

SANDS provides support for bereaved parents and their families when their baby dies at or soon after birth. It has a national helpline and UK-wide network of self-help groups run by and for bereaved parents. Your hospital will probably give you the contact for your local support group as hospitals have strong links with SANDS. The society also publishes a range of books and leaflets.

FSID (Foundation for the Study of Infant Deaths)
www.sids.org.uk/fsid/ fsid@sids.org.uk
Artillery House, 11-19 Artillery Row,
London SW1P 1RT
Helpline: 020 7233 2090 (24 hours)

FSID aims to prevent sudden infant death and raises funds for research into causes and prevention of cot death. It publishes a range of leaflets and other publications, and has a network of befrienders. It also runs the Care of the Next Infant (CONI) scheme in partnership with the NHS.

Miscarriage Association
www.miscarriageassociation.org.uk
c/o Clayton Hospital, Northgate,
Wakefield, West Yorks WF1 3JS
Helpline: 01924 200799 (Mon–Fri 9am–4pm)

Maintains a UK-wide network of phone counsellors and support groups, and issues a range of publications.

When a Baby Suddenly Dies: Cot Death, the Impact and Effects by Janet Deveson Lord, Michelle Anderson Publishing, US, 1994.
A book for parents, siblings, relatives, friends and health workers about what happens after a sudden infant death.

Beginnings and Endings with Lifetimes in Between: A Beautiful Way to Explain Life and Death to Children by Bryan Mellonie and Robert Ingpen, Belitha Press, UK, 1997.
A picture book for children.

IMMUNISATION ───────

Your GP and health visitor will provide immunisation schedule pamphlets – and appointments will arrive for your child in the post. Vaccines are free and most health professionals strongly encourage you to have them.

Given recent controversies, in particular over possible side effects of the combined MMR (Measles, Mumps, Rubella) vaccine, you may want to research the issues before taking a decision. A good place to start, if you have Internet access, is the Families Online Web site (*www.familiesonline.co.uk*) which, unusually, includes good material from both sides of the debate.

THE CASE FOR:

NHS Immunisation
www.immunisation.org.uk

This NHS site is a useful resource on all immunisations offered in the UK, with extensive information on childhood, pre-school and school immunisations.

Institute of Vaccine Safety
www.vaccinesafety.edu

This US Insititute, based at Johns Hopkins University, has an informative Web site with well-presented news, articles and research.

Childhood Immunisation: A Review for Parents and Carers by Dr Richard Elliman, HEA/Marston Book Services, UK, 1998.

Dr Elliman is a Consultant in Community Child Health at St George's Hospital, London. His book is clear, jargon-free and useful in helping you make your decision.

THE CASE AGAINST:

There is anti-immunisation material to be found all over the place – and especially on the Internet. Much of this material is presented emotively and with little regard for the dating of statistics and supporting evidence. The name that crops up all over the Web is Alan Phillips, who wrote a 1996 copyright-free paper in the US ('Dispelling Vaccination Myths') that is constantly re-posted on websites.

The Vaccination Bible by Lynne McTaggart, A What Doctors Don't Tell You Publication (4 Wallace Road, London N1 2PG, UK), 1998.

This is definitively *not* a bible. Read it with caution, but don't be afraid to raise the issues with your GP or health visitor. Much of the material is available on the What Doctors Don't Tell You Web site (*www.wddty.co.uk*), a site run by people who mistrust conventional medicine. Doctors strenuously dispute many of the claims they make against vaccination.

MIDWIVES

You will be referred to NHS hospital midwives through your GP (see p.57 & p.93). If you want to look at using an independent midwife, you may want to contact:

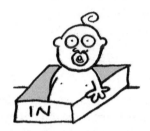

Independent Midwives Association
www.independentmidwives.org.uk
1 The Great Quarry, Guildford, Surrey
GU1 3XN; Tel: 01483 821104

Send an A5 SAE for the IMA's register of midwives offering private care and a list of the various birthing centres available. They offer free advice to women thinking about a home birth.

NATURAL HEALTH

Institute for Complementary Medicine
www.i-c-m.org.uk info@i-c-m.org.uk
PO Box 194, London SE16 7QZ
Tel: 020 7237 5165

A charity providing information on complementary medicine and referrals to qualified practitioners or helpful organisations.

PARENTING AND PREGNANCY HELP

These organisations offer a range of information and support during pregnancy and/or parenthood.

National Childbirth Trust

www.nct.org.uk
Head Office: Alexander House, Oldham Terrace, Acton, London W3 6NH
Tel: 0870 444 8707

The NCT (see p.60) is a charity that offers support and information for expectant and new parents. They run excellent local groups with antenatal preparation classes, postnatal support groups and breastfeeding counsellors. The NCT also publish books and pamphlets with expert advice on baby-care, sleeping, crying and other issues. Its website is reviewed on p.414.

Disability, Pregnancy and Parenthood International (DPPI)

www.dppi.org.uk

The DPPI aims to network information and experience on all aspects of pregnancy and parenthood among disabled parents, potential parents and healthcare professionals.

Disabled Parents Network

www.disabledparentsnetwork.org.uk
Unit F9, 89-93 Fonthill Road, London, N4 3JH
Helpline: 0800 018 4730

Network for disabled parents, offering support in pregnancy, childbirth and parenting.

Gingerbread

www.gingerbread.org.uk
Freephone Advice Line: 0800 018 4318
(Mon–Fri 10am–4pm)

A support group for single parents offering an advice line, fact sheets, discussion groups, and help on a whole range of issues.

35-Plus

www.mothers35plus.co.uk

A Web site for older mothers with 'news', information, stories from mothers and links to other sites.

Fathers Direct

www.fathersdirect.com

Fathers Direct aims to promote close relationships between men and their children, from day one.

POSTNATAL DEPRESSION

If you feel you may have postnatal depression, ask your GP to refer you to a specialist counsellor or centre, or contact your health visitor who will be trained in the care and support of mothers suffering from PND. (Also, read the section on p.377).

The following organisations are also there to help.

Association for Post-Natal Illness

www.apni.org   info@apni.org
145 Dawes Road, London SW6 7EB
Tel: 020 7386 0868

One-to-one advice (by phone, post or email), information and support for mothers who have or think they may have PND. Also publishes leaflets.

Parentline Plus
Tel: 0808 800 2222
http://www.parentlineplus.org.uk/

A national helpline (and useful website) for anyone parenting a child who needs help.

MAMA (Meet-a-Mum Association)
www.mama.co.uk
Helpline: 0845 120 3746 (Mon-Fri 7pm–10pm)

MAMA aims to provide friendship and support to mothers and mothers-to-be who are lonely or isolated after the birth of a baby or following a move to a new area.

Antenatal and Postnatal Depression
by S. Curham, Vermilion, UK, 2000
This valuable book provides information on the probable causes of depression, along with practical advice. It offers support and reassurance by including case histories of many women who have suffered from this form of depression, assuring you that you are not alone (and that it doesn't last forever).

The National Childbirth Trust Book of Postnatal Depression by Heather Welford, NCT, UK, 2002.
A practical and sympathetic little book full of case studies, guidance and clear explanations of causes.

PREMATURE BABIES ——

You may want to ask your paediatrican, midwife or hospital to put you in touch with a local support group.

BLISS (Baby Life Support Systems)
www.bliss.org.uk
68 South Lambeth Rd, London
SW8 1RL   Tel: 020 7820 9471
Helpline 0500 618140 (Mon–Fri 10am–5pm; freephone)

A helpline for parents of premature babies, offering advice and help in understanding and securing the best quality care for their needs.

SCREENING AND BLOOD TESTS ——

The organisations below provide information and support.

ARC (Antenatal Results and Choices)
www.arc-uk.org
Helpline: 0207 631 0280 (Mon–Fri 10am–5.30pm)

ARC is a non-judgmental and non-directive charity organisation that may be helpful with decision making if a serious abnormality is diagnosed in your unborn baby. It is staffed by volunteer counsellors who aim to give continued support to parents who terminate a pregnancy following a diagnosis of serious foetal abnormality.

Thalassaemia Society
www.ukts.org
19 The Broadway, Southgate Circus, London N14 6PH
Information line: 0800 731 1109

Advice for parents and families.

Toxoplasmosis Trust
www.tommys.org
0870 777 3060
Information, support and counselling for sufferers, or those concerned they might have the condition.

Sickle Cell Society
www.sicklecellsociety.org
54 Station Road, Harlesden, London NW10 4UA; Tel: 020 8961 7795/4006

Advice and support line for parents affected by this blood disorder.

SLEEP

It's amazing how a sleep routine can change your life for the better. You may have a baby who won't nap during the day, or one who wakes up often at night, perhaps wanting to be fed every two hours even when a few months old. Many people now seek help with such problems from sleep clinics, which can be arranged through your health visitor.

Solve Your Child's Sleep Problems by Dr Richard Ferber, Dorling Kindersley, UK, 1999.
Dr Ferber is the Big Cheese at the Boston Children's Hospital Center for Pediatric Sleep Disorders and his thesis is the basis for many of the sleep clinics run for mothers and babies in the UK. He has convincing views on what children associate with sleep, and suggests how to build up periods of leaving a child crying and shutting the door behind you. The book also covers night-time disturbances, the importance of a daily schedule, and how to stop night feeding.

The Contented Little Baby Book by Gina Ford, Vermilion, UK, 2002.
This might help, too. See p.396 for a review.

TWINS AND MULTIPLE BIRTHS

If you are having twins (or more) you will receive closer pregnancy care (see p.61), and you may want to get in touch with TAMBA or MBF to prepare for what's in store.

TAMBA (Twins and Multiple Births Assocation)
www.tamba.org.uk
2 The Willows, Gardner Rd, Guildford GU1 4PG
Helpline: 0800 138 0509 (daily 10am–1pm & 7–10pm)

Information and mutual support networks for families of twins, triplets and more, highlighting their unique needs to all involved with their care. There is a confidential helpline and they have specialist local support groups. TAMBA organises study days, conferences and twin clubs.

MBF (Multiple Births Foundation)
www.multiplebirths.org.uk
Queen Charlotte's and Chelsea Hospital,
Hammersmith House, Level Four, Du
Cane Rd, London W12 OHS
Tel: 020 8383 3519

Professional support for families with
twins and multiple births.

**Twins and Multiple Birth – The
Essential Parenting Guide** by Dr Carol
Cooper Assisted by TAMBA, 1997
This is a really great book to get if you are
expecting more than one baby, written
by a GP and mother of twins (see p.63 for
review).

MORE INFO ON THE INTERNET

If you have access to the Internet,
you can browse heaps of Web sites
about all aspects of pregnancy and
parenthood. Many of the most
useful are detailed in the sections
above, and throughout this book,
but there are a number of general
sites that you may well want to
browse, as well as a myriad of
single-issue sites (which you can
access by typing a key word into
your search engine – and trying to
avoid the pesky porno material).
The major pregnancy and baby
sites are good resources in that they
often have chat-rooms or discussion
forums, where you can discuss (or
just browse) problems and stages,
and they often provide a range of
links to further your researches.

There's also no shortage of
commercial sites, selling everything
you could conceivably want during
and after pregnancy (except sleep).

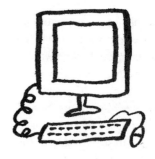

If you can't face getting round the
shops, these can be handy. With a
couple of exceptions (where they
have useful info as well as product),
shops are not detailed below,
but they advertise on the main
pregnancy and baby sites, so they're
easy enough to find.

If you are buying products on
the Web, it's best to do so using a
credit card (and certainly not on
your regular bank/cheque card),
which should cover you in the
(unlikely) case of fraud.

RECOMMENDED SITES

Baby Centre
www.babycentre.co.uk

An impressive UK adaptation of the American parent Web site: everything from advice on conceiving, baby-care and lullaby lyrics to excerpts from Penelope Leach's book on toddlers, and good stuff on sleep routines. Thoughtfully designed and easy to navigate, with a fine search facility, and chat-rooms.

Baby Directory
www.babydirectory.com

A commercial site that, when you join, gives you access to listings for baby and kid-oriented services and shops in your area. It may make you cross that you can't afford all the glam products, but it's a useful site if you need to do some research into where to find things.

Baby Registry
www.thebaby.registry.co.uk

The best feature here is the 'advice directory' which links to helpful organisations concerned with all sorts of subjects. There are decent features, too, with info on pregnancy, babies, toddlers, advice for dads, and contraception fact sheets if you've decided the family's big enough.

Babyworld
www.babyworld.co.uk

The Web site of *Babyworld* magazine features chat-rooms, birth stories

(somehow always compelling reading when you're pregnant), pregnancy diaries, shopping and an ask-their-expert section. There's an antenatal club you can join for online classes and camaraderie. You must register with the site to enter competitions, give-away offers and discussion groups.

Families Online
www.familiesonline.co.uk

No – the name didn't appeal to me either, but this is actually a really good, clear, useful Web site, produced as an extension of the *Families* newsletters, published in London and Edinburgh. The site covers babies, children and children-related issues like health, schools, childcare, plus topical news items (they're excellent on vaccination advice) and a monthly what's on section.

Home Birth
www.homebirth.org.uk

A well-maintained and thorough Web site run by a home-birth advocate. Birth stories, pain-relief options, recommended books and DVDs, articles, and what to do if your GP opposes home birth.

Sheila Kitzinger
www.sheilakitzinger.com

Okay, we've made a lot of jokes about Sheila comparing the size of a developing foetus to various fruits and vegetables, but she's actually pretty fab. Big on helping mothers and babies whether in a town house or in prison, this site is packed with info on home births, water births, breastfeeding, news and recent articles and a 'reflective listening' service for women who have had a bad birth experience such as an emergency caesarean. The picture of 'Sheila demonstrating how not to push a baby out' is hilarious.

Mother and Baby

www.motherandbabymagazine.com

The Web site of this long-established magazine includes an impressive host of features: DVDs of different births (if your computer is up to it – you can download the necessary software free of charge); a virtual hospital tour; chat-rooms; free weekly emails on each week of your pregnancy; a dad's section, and an efficient search facility that takes you to articles in the substantial archive.

Mothercare

www.mothercare.co.uk

Although clearly dominated by the commercial angle, selling you stuff from Mothercare shops, the site also has a library of articles on pregnancy, baby and toddler subjects.

NCT

www.nctpregnancyandbabycare.com

The site will help you locate your nearest branch of the National Childbirth Trust, or nearest antenatal (pre-birth) class, find a breastfeeding counsellor or a chatroom with other expectant mums, or new mums. There's also a section for dads. Info on pregnancy, baby and toddler care.

Net Doctor

www.netdoctor.co.uk

This is an extensive, independent, UK-based health Web site. It has very useful articles by experienced and respected doctors, without the mystifying doctor-speak, on heaps of pregnancy-related subjects and an impressive cross-referencing, hypertext feature lets you zoom from one subject to another. Refreshingly, it doesn't try to sell you anything.

NHS Direct website

www.nhsdirect.nhs.uk
Helpline 0845 4647 (24 hours)

An easy to navigate site with useful information and advice – and a 24-hour helpline.

Tommy's, The Baby Charity

www.tommys.org

Tommy's is a charity committed to funding medical research and providing information to help healthy pregnancies and birth. Its website is an excellent resource, especially for any pregnancy problems, and it runs an information line staffed by midwives, which you can email (info@tommys.org) or phone (0870 777 3060).

index

acknowledgements

I would like to thank many dedicated people who helped to adapt this new UK edition from its original (Australian) incarnation, especially Teresa Driver RM, who lent us all her midwifery expertise and experience, and worked hard and cheerfully to make the book relevant to the British NHS system. Deborah Bosley helped move the diary stories to South London; Peter Buckley contributed new book reviews and helpful suggestions; and obstetricians Jane Wilson MD FRCOG and Sarah Reynolds MMBS MRCOG checked all the medical palaver; Elaine Pollard proofread; Link Hall sorted out all the typesetting squiggles. Editor Mark Ellingham co-ordinated the lot without once resorting to firearms or hissy fits.

On the original edition, a ruly mob of people had already helped to make sure everything was present and correct, especially Dr Maria Dziardek, developmental biologist; midwife and herbalist Ruth Trickey; Mr Len Kliman, obstetrician and gynaecologist; and a bevy of midwives from private practice and hospital staff. The meticulously rigorous Lesley Dunt knocked it into shape. (A complete list of specialist consultants is in the original book, Up The Duff, published by Penguin Australia.)

By its nature this book is subjective, as well as including about a gerzillion facts. Those acknowledged here are not reponsible for errors, or current advice and accepted statistics which may change in an inkling. Nor are they responsible for any of the author's own ludicrously flighty opinions.

And just one final point. When authors compare producing a book to having a baby, they need a damned good slapping.

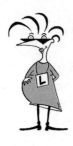

Kaz Cooke is an author, cartoonist and mum. She does not holiday in a rustic French farmhouse with a frightfully artistic husband, and what's more there appears to be some mashed banana in her hair.

we'd love to hear from you

Please write to us about:

⊚ your experiences of any aspect of pregnancy, birth and the first few weeks of caring for your newborn baby

⊚ anything covered in the book that you'd like to comment on or share your feelings about.

Kaz Cooke, Rough Guides
80 Strand, London WC2R 0RL mail@roughguides.com